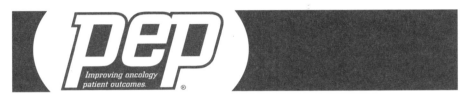

PUTTING
EVIDENCE
INTO
PRACTICE *IMPROVING ONCOLOGY*
PATIENT OUTCOMES

Edited by
Linda H. Eaton, MN, RN, AOCN®
Janelle M. Tipton, MSN, RN, AOCN®

Paula Nelson-Marten
8/2010

Oncology Nursing Society
Pittsburgh, Pennsylvania

ONS Publishing Division
Publisher: Leonard Mafrica, MBA, CAE
Director, Commercial Publishing: Barbara Sigler, RN, MNEd
Managing Editor: Lisa M. George, BA
Staff Editor: Amy Nicoletti, BA
Copy Editors: Sharon Padezanin, BA, Laura Pinchot, BA
Graphic Designer: Dany Sjoen

Putting Evidence Into Practice: Improving Oncology Patient Outcomes

First printing, April 2009
Second printing, October 2009

Library of Congress Control Number: 2009926935
ISBN: 978-1-890504-84-7

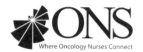

Oncology Nursing Society
Integrity • Innovation • Stewardship • Advocacy • Excellence • Inclusiveness

Printed in the United States of America

Contributors

Editors

Linda H. Eaton, MN, RN, AOCN®
Research Associate
Oncology Nursing Society
Pittsburgh, Pennsylvania
Author (Chapters 2, 4, 5, 8, 10, 11, 12, 14, 18, 19)

Janelle M. Tipton, MSN, RN, AOCN®
Oncology Clinical Nurse Specialist
University of Toledo Medical Center
Toledo, Ohio
Author (Chapters 1, 2, 3, 6, 7, 9, 13, 15, 16, 17, 19)
Chemotherapy-Induced Nausea and Vomiting PEP Resource

Authors

Linda I. Abbott, RN, MSN, AOCN®, CWON
Advanced Practice Nurse
Holden Comprehensive Cancer Center
University of Iowa Hospitals & Clinics
Iowa City, Iowa
Peripheral Neuropathy PEP Resource

Lynn A. Adams, RN, MS, ANP, AOCN®
Nurse Practitioner
Memorial Sloan-Kettering Regional Network
Commack, New York
Anorexia PEP Resource

Lisa B. Aiello-Laws, RN, MSN, APNG, AOCNS®
Knowledge Base Manager
ITA Partners
Philadelphia, Pennsylvania
Pain PEP Resource

Suzanne W. Ameringer, PhD, RN
Assistant Professor, School of Nursing
Virginia Commonwealth University
Richmond, Virginia
Pain PEP Resource

Felicia Andrews, BSN
Nurse Manager
National Institutes of Health
Bethesda, Maryland
Prevention of Infection PEP Resource

Jane M. Armer, RN, PhD, FAAN
Professor, Sinclair School of Nursing
University of Missouri, Columbia
Director of Nursing Research
Ellis Fischel Cancer Center
Columbia, Missouri
Lymphedema PEP Resource; Mucositis PEP Resource

Julie A. Aschenbrenner, RN, BSN, OCN®
Assistant Nurse Manager
Adult Leukemia/Bone Marrow Transplant
University of Iowa Hospitals & Clinics
Iowa City, Iowa
Peripheral Neuropathy PEP Resource

Terry A. Badger, PhD, PMHCNS-BC, FAAN
Professor and Division Director
University of Arizona, College of Nursing
Tucson, Arizona
Anxiety PEP Resource; Depression PEP Resource

Kristen Baileys, RN, MSN, CRNP, AOCNP®
Project Manager
ONS Education Team
Oncology Nursing Society
Pittsburgh, Pennsylvania
Diarrhea PEP Resource; Peripheral Neuropathy PEP Resource

Marie A. Bakitas, DNSc, ARNP, AOCN®, FAAN
Assistant Professor
Clinical Researcher
Adult Nurse Practitioner, Palliative Care Section of Palliative Medicine
Dartmouth-Hitchcock Medical Center
Lebanon, New Hampshire
Pain PEP Resource

Laurel A. Barbour, RN, MSN, APN, AOCN®
Biotherapy Care Manager
Advocate Lutheran General Hospital
Park Ridge, Illinois
Chemotherapy-Induced Nausea and Vomiting PEP Resource

Susan L. Beck, APRN, PhD, AOCN®, FAAN
Professor and Carter Endowed Chair in Nursing
University of Utah, College of Nursing
Salt Lake City, Utah
Fatigue PEP Resource

Heather Belansky, RN, MSN
Project Manager
ONS Education Team
Oncology Nursing Society
Pittsburgh, Pennsylvania
Anorexia PEP Resource; Caregiver Strain and Burden PEP Resource; Depression PEP Resource; Diarrhea PEP Resource; Dyspnea PEP Resource; Lymphedema PEP Resource; Peripheral Neuropathy PEP Resource; Prevention of Bleeding PEP Resource; Prevention of Infection PEP Resource

Ann M. Berger, PhD, RN, AOCN®, FAAN
Professor and Dorothy Hodges Olson Endowed Chair in Nursing, Advanced Practice Nurse
Director, PhD Program, College of Nursing
University of Nebraska Medical Center, College of Nursing
Omaha, Nebraska
Sleep-Wake Disturbances PEP Resource

Annette Kay Bisanz, RN, BSN, MPH
Clinical Nurse Specialist
University of Texas M.D. Anderson Cancer Center
Houston, Texas
Constipation PEP Resource

Jeannine M. Brant, PhD, APRN, AOCN®
Clinical Nurse Specialist and Nurse Scientist
Billings Clinic
Billings, Montana
Prevention of Bleeding PEP Resource

Ruth Ann Brintnall, RN, PhD, AOCN®, APRN-BC
Associate Professor
Grand Valley State University
Kirkhof College of Nursing
Grand Rapids, Michigan
Caregiver Strain and Burden PEP Resource

Annette Parry Bush, RN, BSN, MBA, OCN®
Certification Programs Manager
Oncology Nursing Certification Corporation
Pittsburgh, Pennsylvania
Prevention of Bleeding PEP Resource

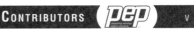

Rose Ann Caruso, RN, OCN®
Staff Registered Nurse
Memorial Sloan-Kettering Cancer Center
Commack, New York
Anorexia PEP Resource

Barbara J. Cashavelly, MSN, RN, AOCN®
Nurse Director of Clinical Practices
Massachusetts General Hospital Cancer
   Center
Boston, Massachusetts
Mucositis PEP Resource

Deirdre B. Colao, RN, BSN, OCN®
Manager of Clinical Operations
Arizona Pulmonary Specialists Ltd.
Phoenix, Arizona
Caregiver Strain and Burden PEP Resource

Mary L. Collins, RN, MSN, OCN®
Clinical Educator
Carle Clinic Cancer Center
Urbana, Illinois
Peripheral Neuropathy PEP Resource

Regina S. Cunningham, PhD, RN, AOCN®
Senior Director, Oncology
The Tisch Cancer Institute
Mount Sinai Medical Center
New York, New York
Anorexia PEP Resource

Ann E. Culkin, RN, OCN®
Clinical Nurse
Memorial Sloan-Kettering Cancer Center
New York, New York
Dyspnea PEP Resource

Barbara I. Damron, PhD, RN
Director of Oncology Nursing Research and
   Government and Community Advocacy
University of New Mexico Cancer Center
Albuquerque, New Mexico
Prevention of Bleeding PEP Resource

Arlene B. Davis, RN, MSN, AOCN®
Oncology Clinical Specialist
Gainesville VA Medical Center
Gainesville, Florida
Diarrhea PEP Resource

Nancy A. Delzer, MSN, MBA, AOCN®, BC-PCM
Director, Cancer Clinical Services
Columbia St. Mary's
Milwaukee, Wisconsin
Pain PEP Resource

Wendye M. DiSalvo, MSN, ARNP, AOCN®
Advanced Registered Nurse Practitioner
Dartmouth-Hitchcock Medical Center
Lebanon, New Hampshire
Dyspnea PEP Resource

Amy H. Dolce, RN, APN, MS, AOCN®, CHPN
Oncology Clinical Nurse Specialist
Northwest Community Hospital
Arlington Heights, Illinois
Anxiety PEP Resource

Rachael Christine Drabot, MPH, CNSD, RD
Clinical Research Dietitian
National Institutes of Health
Bethesda, Maryland
Diarrhea PEP Resource

June G. Eilers, PhD, APRN-CNS, BC
Clinical Nurse Researcher
Oncology Clinical Nurse Specialist
The Nebraska Medical Center
Omaha, Nebraska
Mucositis PEP Resource

Patricia J. Friend, PhD, APRN, AOCN®
Assistant Professor
Niehoff School of Nursing
Loyola University Chicago
Maywood, Illinois
*Chemotherapy-Induced Nausea and Vomit-
   ing PEP Resource; Prevention of Bleeding
   PEP Resource*

Christopher R. Friese, RN, PhD, AOCN®
Assistant Research Scientist
University of Michigan, School of Nursing
Ann Arbor, Michigan
Prevention of Infection PEP Resource

Caryl D. Fulcher, RN, MSN, CNS-BC
Clinical Nurse Specialist
Duke University Hospital
Durham, North Carolina
Depression PEP Resource

Stephanie Fulton, MSIS
Assistant Director of the Research Medical
    Library
University of Texas M.D. Anderson Cancer
    Center
Houston, Texas
Constipation PEP Resource

Lindsay Gaido, MSN, RN
Clinical Nurse Specialist
University of Texas M.D. Anderson Cancer
    Center
Houston, Texas
Constipation PEP Resource

Barbara A. Given, PhD, RN, FAAN
University Distinguished Professor
Associate Dean for Research and Doctoral
    Program
Michigan State University
East Lansing, Michigan
Caregiver Strain and Burden PEP Resource

Barbara Holmes Gobel, MS, RN, AOCN®
Oncology Clinical Nurse Specialist
Northwestern Memorial Hospital
Chicago, Illinois
*Chapter 1; Prevention of Infection PEP
    Resource*

Ashley K. Gunter, RN, BSN, OCN®
Clinical Nurse III
Duke University Medical Center
Durham, North Carolina
Depression PEP Resource

Amber Harriman, RN
Staff Nurse
Oregon Health & Science University
Portland, Oregon
Mucositis PEP Resource

Debra J. Harris, RN, MSN, OCN®
Nursing Practice and Education Coordinator
Oregon Health & Science University
Portland, Oregon
Mucositis PEP Resource

Connie Hart, RN, BSN, OCN®
Clinical Educator
Carle Foundation Hospital
Urbana, Illinois
Peripheral Neuropathy PEP Resource

Jody Hauser, RN, MS, AOCNP®
Oncology Nurse Practitioner
San Francisco Oncology Associates
San Francisco, California
Prevention of Infection PEP Resource

Norissa J. Honea, PhD(c), MSN, RN, AOCN®,
    CCRP
Clinical Research Nurse
Arizona Oncology Services Foundation
Phoenix, Arizona
Caregiver Strain and Burden PEP Resource

Linda Edwards Hood, RN, MSN, AOCN®
Duke Cancer Palliative Care Research Nurse
Duke University Medical Center
Durham, North Carolina
Fatigue PEP Resource

Lauran B. Johnson, RN, BSN, MSN
Bone Marrow Transplant Coordinator
University of California at San Francisco
    Medical Center
San Francisco, California
Sleep-Wake Disturbances PEP Resource

Mary Pat Johnston, RN, MS, AOCN®
Oncology Clinical Nurse Specialist
ProHealth Care, Regional Cancer Center
Waukesha Memorial Hospital
Waukesha, Wisconsin
*Chemotherapy-Induced Nausea and Vomit-
    ing PEP Resource*

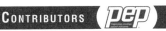

Margaret M. Joyce, PhD(c), RN, MSN, AOCN®
Advanced Practice Nurse
Cancer Institute of New Jersey
New Brunswick, New Jersey
Dyspnea PEP Resource

Marilyn K. Kayne, BSN, RN, OCN®
Staff Nurse, Clinical Nurse IV
University of Toledo Medical Center
Toledo, Ohio
Chemotherapy-Induced Nausea and Vomiting PEP Resource

Elizabeth S. Kiker, RN, BN, OCN®
Charge Nurse, Chemotherapy Clinic
Gainesville VA Medical Center
Gainesville, Florida
Diarrhea PEP Resource

Michele M. Lacher, RN, OCN®
Clinical Resource Nurse
Hematology-Oncology Centers of the
    Northern Rockies
Billings, Montana
Prevention of Bleeding PEP Resource

Kristine B. LeFebvre, MSN, RN, AOCN®
Project Manager
ONS Education Team
Oncology Nursing Society
Pittsburgh, Pennsylvania
Pain PEP Resource

Barbara G. Lubejko, RN, MS
Project Manager
ONS Education Team
Oncology Nursing Society
Pittsburgh, Pennsylvania
*Dyspnea PEP Resource; Lymphedema PEP
    Resource; Prevention of Infection PEP
    Resource*

Hannah F. Lyons, RN, MSN, AOCN®, BC
Oncology Clinical Nurse Specialist
Massachusetts General Hospital
Boston, Massachusetts
Constipation PEP Resource

Kathleen Mackay, RN, BSN, OCN®
Phase I Research Nurse
Dartmouth-Hitchcock Medical Center
Lebanon, New Hampshire
Dyspnea PEP Resource

Gail Mallory, PhD, RN, NEA-BC
Director of Research
Oncology Nursing Society
Pittsburgh, Pennsylvania
*Caregiver Strain and Burden PEP Resource;
    Chemotherapy-Induced Nausea and Vomiting PEP Resource*

Joyce A. Marrs, MS, FNP-BC, AOCNP®
Nurse Practitioner
Dayton Physicians, Hematology & Oncology
Dayton, Ohio
Depression PEP Resource

Kathy Marsh, BA, RN, OCN®
Staff Nurse
Northwest Community Hospital
Arlington Heights, Illinois
Anxiety PEP Resource

Cathy L. Maxwell, RN, OCN®
Director of Clinical Operations
Advanced Medical Specialties
Miami, Florida
Mucositis PEP Resource

Roxanne W. McDaniel, PhD, RN
Associate Dean
Sinclair School of Nursing
University of Missouri, Columbia
Columbia, Missouri
Chemotherapy-Induced Nausea and Vomiting PEP Resource

Christine A. Miaskowski, RN, PhD, FAAN
Professor and Associate Dean for Academic
    Affairs
Sharon A. Lamb Endowed Chair
Department of Physiological Nursing
University of California, San Francisco
San Francisco, California
Pain PEP Resource

Sandra A. Mitchell, PhD, CRNP, AOCN®
Research and Practice Development Service
National Institutes of Health Clinical Center
Oncology Nurse Practitioner, National Cancer Institute
Bethesda, Maryland
Fatigue PEP Resource; Prevention of Bleeding PEP Resource

Katen Moore, MSN, APN-C, AOCN®
Nurse Practitioner
Cancer Institute of New Jersey
New Brunswick, New Jersey
Fatigue PEP Resource

Paula Muehlbauer, RN, MSN, OCN®
Clinical Nurse Specialist/Academic Educator
VA Healthcare San Diego/San Diego State University
San Diego, California
Diarrhea PEP Resource

Martha J. Norling, RN, OCN®
Staff Nurse
California Cancer Care
Greenbrae, California
Anorexia PEP Resource

Laurel L. Northouse, RN, PhD, FAAN
Mary Lou Willard French Professor of Nursing
University of Michigan, School of Nursing
Ann Arbor, Michigan
Caregiver Strain and Burden PEP Resource

Colleen O'Leary, RN, MSN, AOCNS®
Registered Nurse, Staff Educator
Northwestern Memorial Hospital
Chicago, Illinois
Prevention of Infection PEP Resource

Margaretta S. Page, RN, MS
Clinical Nurse Specialist
University of California, San Francisco
San Francisco, California
Sleep-Wake Disturbances PEP Resource

Mary E. Peterson, RN, ANP-BC, OCN®
Nurse Practitioner
Bone Marrow Transplant Program
Mayo Clinic Hospital
Phoenix, Arizona
Pain PEP Resource

Ellen Gordon Poage, MSN, ARNP, MPH, CLT-LANA
Certified Lymphedema Therapist and Nurse Practitioner
Rehabilitation Associates of Naples
Naples, Florida
Lymphedema PEP Resource

Melanie D. Poundall, RN, OCN®
Infusion Nurse
Y8 Cancer Center
Massachusetts General Hospital
Boston, Massachusetts
Lymphedema PEP Resource

Barbara L. Rawlings, RN, BSN
Senior Clinical Research Nurse
National Institutes of Health Clinical Center
Bethesda, Maryland
Diarrhea PEP Resource

Jill M. Reese, RN, BSN, OCN®
Clinical Nurse Educator
Dayton Physicians, Hematology & Oncology
Dayton, Ohio
Depression PEP Resource

Janice K. Reynolds, RN, BC, OCN®, CHPN
Staff Nurse
Mid Coast Hospital
Brunswick, Maine
Pain PEP Resource

Marita L. Ripple, RN, OCN®
Staff Nurse Clinician
Advocate Lutheran General Hospital 8 Center
Park Ridge, Illinois
Chemotherapy-Induced Nausea and Vomiting PEP Resource

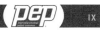

Susan M. Samsonow, RN, OCN®
Staff Nurse/Clinical Education Support
Dartmouth-Hitchcock Medical Center
Lebanon, New Hampshire
Prevention of Bleeding PEP Resource

Anna D. Schaal, RN, BScN, MS, ARNP
Hematology Nurse Practitioner
Dartmouth-Hitchcock Medical Center
Lebanon, New Hampshire
Prevention of Bleeding PEP Resource

Lisa Kennedy Sheldon, PhD, APRN-BC,
    AOCNP®
Assistant Professor
University of Massachusetts–Boston
Oncology Nurse Practitioner
St. Joseph Hospital
Nashua, New Hampshire
Anxiety PEP Resource

M. Jeanne Shellabarger, RN, MSN
Breast Clinic Coordinator
University of Missouri, Columbia
Ellis Fischel Cancer Center
Columbia, Missouri
Lymphedema PEP Resource

Nancy Shepard, RN, MS, AOCN®
Oncology Nurse Practitioner
California Cancer Care, Inc.
Greenbrae, California
Anorexia PEP Resource

Paula R. Sherwood, RN, PhD, CNRN
Assistant Professor
School of Nursing; School of Medicine,
    Department of Neurosurgery
University of Pittsburgh
Pittsburgh, Pennsylvania
Caregiver Strain and Burden PEP Resource

Marybeth Singer, MS, APN-BC, AOCN®,
    ACHPN
Nurse Practitioner, Gillette Center for Breast
    Oncology
Massachusetts General Hospital Cancer
    Center
Boston, Massachusetts
Lymphedema PEP Resource

Susan Claire Somers, RN, BSN, OCN®
Oncology Staff Nurse
Spectrum Health
Grand Rapids, Michigan
Caregiver Strain and Burden PEP Resource

Patricia Starr, RN, MSN, OCN®
Neuro-Oncology/CyberKnife® Care Coordinator
Waukesha Memorial Hospital
Waukesha, Wisconsin
*Chemotherapy-Induced Nausea and Vomit-
    ing PEP Resource*

Julie A. Summers, RN, BSN
Nursing Supervisor
Texas Health Harris Methodist Hospital of
    Fort Worth
Fort Worth, Texas
Anxiety PEP Resource

Susan A. Swanson, RN, MS, AOCN®
Oncology Clinical Nurse Specialist, Charge
    Nurse Anschutz Cancer Pavilion
University of Colorado Hospital
Denver, Colorado
Anxiety PEP Resource

Ellen R. Tanner, RN, BSN, OCN®
Staff Nurse
Penn State Cancer Institute Milton S.
    Hershey Medical Center
Hershey, Pennsylvania
Fatigue PEP Resource

Robi Thomas, PhD, RN
Associate Professor of Nursing, Chair of
    Grand Rapids Campus
McAuley School of Nursing
University of Detroit Mercy
Grand Rapids, Michigan

Deborah Thorpe, PhD, APRN, AOCNS®,
    ACHPN
Pain Medicine and Palliative Care
Huntsman Cancer Institute
University of Utah
Salt Lake City, Utah
Diarrhea PEP Resource

Leslie B. Tyson, MS, APRN-BC, OCN®
Nurse Practitioner
Memorial Sloan-Kettering Cancer Center
New York, New York
Dyspnea PEP Resource

Mary Yenulevich, RN, BSN, OCN®
Charge Nurse
Dana-Farber Cancer Institute
Boston, Massachusetts
Constipation PEP Resource

Constance Visovsky, RN, PhD, ACNP
Associate Professor, College of Nursing
University of Nebraska Medical Center
Omaha, Nebraska
Peripheral Neuropathy PEP Resource

Laura Zitella, RN, MS, NP, AOCN®
Nurse Practitioner
Stanford Hospital and Clinics
Stanford, California
Prevention of Infection PEP Resource

Myra J. Woolery, MN, RN, CPON®
Pediatric Clinical Nurse Specialist
National Institutes of Health
Bethesda, Maryland
Constipation PEP Resource
Prevention of Infection PEP Resource

Reviewers

Linda Lillington, DNSc, RN, CCRC
Research Program Director
Division of Endocrinology
Department of Medicine
Los Angeles Biomedical Research Institute
Harbor-UCLA Medical Center
Torrance, California

Dana N. Rutledge, PhD, RN
Professor of Nursing
California State University, Fullerton
Fullerton, California

Gail Mallory, PhD, RN, NEA-BC
Director of Research
Oncology Nursing Society
Pittsburgh, Pennsylvania

Disclosure

Editors and authors of books and guidelines provided by the Oncology Nursing Society are expected to disclose to the participants any significant financial interest or other relationships with the manufacturer(s) of any commercial products.

A vested interest may be considered to exist if a faculty member is affiliated with or has a financial interest in commercial organizations that may have a direct or indirect interest in the subject matter. A "financial interest" may include, but is not limited to, being a shareholder in the organization; being an employee of the commercial organization; serving on an organization's speakers bureau; or receiving research from the organization. An "affiliation" may be holding a position on an advisory board or some other role of benefit to the commercial organization. Vested interest statements appear in the front matter for each publication.

Contributors are expected to disclose any unlabeled or investigational use of products discussed in their content. This information is acknowledged solely for the information of the readers.

The contributors provided the following disclosure and vested interest information:

Kristen Baileys, RN, MSN, CRNP, AOCNP®, Oncology Nursing Society, employee

Heather Belansky, RN, MSN, Oncology Nursing Society, employee

Jeannine M. Brant, PhD, APRN, AOCN®, IMER, M-K Medical Communications, speaker

Annette Parry Bush, RN, BSN, MBA, OCN®, Oncology Nursing Society, employee

Ann E. Culkin, RN, OCN®, Lilly, Genentech, Inc., speakers bureaus

Nancy A. Delzer, MSN, MBA, AOCN®, BC-PCM, Roche Pharmaceuticals, Sanofi-Aventis, speakers bureaus

Linda H. Eaton, MN, RN, AOCN®, Oncology Nursing Society, employee

June G. Eilers, PhD, APRN-CNS, BC, Cytogen, Amgen Inc., Endo, advisory board and speakers bureaus; EUSA Pharma, speakers bureau

Christopher R. Friese, RN, PhD, AOCN®, Amgen Inc., speakers bureau, consultant

Kristine B. LeFebvre, MSN, RN, AOCN®, Oncology Nursing Society, employee

Barbara G. Lubejko, RN, MS, Oncology Nursing Society, employee

Joyce A. Marrs, MS, FNP-BC, AOCNP®, Genentech, Inc., Pfizer Inc., speakers bureaus

Cathy L. Maxwell, RN, OCN®, Novartis, Amgen Inc., Merck, Roche Pharmaceuticals, Sanofi-Aventis, Pfizer Inc., MGI, AstraZeneca, nurse speaker, nurse adviser, research

Christine A. Miaskowski, RN, PhD, FAAN, Endo, Cephalon, PriCara, consultant

Janice K. Reynolds, RN, BC, OCN®, CHPN, MEDA Pharmaceuticals, advisory board for new drug not yet on the market

Deborah Thorpe, PhD, APRN, AOCNS®, ACHPN, Wyeth Pharmaceuticals, speakers bureau

Janelle M. Tipton, MSN, RN, AOCN®, Amgen Inc., ProStrakan, speakers bureaus

Laura Zitella, RN, MS, NP, AOCN®, ProStrakan, Schering-Plough, consultant

Contents

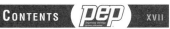

PEP Up Your Practice:

An Introduction to the Oncology Nursing Society Putting Evidence Into Practice Resources

Barbara Holmes Gobel, MS, RN, AOCN®, and Janelle M. Tipton, MSN, RN, AOCN®

Introduction

The goal of *Putting Evidence Into Practice: Improving Oncology Patient Outcomes* is to provide a single publication of the updated Oncology Nursing Society (ONS) Putting Evidence Into Practice (PEP) Resources, assessment and measurement tools, ideas for patient care and organizational use, and case studies to illustrate application of the tools. The inclusion of the assessment and measurement tools will provide all of the resources to guide oncology nurses in the nursing process. These tools and references then can be used to begin to measure application of the interventions in practice. Ultimately, the measurement of patient outcomes will assist nurses, their clients, organizations, and regulators and insurers of health care to document and validate the impact of nursing interventions on patient outcomes. The measurement of outcomes may translate into more cost-effective care, improved patient satisfaction, recognition of a professional approach to care, increased collaboration with physicians and other healthcare professionals, and optimal patient outcomes.

Overview of the PEP Resources

The mission of ONS is to promote excellence in oncology nursing. Excellence in oncology nursing supports the quality of nursing care that is delivered to individuals and their families affected by cancer. One of ONS's strategic goals is to drive quality oncology care through practice, research, education, and policy. In recent years, a major initiative of the Society in supporting its mission and strategic goals has been the development of the ONS PEP Resources. These resources help oncology nurses use evidence-based interventions in their practice, thereby improving nursing-sensitive patient outcomes (NSPOs).

Evidence-Based Practice

Evidence-based practice (EBP) is a concept that is integral within today's healthcare environment. Nurses and other healthcare providers must be able to provide care that is based on the best available evidence in order to effect the best possible patient outcomes. According to Rutledge and Grant (2002), EBP "defines care that integrates best scientific evidence with clinical expertise, knowledge of pathophysiology, knowledge of psychosocial issues, and decision making preferences of patients" (p. 1). Although EBP relies heavily on evidence available through science and research, it also includes the preferences and values of patients and families. Thus, the application of evidence and patient outcomes will differ based on patients' values, concerns, expectations, and preferences. The ability to provide evidence for nursing interventions and outcomes is critical to all aspects of patient care, including patient teaching, provision of patient care, development of standards of care, development of policies and procedures, and development of telephone triage protocols.

Nursing-Sensitive Patient Outcomes

The term *outcomes* can have diverse meaning in many situations. Donabedian (1980) defined outcomes related to health care as favorable or adverse changes in health status due to prior or concurrent care. Outcomes are the way by which we validate the effectiveness and quality of our care (Donabedian). Classification of outcomes can be broad-based indicators, including cost, access to care, patient satisfaction, and quality of care provided. Outcomes also can relate to specific indicators, such as relief of nausea and vomiting, prevention of infection, or comfort during palliative care. Both broad-based and specific indicators are applicable outcomes in cancer care.

NSPOs are outcomes that are amenable to nursing intervention. NSPOs must be within the scope of nursing practice and integral to the processes of nursing care (Given & Sherwood, 2005). NSPOs represent the effects of nursing interventions and result in changes in patient safety, symptom experience, functional status, psychological distress, and/or healthcare costs (Gobel, Beck, & O'Leary, 2006). These outcomes are not always accomplished by nursing alone—they also may be affected by other healthcare professionals such as physicians, chaplains, social workers, and physical and occupational therapists.

History of the ONS PEP Project

ONS held a state-of-the-science conference on NSPOs in 1998 to define NSPOs as they relate to oncology nursing care and to provide direction for research and clinical practice in the promotion of evidence-based care. Although no definitive list of oncology NSPOs was identified, the consensus from the conference was that NSPOs are measurable effects of care that can be attributed to nurses and that the creation of a framework to guide efforts in NSPOs in cancer care was needed (Given & Sherwood, 2005). In 2000, ONS convened an expert panel on NSPOs to identify gaps and goals for outcomes research. Goals that were identified by the panel included identifying NSPOs in oncology care, commissioning a compendium of appropriate research instruments to study NSPOs, and providing support for clinical trials nurses to include NSPOs in research. The 2003–2005 ONS Research Agenda identified NSPOs as one of the Society's top research priorities (ONS, 2003).

In 2003, ONS funded an Outcomes Project Team to develop a strategic plan regarding NSPOs. The Outcomes Project Team developed a statement on and definition of NSPOs, as well as a list of NSPOs to be examined (see Figure 1-1). Outcomes chosen for initial review included fatigue, nausea and vomiting, prevention of infection, and return to usual function. The initial phase of examination of these outcomes included an evidence-based summary of each outcome developed by a nurse scientist that included definitions, references and links to integrated reviews, meta-analyses, clinical guideline tables related to each outcome, key points relating to the research regarding the outcome, and a summary of available instruments/tools to measure the outcome (see www.ons.org/outcomes). The nurse scientists subsequently met with a group of advanced practice nurses (APNs) at the 2004 Advanced Practice Nursing Retreat to discuss the summaries. The APN group requested that more clinical guidance be provided throughout the summaries for nurses in clinical practice and recommended that a comprehensive list of interventions be developed for each outcome, including the level of evidence, or strength of evidence, to support various nursing interventions.

Figure 1-1. Outcome Exemplars From the Oncology Nursing Society Outcomes Project Team

Symptom Control and Management
- Pain
- Peripheral neuropathy
- Fatigue
- Insomnia
- Nausea
- Constipation
- Anorexia
- Breathlessness
- Diarrhea
- Altered skin or mucous membrane
- Neutropenia

Functional Status
- Activities of daily living
- Instrumental activities of daily living
- Role functioning
- Activity tolerance
- Ability to carry out usual activities
- Nutritional status

Psychological Health Status
- Anxiety
- Depression
- Spiritual distress
- Coping

Economic (Incorporate this category into all categories.)
- Length of stay
- Unexpected readmissions
- Emergency room visits
- Out-of-pocket costs (family)
- Homecare visits
- Costs per day per episode

Note. Based on information from Oncology Nursing Society, 2004.

ONS PEP Resource Development

The goal of the ONS PEP Resources is to facilitate application of current available evidence into everyday cancer care. The intent of this goal is to provide the level of evidence for interventions that can be integrated into the management of specific oncology problems. All of the ONS PEP Resources have been developed by teams of oncology APNs, staff nurses, and nurse scientists. The development process that each team has followed is the EBP model of problem identification, evidence search, critique of the research, synthesis of the research, and summary of the strength of the evidence (see Figure 1-2). Each team performed exhaustive reviews of the available intervention research for each outcome, including case studies and expert opinion. ONS set a predetermined date to which the literature would be reviewed, with a commitment to continue with updates of the literature every two to three years beyond the original review date. These dates are published on all of the ONS PEP Resources. See Figure 1-3 for a list of available ONS PEP Resources.

Figure 1-2. Evidence-Based Practice Model of Research Review

- Problem identification
- Evidence search
- Critique of the research
- Synthesis of the research
- Summary of the strength of the evidence

Figure 1-3. Available ONS PEP Resources

- Guidelines tables
- Tables of evidence
- Meta-analyses/systematic reviews tables
- Definitions related to each outcome area
- ONS PEP resources (volumes 1–4)
- ONS PEP detailed resources (available for volumes 1–3)

Review of the Research

The development of clinical questions guided the review of the literature. For example, the team that originally developed the ONS PEP Resources regarding the outcome of pain decided to narrow its literature review by asking the following question: What are the pharmacologic interventions for nociceptive and neuropathic cancer pain in adults? The following elements were then documented based on the review of the literature: author and year; characteristics of the intervention; sample characteristics, setting characteristics, study design, and conceptual model; measures; results and conclusions; limitations, major and minor flaws, cautions or contraindications, special training needs and costs; and the ONS Levels of Evidence and comments. The tables of evidence for each outcome are available at www.ons.org/outcomes.

The *ONS Levels of Evidence* (Hadorn, Baker, Hodges, & Hicks, 1996; Ropka & Spencer-Cisek, 2001) were chosen to rate the level of evidence, or strength of the evidence, for each research article included in volumes 1–3 (see Table 1-1). The *Evidence Rating System for the Hierarchy of Evidence* was used to rate the level of evidence for volume 4 (Melnyk & Fineout-Overholt, 2005). For resources beyond the first four volumes, ONS decided to no longer continue with the levels of evidence for each study and instead rely on the review of the study design and study limitations to help to identify the weight of evidence for each intervention. The levels of evidence and the subsequent identification of the weight-of-evidence classification of nursing interventions were peer reviewed in each group, between groups, and by a field review process.

Putting Evidence Into Practice: Weight-of-Evidence Classification Model

After the research reviews were completed, the team categorized the interventions using a classification system that had been designed to provide evidence-based guidance in the choice of interventions. The classification model was based on the *BMJ* model (BMJ Publishing Group, 2002) but was modified to reflect the ONS Levels of Evidence. One of the identified drawbacks of using the *BMJ* model is that only systematic reviews and meta-analyses are included. Another model that was initially considered for classifying the weight of evidence was the U.S. Preventive Services Task Force classification model (Harris et al., 2001). This model has been used primarily to classify public health interventions and does not provide clinical guidance in the choice of nursing interventions. The ONS weight-of-evidence classifications are color-coded on the ONS PEP pocket resources (and the previously developed ONS PEP detailed resources) to enable nurses to quickly determine the level of evidence for each intervention.

Table 1-1. ONS PEP Resources: Volumes 1–4	
ONS PEP Volume	**Outcomes**
1	• Fatigue • Nausea and vomiting • Prevention of infection • Sleep-wake disturbances
2	• Caregiver strain and burden • Constipation • Depression • Dyspnea • Mucositis • Peripheral neuropathy
3	• Pain • Prevention of bleeding
4	• Anorexia • Anxiety • Diarrhea • Lymphedema

- Interventions that are color-coded green are of the highest level of evidence, in which the evidence supports consideration of these interventions in practice and are labeled either *Recommended for Practice* or *Likely to Be Effective.*
- Yellow color-coded interventions have less research to support their use and are labeled *Benefits Balanced With Harms* or *Effectiveness Not Established.*
- Red color-coded interventions either have very little research to support their practice, labeled *Effectiveness Unlikely,* or have been found to be ineffective or even harmful, labeled *Not Recommended for Practice.*

See Table 1-2 for a detailed description of the ONS Weight-of-Evidence Classification Model.

Table 1-2. ONS PEP Weight-of-Evidence Classification Model	
Classification	**Definition**
Recommended for practice	Interventions for which effectiveness has been demonstrated by strong evidence from rigorously conducted studies, meta-analyses, or systematic reviews and for which expectation of harms is small compared with the benefits
Likely to be effective	Interventions for which effectiveness has been demonstrated by supportive evidence from a single rigorously conducted controlled trial, consistent supportive evidence from well-designed controlled trials using small samples, or guidelines developed from evidence and supported by expert opinion
Benefits balanced with harms	Interventions for which clinicians and patients should weigh the beneficial and harmful effects according to individual circumstances and priorities
Effectiveness not established	Interventions for which insufficient or conflicting data or data of inadequate quality currently exist, with no clear indication of harm
Effectiveness unlikely	Interventions for which lack of effectiveness has been demonstrated by negative evidence from a single rigorously conducted controlled trial, consistent negative evidence from well-designed controlled trials using small samples, or guidelines developed from evidence and supported by expert opinion
Not recommended for practice	Interventions for which lack of effectiveness or harmfulness has been demonstrated by strong evidence from rigorously conducted studies, meta-analyses, or systematic reviews, or interventions where the costs, burden, or harms associated with the intervention exceed anticipated benefit
Expert opinion	Low-risk interventions that are (1) consistent with sound clinical practice, (2) suggested by an expert in a peer-reviewed publication (journal or book chapter), and (3) for which limited evidence exists. An expert is an individual who has published articles in a peer-reviewed journal in the domain of interest.

Applying ONS PEP Resources to Practice

The ONS PEP Resources provide significant benefits for oncology nursing in the areas of clinical practice, education, and research. The ONS PEP Resources and tools have been developed because EBP is essential to the delivery of high-quality cancer care. As oncology nurses, recognizing the evidence equation is important: clinician experience + patient preference + scientific findings = evidence-based practice (DePalma, 2000). EBP-based strategies can promote change and better practice in any cancer-care setting. Institutional uses of PEP Resources may include updating standard chemotherapy order sets based on current evidence of the management of nausea and vomiting, developing evidence-based standards of practice, and supporting activities related to acquisition of resources to utilize interventions that have strong evidence to support their use. From an education standpoint, the ONS PEP

Resources could be used for oncology nursing orientation and support of standards of practice; additional education resources for the ONS Chemotherapy and Biotherapy Course; and ongoing education of relevant topics through nursing grand rounds, nursing in-services, and journal clubs. Nursing research also may be an outcome of the resources. For some ONS PEP Resources, the evidence available to provide clinical guidance is scant and requires more study in order for interventions to be recommended for practice. Further discussion regarding the evidence presented in the ONS PEP Resources is presented in articles published in the *Clinical Journal of Oncology Nursing* for each ONS PEP outcome. Presentations at the ONS Institutes of Learning and ONS Congress, as well as local chapter presentations by the ONS PEP Chapter Champions program, provide education on the ONS PEP Resources and applications to clinical practice situations. The ONS PEP Chapter Champions program is an educational program that is offered to ONS chapters throughout the United States that highlights the development, clinical application, and potential outcomes of the ONS PEP Resources.

The ONS PEP Resources are available on the ONS Web site at www.ons.org/outcomes. The Web-based resources provide comprehensive information, including tables of evidence and references. The materials can be printed or bookmarked for use. In addition, the resources are available in PDA format through Pepid® (www.pepid.com).

Summary

An increasingly robust body of evidence exists on which to base nursing practice. It is critical for oncology nurses to seek out evidence so they can provide the best possible care for patients and their families. ONS has developed the ONS PEP Resources to provide oncology nurses with current evidence to help to guide their nursing practice. These resources can be used by novice as well as experienced oncology nurses, APNs, and nurse scientists. In today's healthcare environment, nurses need to be able to articulate the evidence base for oncology nursing practice to patients, families, and nursing and other professional colleagues. This articulation of evidence and outcomes also will help to validate oncology nursing practice for healthcare organizations, regulators and insurers of health care, and policy makers.

References

BMJ Publishing Group. (2002). *Clinical evidence concise* (7th ed.). London: Author.

DePalma, J. (2000). Evidence-based clinical practice guidelines. *Seminars in Perioperative Nursing, 9*(3), 115–120.

Donabedian, A. (1980). *The definition of quality and approaches to its assessment.* Ann Arbor, MI: Health Administration Press.

Given, B.A., & Sherwood, P.R. (2005). Nursing-sensitive patient outcomes—A white paper. *Oncology Nursing Forum, 32*(4), 773–784.

Gobel, B.H., Beck, S.L., & O'Leary, C. (2006). Nursing-sensitive patient outcomes: The development of the Putting Evidence Into Practice resources for nursing practice. *Clinical Journal of Oncology Nursing, 10*(5), 621–624.

Hadorn, D.C., Baker, D., Hodges, J.S., & Hicks, N. (1996). Rating the quality of evidence for clinical practice guidelines. *Journal of Clinical Epidemiology, 49*(7), 749–754.

Harris, R.P., Helfand, M., Woolf, S.H., Lohr, K.N., Mulrow, C.D., Teutsch, S.M., et al. (2001). Current methods of the U.S. Preventive Services Task Force: A review of the process. *American Journal of Preventive Medicine, 20*(Suppl. 3), 21–35.

Melnyk, B., & Fineout-Overholt, E. (2005). *Evidence-based practice in nursing and healthcare: A guide to best practice.* Philadelphia: Lippincott Williams & Wilkins.

Oncology Nursing Society. (2003). *Oncology Nursing Society 2003–2005 research agenda.* Retrieved May 25, 2008, from http://www.ons.org/research/information/agenda.shtml

Oncology Nursing Society. (2004). *Nursing-sensitive patient outcomes—Description and framework.* Retrieved May 25, 2008, from http://www.ons.org/outcomes/measures/framework.shtml

Ropka, M.E., & Spencer-Cisek, P. (2001). PRISM: Priority Symptom Management project phase I: Assessment. *Oncology Nursing Forum, 28*(10), 1585–1594.

Rutledge, D.N., & Grant, M. (2002). Introduction. *Seminars in Oncology Nursing, 18*(1), 1–2.

CHAPTER 2

Assessment and Measurement

Linda H. Eaton, MN, RN, AOCN®,
and Janelle M. Tipton, MSN, RN, AOCN®

Integration of the Putting Evidence Into Practice Resources With the Nursing Process

Since the first Oncology Nursing Society (ONS) Putting Evidence Into Practice (PEP) Resources debuted at the ONS Congress in May 2006, the demand for and use of the resources have increased considerably. To date, more than 140,000 volumes of ONS PEP Resources have been distributed. Many steps have been taken to educate nurses about the resources through articles, case studies, and presentations. Consolidating and synthesizing the evidence into a resource that can assist nurses in everyday practice is valuable. Because nurses provide extensive interventions with and for patients, it became apparent fairly quickly that the ONS PEP Resources are useful in practice. However, to better implement the interventions, it is important to go back a step or two in the nursing process. Two parts of the nursing process, assessment and analysis/planning, are important to review before selecting interventions. These steps are critical to best know the patient, risk factors, and preferences. A good nursing assessment will assist in planning the appropriate interventions, guided by the evidence categories in the ONS PEP Resources. Inadequate assessment is a barrier to effective management of symptoms (National Institutes of Health [NIH], 2002), and inadequate management of symptoms and toxicities can have negative consequences. For example, this is especially relevant with chemotherapy toxicities, when morbidity and life-threatening complications occur. Febrile neutropenia can contribute to morbidity, mortality, and healthcare costs. Nursing education should emphasize the risk factors for febrile neutropenia and its consequences, patient assessment, and documentation of interventions, as well as patient response (Maxwell & Stein, 2006).

Nursing Assessment

The nursing process is described as an organized sequence of problem-solving steps used to identify and manage health problems of clients. The sequential steps of the nursing process are assessment, nursing diagnosis, analysis/planning, implementation, and evaluation. As an organized framework for the practice of nursing, the process is orderly, systematic, and central to all nursing care and encompasses all steps taken by the nurse in caring for a patient. Benefits of the nursing process are (a) an orderly and systematic method for planning and providing care, (b) enhancement of nursing efficiency by standardizing nursing practice, (c) facilitation of documentation of care, (d) unity of language for the nursing profession, (e) emphasis of independent function of nurses, and (f) improvement of care quality through the use of deliberate actions. The nursing process is based on knowledge requiring critical thinking and requires planning, organization, and systematic actions. The nursing process is client-centered, goal-directed, and dynamic and involves prioritization (Murray & Atkinson, 2000).

Assessment is the critical first step in effective management of the patient and helps to facilitate patient-centered interventions by identifying problems (Ropka & Spencer-Cisek, 2001). Risk assessment prior to treatment helps to evaluate the patient's risk factors for symptoms prior to treatment (Ropka, Padilla, & Gillespie, 2005). Once a symptom or problem has been identified, further assessment and measurements are useful to determine its cause, to guide interventions, and to communicate with the patient. Management is a type of assessment that provides quantifiable data (Marvin, 1995).

Selection of Interventions

When selecting the interventions, the assessment data may provide an insight into the patient's clinical information and preferences. Other critical pieces of information include the best scientific knowledge and the clinician's experience. Consideration and analysis of these three elements will help to lead to nursing diagnosis of a clinical problem and the intervention selection. According to the ONS PEP weight-of-evidence categories, interventions that are color-coded green on the ONS PEP resource show that the intervention is supported by strong research evidence. Interventions that are color-coded yellow may be selected, but with caution, as there may not be sufficient evidence to support the intervention. Interventions that are color-coded red should be avoided because of lack of evidence for effectiveness or possible harm. Figure 2-1 depicts the stoplight weight-of-evidence analogy.

Why Should Nurses Be Concerned About Measurement?

Measurement is relevant to nursing for several reasons. First, in nursing, an innate concern exists for the human condition. Nurses are taught to do no harm and to provide the best quality of care. Second, customers care. The recipients of nursing care—patients and families and nursing colleagues—have high expectations of nursing and consider the profession to be one of the most trusted. Patients and families are increasingly concerned about outcomes of care and have been sensitized to concerns of safety through the media. Other stakeholders concerned

Figure 2-1. ONS PEP Weight-of-Evidence Stoplight Analogy

Green = GO!
The evidence supports the consideration of these interventions in practice.

Yellow = CAUTION!
There is not sufficient evidence to say whether these interventions are effective or not.

Red = STOP!
The evidence indicates that these interventions are either ineffective or may cause harm.

about quality care issues are institutions, accrediting bodies, payers, and regulators of care.

Two very important issues influence nurses' reasons for measuring patient outcomes and documenting nursing interventions and patient response. The first relates to patient safety. It is critical that nurses use the nursing process and document their interventions. As mentioned previously, neutropenia and infection have safety outcomes. For several of the clinical problems presented in the ONS PEP Resources, adverse events can occur that need prompt identification, intervention, and communication. One must be very cautious of utilizing interventions from the categories that have little evidence for effectiveness or may cause harm. In the future, healthcare professionals may be given a report card grading them on impact on patient outcomes.

The second important reason to measure outcomes is patient satisfaction. The patient's perception of the quality of care received can validate nursing's performance and can affect patient outcomes through cooperation with care. Several studies demonstrated predictors for quality of care and satisfaction with care (Avery et al., 2006; Kleeberg, Feyer, Gunther, & Behrens, 2008; Sandoval, Levinton, Blackstien-Hirsch, & Brown, 2006). Improvement in oncology practice also has become relevant to physician colleagues. The American Society of Clinical Oncology's Quality Oncology Practice Initiative was started in 2006 to look at measurement and quality improvement in practice. Insurance providers and other professional organizations will likely recognize and reward those practices where quality initiatives are carried out and show improvements (Jacobson et al., 2008; McNiff, 2006).

For nursing, the National Quality Forum (2008) has begun to set criteria measures. Through a rigorous review process in 2003, 15 items were identified as nursing-sensitive standards for inpatient care. Although not specific to oncology or all settings, the standards are primarily related to patient safety and healthcare outcomes. Limited attention has been given in the past to performance measurement and public reporting; however, initial steps are being taken to support the need for redesign of care processes and the environment of nursing care. The issue of measuring the quality of care is relevant to the evaluation piece of the nursing process. Determining how well the standard of care is being met is critical to identifying areas for performance improvement.

Documentation is very important throughout the nursing process and can provide an increased awareness and rationale for selected interventions. It is crucial for nurses to know the baselines for various symptoms and clinical problems, and these data will become a benchmark for comparison as interventions are implemented. This information can lead to better insight into a patient's clinical problems, selection of evidence-based interventions, and focused patient education.

Measurement Issues

Baseline and routine measurements are important in determining individual response to interventions in addition to disease progression (LaCasse & Beck, 2007). The first step in measuring a clinical problem is to identify an appropriate tool. Several items need to be considered in choosing a tool, including symptom dimensions, symptom clusters, clinical utility, and barriers to effective measurement.

Symptom Dimensions

Several of the PEP topics are related to symptoms, which are clinical problems. *Symptoms* are subjective evidence of an illness or condition, whereas *signs* are objective evidence (Thomas, 1997). Signs often are accompanied by predictable symptoms (Krishnan, Stanton, Collins, Liston, & Jewell, 2001). Patient self-report is the most accurate method for symptom assessment, although self-report may be difficult for patients who are very sick (NIH, 2002). Most nurses in clinical settings screen patients for more than one symptom, and when symptoms are identified, a more in-depth assessment is performed. Symptom screening can be assessed by patients responding "yes" or "no" when asked whether they are experiencing a particular symptom.

The next step is to have the patient rate the dimensions of a symptom using a measurement tool. Unidimensional tools provide measurement of one symptom dimension, whereas multidimensional tools evaluate several dimensions of a symptom. It is important to measure intensity, frequency, distress, location, and onset of a symptom in addition to the outcomes of an intervention, including relief and patient satisfaction (Paice, 2004). Common unidimensional measurement tools include the visual analog scale (VAS) and the numeric rating scale (NRS). The VAS is a 100 mm line (vertical or horizontal) with a descriptor at each end to indicate extremes of the sensation. The VAS score is achieved by measuring the distance from the bottom or left end of the scale to the level indicated by the individual. The NRS requires individuals to rate their sensation on a 0–10 horizontal scale, with 0 being no sensation and 10 being sensation that is as bad as can be. Generally, a score of 1–3 is considered mild, 4–6 indicates a moderate level, and 7–10 is the highest (or severe) level (D'Arcy, 2007). Symptom intensity typically is measured using the VAS or NRS.

Symptom Clusters

Symptoms may present in clusters of two or more (Fan, Filipczak, & Chow, 2007; LaCasse & Beck, 2007). The symptom clusters may be related to disease or treatment or both (Gift, 2007; LaCasse & Beck; Miaskowski, 2006). Some symptom clusters may have a common cause, whereas others may influence one another; for example, pain may disturb sleep, which may result in fatigue (Beck, Dudley, & Barsevick, 2005).

Examples of cancer-related symptom clusters identified in the literature include
- Pain, sleep disturbance, and fatigue (with or without depression) in people with breast cancer (Gaston-Johannson, Fall-Dickson, Bakos, & Kennedy, 1999) and people with bone metastases (Miaskowski & Lee, 1999)
- Fatigue, loss of concentration, and mood disturbance (anxiety, nervousness, depression) in people with breast cancer (Bender, Ergyn, Rosenzweig, Cohen, & Sereika, 2005)
- Fatigue, weakness, nausea, vomiting, loss of appetite, weight loss, and altered taste in people with lung cancer (Gift, Jablonski, Stommel, & Given, 2004)
- Fatigue, frequent pain, and insomnia in people with lung cancer (Sarna, 1993).

Studies are needed to identify which tools will provide the most valid and reliable data to determine the occurrence of clinically relevant symptom clusters and which dimensions of a symptom are important for the measurement of a symptom within a symptom cluster (Miaskowski, 2006). Multi-symptom assessment tools are helpful in assessing the overall symptom experience and emerging symptom patterns, but they are not specific to the assessment of symptom clusters (LaCasse & Beck, 2007).

Several tools have been designed to measure multiple symptoms, including the Edmonton Symptom Assessment System (ESAS), M.D. Anderson Symptom Inventory, Memorial Symptom Assessment Scale (MSAS), Rotterdam Symptom Checklist, and Symptom Distress Scale. All of these tools have strong validity and reliability in measuring cancer-related symptoms and are reported to take no longer than 10 minutes to complete (LaCasse & Beck, 2007; Paice, 2004). The ESAS (see Figure 2-2) is composed of nine VASs that measure pain, activity, nausea, depression, anxiety, drowsiness, lack of appetite, well-being, and shortness of breath. The score is a sum of the nine symptoms (Bruera, Kuehn, Miller, Selmser, & Macmillan, 1991). The MSAS (see Figure 2-3) consists of five-point Likert scales to measure the prevalence, severity, and distress related to 24 physical and psychological symptoms experienced during the prior week. Each symptom score is an average of the three dimensions. The severity and distress of eight additional symptoms are measured. The total MSAS score is the average of all 32 symptom scores (Portenoy et al., 1994).

Clinical Utility

Measurement of clinical problems in daily clinical practice must be practical and easy to do for both clinicians and patients. The same tool should be used to measure

Figure 2-2. Edmonton Symptom Assessment System (ESAS)

Date of completion: _____ Time: _____

Please circle the number that best describes:

```
            0  1  2  3  4  5  6  7  8  9  10
            |__|__|__|__|__|__|__|__|__|__|
No pain                                   Worst possible pain

            0  1  2  3  4  5  6  7  8  9  10
            |__|__|__|__|__|__|__|__|__|__|
Not tired                                 Worst possible tiredness

            0  1  2  3  4  5  6  7  8  9  10
            |__|__|__|__|__|__|__|__|__|__|
Not nauseated                             Worst possible nausea

            0  1  2  3  4  5  6  7  8  9  10
            |__|__|__|__|__|__|__|__|__|__|
Not depressed                             Worst possible depression

            0  1  2  3  4  5  6  7  8  9  10
            |__|__|__|__|__|__|__|__|__|__|
Not anxious                               Worst possible anxiety

            0  1  2  3  4  5  6  7  8  9  10
            |__|__|__|__|__|__|__|__|__|__|
Not drowsy                                Worst possible drowsiness

            0  1  2  3  4  5  6  7  8  9  10
            |__|__|__|__|__|__|__|__|__|__|
Best appetite                             Worst possible appetite

            0  1  2  3  4  5  6  7  8  9  10
            |__|__|__|__|__|__|__|__|__|__|
Best feeling of                           Worst possible feeling
well-being                                of well-being

            0  1  2  3  4  5  6  7  8  9  10
            |__|__|__|__|__|__|__|__|__|__|
No shortness of                           Worst possible shortness
breath                                    of breath

            0  1  2  3  4  5  6  7  8  9  10
            |__|__|__|__|__|__|__|__|__|__|
Other problem
```

ESAS completed by:
__ Patient__ Health professional
__ Family __ Assisted by family or health professional

Note. From "The Edmonton Symptom Assessment System (ESAS): A Simple Method for the Assessment of Palliative Care Patients," by E. Bruera, N. Kuehn, M. Miller, P. Selmser, and K. Macmillan, 1991, *Journal of Palliative Care, 7*(2), p. 7. Copyright 1991 by Centre for Bioethics. Reprinted with permission.

Figure 2-3. Memorial Symptom Assessment Scale

Name   Date

Section 1

Instructions: We have listed 24 symptoms below. Read each one carefully. If you have had the symptom during this past week, let us know how <u>OFTEN</u> you had it, how <u>SEVERE</u> it was usually and how much it <u>DISTRESSED or BOTHERED</u> you by circling the appropriate number. If you <u>DID NOT HAVE</u> the symptom, make an "X" in the box marked "<u>DID NOT HAVE</u>."

<u>DURING THE PAST WEEK</u> Did you have any of the following symptoms?	DID NOT HAVE	IF YES How OFTEN did you have it?				IF YES How SEVERE was it usually				IF YES How much did it DISTRESS or BOTHER you?				
		Rarely	Occasionally	Frequently	Almost Constantly	Slight	Moderate	Severe	Very Severe	Not at all	A Little Bit	Somewhat	Quite a Bit	Very Much
Difficulty concentrating		1	2	3	4	1	2	3	4	0	1	2	3	4
Pain		1	2	3	4	1	2	3	4	0	1	2	3	4
Lack of energy		1	2	3	4	1	2	3	4	0	1	2	3	4
Cough		1	2	3	4	1	2	3	4	0	1	2	3	4
Feeling nervous		1	2	3	4	1	2	3	4	0	1	2	3	4
Dry mouth		1	2	3	4	1	2	3	4	0	1	2	3	4
Nausea		1	2	3	4	1	2	3	4	0	1	2	3	4
Feeling drowsy		1	2	3	4	1	2	3	4	0	1	2	3	4
Numbness/tingling in hands/feet		1	2	3	4	1	2	3	4	0	1	2	3	4
Difficulty sleeping		1	2	3	4	1	2	3	4	0	1	2	3	4
Feeling bloated		1	2	3	4	1	2	3	4	0	1	2	3	4
Problems with urination		1	2	3	4	1	2	3	4	0	1	2	3	4
Vomiting		1	2	3	4	1	2	3	4	0	1	2	3	4
Shortness of breath		1	2	3	4	1	2	3	4	0	1	2	3	4
Diarrhea		1	2	3	4	1	2	3	4	0	1	2	3	4
Feeling sad		1	2	3	4	1	2	3	4	0	1	2	3	4
Sweats		1	2	3	4	1	2	3	4	0	1	2	3	4
Worrying		1	2	3	4	1	2	3	4	0	1	2	3	4
Problems with sexual interest or activity		1	2	3	4	1	2	3	4	0	1	2	3	4
Itching		1	2	3	4	1	2	3	4	0	1	2	3	4
Lack of appetite		1	2	3	4	1	2	3	4	0	1	2	3	4
Dizziness		1	2	3	4	1	2	3	4	0	1	2	3	4
Difficulty swallowing		1	2	3	4	1	2	3	4	0	1	2	3	4
Feeling irritable		1	2	3	4	1	2	3	4	0	1	2	3	4

(Continued on next page)

Figure 2-3. Memorial Symptom Assessment Scale *(Continued)*

Section 2

INSTRUCTIONS: We have listed 8 symptoms below. Read each one carefully. If you have had the symptom during this past week, let us know how SEVERE it was usually and how much it DISTRESSED or BOTHERED you by circling the appropriate number. If you DID NOT HAVE the symptom, make an "X" in the box marked "DID NOT HAVE."

DURING THE PAST WEEK, Did you have any of the following symptoms?	DID NOT HAVE	IF YES How SEVERE was it usually?				IF YES How much did it DISTRESS or BOTHER you?				
		Slight	Moderate	Severe	Very Severe	Not at all	A little bit	Somewhat	Quite a bit	Very much
Mouth sores		1	2	3	4	0	1	2	3	4
Change in the way food tastes		1	2	3	4	0	1	2	3	4
Weight loss		1	2	3	4	0	1	2	3	4
Hair loss		1	2	3	4	0	1	2	3	4
Constipation		1	2	3	4	0	1	2	3	4
Swelling of arms or legs		1	2	3	4	0	1	2	3	4
"I don't look like myself"		1	2	3	4	0	1	2	3	4
Changes in skin		1	2	3	4	0	1	2	3	4

IF YOU HAD ANY OTHER SYMPTOMS DURING THE PAST WEEK, PLEASE LIST BELOW AND INDICATE HOW MUCH THE SYMPTOM HAS DISTRESSED OR BOTHERED YOU.

Other:						0	1	2	3	4
Other:						0	1	2	3	4
Other:						0	1	2	3	4

Note. Figure courtesy of Russell Portenoy, MD. Used with permission.

the severity of a patient's clinical problem at different points in time in order to collect comparable data. Tools must be short, easy to read and score, and have clear instructions. This is particularly important for patients with considerable symptom burden (Paice, 2004). The clinician at the bedside often does not have easy access to measurement tools, or the cost of a tool may be prohibitive; however, many free tools are available. If a tool is copyrighted, one must obtain permission before use, which sometimes is an arduous process.

NIH, through the NIH Roadmap Initiative, provides a publicly available resource of standardized, accurate, and efficient measures for physical function, fatigue, pain, emotional distress (including depression and anxiety), global health, and social health (social function and social support). NIH's Patient-Reported Outcomes Measurement Information System (PROMIS) is available at www.nihPROMIS.org and is intended for a variety of chronic diseases, including cancer. PROMIS is developing measures specifically for cancer care, such as sleep-wake function, sexual function, cognitive function, and the psychosocial impacts of the illness experience (i.e., stress response and coping, shifts in self-concept, social interactions, spirituality) (Garcia et al., 2007; NIH, 2008).

Barriers to Effective Symptom Measurement

Barriers to clinical measurement of symptoms are related to the healthcare provider, the patient, and the healthcare system. Healthcare provider barriers are considerable and include lack of awareness, limited time, the subjective nature of cancer-related symptoms, and assumptions that patients will voluntarily report these symptoms. A patient-related barrier to effective measurement is the assumption that healthcare providers "know" when the patient experiences symptoms so reporting them is not necessary. In addition, patients may be reluctant to report symptoms because they do not want to bother their healthcare providers or family members (Paice, 2004). A study investigating pain found that patients are reluctant to report pain and other symptoms because it may make them ineligible for participation in a clinical trial (Cleeland, 2002). Healthcare system barriers include lack of time for trained healthcare professionals to perform clinical measurements because of decreased staffing and increased patient acuity. Lack of clinical measurement tools with established reliability, validity, and sensitivity in patients with cancer is also a barrier.

Survey of Clinical Measurement Tools Used to Evaluate Oncology Patient Problems

In July 2008, ONS distributed a 25-item electronic survey to a random sample of advanced practice nurse (APN) members. The purpose of the survey was to determine which clinical measurement tools were being used to measure oncology patient problems. The survey was first pilot-tested with five ONS APN members to determine ease and appropriateness of the questions. The survey then was distributed to 1,800 clinical nurse specialists and nurse practitioners. Almost 300 APN members responded to the survey, yielding a response rate of 17%.

Characteristics and Work Settings of Advanced Practice Nurses Surveyed

The survey gathered details about the characteristics and work settings of the APNs who responded. The APNs worked in the following roles: nurse practitioner (46%), clinical nurse specialist (37%), both nurse practitioner and clinical nurse specialist (11%), manager (3%), educator (2%), and other (2%). The APNs worked in a variety of settings: community (27%), academic (25%), comprehensive cancer center (23%), major medical center (12%), and private practice (12%). Within these settings, 37% of the APNs worked in an outpatient hospital-based clinic (n = 109), 21% worked in an outpatient physician office/infusion center (n = 64), and 24% worked on an inpatient medical oncology unit (n = 43). The remaining APNs worked in a variety of inpatient and outpatient settings, including "other settings" such as home infusion pharmacy, palliative care unit, and outpatient rehabilitation center for lymphedema. The majority of the APNs (n = 254, 85%) reported that the nurses in their workplaces cared for patients on clinical trials. The percentage of patients on clinical trials ranged from less than 5% to 100%, and the greatest number of APNs (n = 74, 25%) indicated that 6%–10% of patients were on clinical trials. The top three cancers seen in the APNs' work settings were breast (n = 124, 42%), lung (n = 65, 22%), and colorectal (n = 46, 15%). The top three most common treatments or types of care received by patients in the APNs' primary work settings were chemotherapy (n = 206, 69%), surgery (n = 42, 14%), and radiation therapy (n = 24, 8%).

Clinical Measurement Tools

The APNs identified the clinical measurement tools used by the nurses in their workplace to evaluate the 16 oncology problems addressed by the ONS PEP Resources (see Table 2-1). The APNs selected the tools from a list of three tools, entered a different tool used in their workplace, or indicated that a clinical measurement tool was not used. The majority of APNs reported that a clinical measurement tool was not used by the nurses in their workplace to measure 10 of the oncology problems. The six oncology problems for which the majority of nurses did use a clinical measurement tool were diarrhea, fatigue, lymphedema, mucositis, pain, and peripheral neuropathy. The National Cancer Institute (NCI) Cancer Therapy Evaluation Program's (CTEP's) Common Terminology Criteria for Adverse Events (CTCAE) was the tool used most commonly for measuring severity of diarrhea, fatigue, mucositis, pain, and peripheral neuropathy. This may have been related to the high number of nurses caring for patients on clinical trials.

The CTCAE (version 3.0) is a well-known tool that provides a standard language for reporting adverse events in patients participating in clinical trials. A grading scale with specific criteria for each adverse event is used to determine the severity of the symptom (NCI CTEP, 2006). The CTCAE is a good tool for symptom screening, but it appears to be sensitive to the measurement of only significant changes in a symptom (Rutledge & McGuire, 2004). Thus, the tool may not be ideal for determining individual responses to nursing interventions. Reliability, validity, and sensitivity testing of the CTCAE have not been published.

Reasons for Not Using a Clinical Measurement Tool

The most frequently reported reason for not using a clinical measurement tool was lack of knowledge about clinical measurement tools (58%). Lack of availability of clinical measurement tools (47%) and not enough time to use clinical measurement tools (34%) also were reported. The expense of clinical measurement tools was a factor for a small number of APNs (5.4%). Only 20 APNs (7%) reported that the nurses in their work setting do use clinical measurement tools to measure all 16 oncology problems addressed by the ONS PEP Resources.

Selection of Tools for This Book

The focus of chapters 3–18 is on the specific ONS PEP Resources for the identified clinical problem or symptom. The authors of the ONS PEP Resources have

Table 2-1. Use of Clinical Measurement Tools

Symptom	Measurement Tools	n	%
1. Anorexia	NCI CTCAE	81	27%
	PG-SGA	19	6%
	Malnutrition Screening Tool	18	6%
	Other: Body weight, dietitian consult, ESAS, PCM	20	7%
	No clinical measurement tool used	179	60%
2. Anxiety	NCCN Distress Thermometer	40	13%
	Beck Anxiety Inventory	15	5%
	HADS	13	4%
	Other: BSI, ESAS, NCI CTCAE, NRS, PCM, PHQ-9	25	8%
	No clinical measurement tool used	211	71%
3. Bleeding	NCI CTCAE	116	39%
	FACT-Thrombocytopenia	12	4%
	Other: Laboratory values	7	2%
	No clinical measurement tool used	168	56%
4. Caregiver strain and burden	Caregiver Strain Index	8	3%
	Caregiver Reaction Assessment	8	3%
	Zarit Burden Inventory	1	0.34%
	Other: Social service consult	3	1%
	No clinical measurement tool used	280	94%
5. Chemotherapy-induced nausea and vomiting	Likert scale	46	15%
	VAS	27	9%
	Index of Nausea, Vomiting, and Retching–2	26	9%
	Other: ESAS, NCI CTCAE, NCCN guidelines, NRS, PCM, Rhodes Index of Nausea and Vomiting	57	19%
	No clinical measurement tool used	149	50%
6. Constipation	NCI CTCAE	110	37%
	Constipation Assessment Scale	18	6%
	Other: ESAS, NCI CTCAE, NRS, PCM	18	6%
	No clinical measurement tool used	161	54%
7. Depression	Beck Depression Inventory	32	11%
	HADS	26	9%
	Brief Zung Self-Rating Depression Scale	14	4%
	Other: BSI, CES-D, NCCN Distress Thermometer, PHQ-9, psychologist	32	11%
	No clinical measurement tool used	199	67%

(Continued on next page)

Table 2-1. Use of Clinical Measurement Tools *(Continued)*

Symptom	Measurement Tools	n	%
8. Diarrhea	NCI CTCAE	155	52%
	National Surgical Adjuvant Breast and Bowel Project toxicity rating	3	1%
	Other: ESAS, graft-versus-host disease score, NCCN guidelines, PCM	18	6%
	No clinical measurement tool used	131	44%
9. Dyspnea	NRS	36	12%
	Dyspnea VAS	14	5%
	Cancer Dyspnea Scale	7	2%
	Other: ESAS, NCI CTCAE	27	9%
	No clinical measurement tool used	218	73%
10. Fatigue	NCI CTCAE	97	33%
	NRS	64	21%
	Brief Fatigue Inventory	21	7%
	Other: ESAS, FACT-Fatigue, NCI CTCAE	17	6%
	No clinical measurement tool used	112	38%
11. Infection	NCI CTCAE	123	41%
	FACT-Neutropenia	18	6%
	Other: Laboratory values, NCCN guidelines	10	3%
	No clinical measurement tool used	155	52%
12. Lymphedema	Circumferential measurement	140	47%
	Lymphedema and Breast Cancer Question-naire	12	4%
	Impedance	10	3%
	Other: NCI CTCAE	8	3%
	No clinical measurement tool used	148	50%
13. Mucositis	NCI CTCAE	138	46%
	Oral Assessment Guide	72	24%
	World Health Organization Oral Toxicity Scale	21	7%
	Other: Radiation Therapy Oncology Group Assessment, Walsh Modified Oral Score	10	3%
	No clinical measurement tool used	83	28%
14. Pain	Numeric Pain Intensity Scale	248	83%
	Pain VAS	87	29%
	Brief Pain Inventory	27	9%

(Continued on next page)

Table 2-1. Use of Clinical Measurement Tools *(Continued)*			
Symptom	**Measurement Tools**	**n**	**%**
	Other: ESAS, FACES Pain Rating Scale, PCM, University of Rochester Nonverbal Pain Scale	16	5%
	No clinical measurement tool used	17	6%
15. Peripheral neuropathy	NCI CTCAE	127	43%
	Eastern Cooperative Oncology Group Rating Scale	32	11%
	FACT–Gynecologic Oncology Group-Neurotoxicity	10	3%
	Other: DN4, PCM, NRS	12	3%
	No clinical measurement tool used	135	45%
16. Sleep-wake disturbances	Insomnia Severity Index	8	3%
	Epworth Sleepiness Scale	3	1%
	Pittsburgh Sleep Quality Index	1	0.34%
	Other: ESAS, NCI CTCAE, PCM	12	4%
	No clinical measurement tool used	278	93%

N = 298 (*Note.* Numbers will not equal the total sample size because more than one tool may be used.)

BSI—Brief Symptom Inventory; CES-D—Center for Epidemiologic Studies Depression Scale; DN4—Douleur Neuropathique, 4-item questionnaire for neuropathic pain; ESAS—Edmonton Symptom Assessment System; FACT—Functional Assessment of Cancer Therapy; HADS—Hospital Anxiety and Depression Scale; NCCN—National Comprehensive Cancer Network; NCI CTCAE—National Cancer Institute Common Terminology Criteria for Adverse Events; NRS—numeric rating scale; PCM—Patient Care Monitor; PG-SGA—Patient-Generated Subjective Global Assessment; PHQ—patient health questionnaire; VAS—visual analog scale

provided a definition of the problem at the beginning of each chapter. Information on incidence, assessment, and the specific clinical measurement tools are provided as a resource for use in nursing practice. Lastly, each chapter ends with a case study that demonstrates the importance of assessment and measurement, implementation of the evidence-based interventions identified by the specific ONS PEP Resources, and continued measurement of the clinical problem until the problem is either resolved or considered tolerable by the patient with cancer or the caregiver.

The clinical measurement tools listed in the subsequent chapters were selected after much thought and consideration. First, the ONS evidence-based measurement summaries were considered. These documents provide data and recommendations on measurement tools for oncology clinical problems. The summaries can be found online at www.ons.org/outcomes/measures/summaries.shtml. In addition to the evidence-based measurement summary authors' recommendations, the survey data from the

ONS APN group and the literature were evaluated. Many of the tools selected had established reliability and validity and had been studied in the oncology population. Other tools were selected based on access and ease of oncology nurse use. It is our hope that nurses will begin or continue to use a tool that works in individual work settings. Using a tool is better than not using one at all, and as nurses become more familiar with the available tools, further selection criteria can be explored for individual work settings.

References

Avery, K.N., Metcalfe, C., Nicklin, J., Braham, C.P., Alderson, D., Donovan, J.L., et al. (2006). Satisfaction with care: An independent outcome measure in surgical oncology. *Annals of Surgical Oncology, 13*(6), 817–822.

Beck, S.L., Dudley, W.N., & Barsevick, A.M. (2005). Pain, sleep disturbance, and fatigue in patients with cancer: Using a mediation model to test a symptom cluster [Online exclusive]. *Oncology Nursing Forum, 32*(3), E48–E55. Retrieved August 25, 2008, from http://ons.metapress.com/content/122n61u334093256/fulltext.pdf

Bender, C.M., Ergyn, F.S., Rosenzweig, M.Q., Cohen, S.M., & Sereika, S.M. (2005). Symptom clusters in breast cancer across 3 phases of the disease. *Cancer Nursing, 28*(3), 219–225.

Bruera, E., Kuehn, N., Miller, M.J., Selmser, P., & Macmillan, K. (1991). The Edmonton Symptom Assessment System (ESAS): A simple method for the assessment of palliative care patients. *Journal of Palliative Care, 7*(2), 6–9.

Cleeland, C.S. (2002, March). *Pain and symptom burden: Lessons from patients with cancer.* Paper presented at the 21st Annual Scientific Meeting of the American Pain Society, Baltimore, MD.

D'Arcy, Y. (2007). *Pain management: Evidence-based tools and techniques for nursing professionals.* Marblehead, MA: HCPro, Inc.

Fan, G., Filipczak, L., & Chow, E. (2007). Symptom clusters in cancer patients: A review of the literature. *Current Oncology, 14*(5), 173–179.

Garcia, S.F., Cella, D., Clauser, S.B., Flynn, K.E., Lad, T., Lai, J.S., et al. (2007). Standardizing patient-reported outcomes assessment in cancer clinical trials: A patient-reported outcomes measurement information system initiative. *Journal of Clinical Oncology, 25*(32), 5106–5112.

Gaston-Johannson, F., Fall-Dickson, J.M., Bakos, A.B., & Kennedy, M.J. (1999). Fatigue, pain, and depression in pre-autotransplant breast cancer patients. *Cancer Practice, 7*(5), 240–247.

Gift, A.G. (2007). Symptom clusters related to specific cancers. *Seminars in Oncology Nursing, 23*(2), 136–141.

Gift, A.G., Jablonski, A., Stommel, M., & Given, C.W. (2004). Symptom clusters in elderly patients with lung cancer. *Oncology Nursing Forum, 31*(2), 203–209.

Jacobson, J.O., Neuss, M.N., McNiff, K.K., Kadlubek, P., Thacker, L.R., Song, F., et al. (2008). Improvement in oncology practice performance through voluntary participation in the Quality Oncology Practice Initiative. *Journal of Clinical Oncology, 26*(11), 1893–1898.

Kleeberg, U.R., Feyer, P., Gunther, W., & Behrens, M. (2008). Patient satisfaction in outpatient cancer care: A prospective survey using the PASQOC® questionnaire. *Supportive Care in Cancer, 16*(8), 947–954.

Krishnan, L., Stanton, A.L., Collins, C.A., Liston, V.E., & Jewell, W.R. (2001). Form or function? Part 2. Objective cosmetic and functional correlates of quality of life in women treated with breast-conserving surgical procedures and radiotherapy. *Cancer, 91*(12), 2282–2287.

LaCasse, C., & Beck, S.L. (2007). Clinical assessment of symptom clusters. *Seminars in Oncology Nursing, 23*(2), 106–112.

Marvin, J.A. (1995). Pain assessment versus measurements. *Journal of Burn Care and Rehabilitation, 16*(3), 348–357.

Maxwell, C., & Stein, A. (2006). Implementing evidence-based guidelines for preventing chemotherapy-induced neutropenia: From paper to clinical practice. *Community Oncology, 3*(8), 530–536.

McNiff, K. (2006). The Quality Oncology Practice Initiative: Assessing and improving care within the medical oncology practice. *Journal of Oncology Practice, 2*(1), 26–30.

Miaskowski, C. (2006). Symptom clusters: Establishing the link between clinical practice and symptom management research. *Supportive Care in Cancer, 14*(8), 792–794.

Miaskowski, C., & Lee, K.A. (1999). Pain, fatigue, and sleep disturbances in oncology out-patients receiving radiation therapy for bone metastasis: A pilot study. *Journal of Pain and Symptom Management, 17*(5), 320–332.

Murray, M.E., & Atkinson, L.D. (2000). *Understanding the nursing process in a changing healthcare environment.* New York: McGraw-Hill.

National Cancer Institute Cancer Therapy Evaluation Program. (2006). *Common terminology criteria for adverse events* (version 3.0). Bethesda, MD: National Cancer Institute. Retrieved August 28, 2008, from http://ctep.cancer.gov/protocolDevelopment/electronic_applications/docs/ctcaev3.pdf

National Institutes of Health. (2002). *State-of-the-science conference statement. Symptom management in cancer: Pain, depression and fatigue.* Retrieved August 13, 2008, from http://consensus.nih.gov/2002/2002CancerPainDepressionFatiguesos022html.htm

National Institutes of Health. (2008). *Patient-Reported Outcomes Measurement Information System (PROMIS).* Retrieved December 30, 2008, from http://www.nihpromis.org

National Quality Forum. (2008). *Nursing care quality at NQF.* Retrieved August 31, 2008, from http://www.qualityforum.org/nursing

Paice, J.A. (2004). Assessment of a symptom clusters in people with cancer. *Journal of the National Cancer Institute Monographs, 2004*(32), 98–102.

Portenoy, R.K., Thaler, H.T., Kornblith, A.B., Lepore, J.M., Frielander-Klar, H., Kiyasu, E., et al. (1994). The Memorial Symptom Assessment Scale: An instrument for the evaluation of symptom prevalence, characteristics and distress. *European Journal of Cancer, 30A*(9), 1326–1336.

Ropka, M.E., Padilla, G., & Gillespie, T.W. (2005). Risk modeling: Applying evidence-based risk assessment in oncology nursing practice. *Oncology Nursing Forum, 32*(1), 49–56.

Ropka, M.E., & Spencer-Cisek, P. (2001). PRISM: Priority Symptom Management Project phase I: Assessment. *Oncology Nursing Forum, 28*(10), 1585–1594.

Rutledge, D.N., & McGuire, C. (2004). Evidence-based symptom management. In C.H. Yarbro, M.H. Frogge, & M. Goodman (Eds.), *Cancer symptom management* (3rd ed., pp. 3–14). Sudbury, MA: Jones and Bartlett.

Sandoval, G.A., Levinton, C., Blackstien-Hirsch, P., & Brown, A.D. (2006). Selecting predictors of cancer patients' overall perceptions of the quality of care received. *Annals of Oncology, 17*(1), 151–156.

Sarna, L. (1993). Correlates of symptom distress in women with lung cancer. *Cancer Practice, 1*(1), 21–28.

Thomas, C.L. (1997). *Taber's® cyclopedic medical dictionary.* Philadelphia: F.A. Davis.

CHAPTER **3**

Anorexia

Problem

Anorexia is an involuntary loss of appetite that is present in up to one-half of newly diagnosed patients with cancer. Anorexia and eating are regulated by myriad physiologic, gastrointestinal, metabolic, and nutritional factors, as well as neuronal and endocrine mechanisms. Changes in any of these components may result in the development of anorexia. Often accompanied by weight loss and most typically associated with advanced disease, anorexia is a complex clinical problem that may develop as a result of a decrease in the patient's ability to smell or taste food, early satiety, dysfunctional hypothalamic activity, increased brain tryptophan, or increased cytokine production (Tisdale, 2001). Anorexia and weight loss may contribute to the development or exacerbation of other disease- or treatment-related symptoms and affect functional status and quality of life. Although anorexia frequently is associated with cachexia (often referred to as the "anorexia-cachexia syndrome"), it warrants consideration as a unique symptom. For the purpose of the Oncology Nursing Society (ONS) Putting Evidence Into Practice (PEP) resource, anorexia was investigated as an independent symptom. Studies included in this review were those that evaluated anorexia, weight gain, oral intake, or some measure of appetite as primary outcomes variables.

Incidence

The incidence of anorexia has been reported to be as high as 70%–80% in the late stages of cancer (Nelson, 2000). Cancers of the aerodigestive tract are among the highest in frequency in weight loss and malnutrition. The frequency of weight loss and malnutrition can range from 30%–80%, depending on the type of tumor and stage (Dewys et al., 1980). Patients receiving multimodality therapies that can result in difficulties with ingestion, digestion, or nutrient absorption are also at high risk (Huhmann & Cunningham, 2005). This has clinical significance because poor nutritional status has been linked to adverse clinical outcomes. For example, malnutrition has been associated with reduced response to treatment, decreased quality of life, and poor survival (Dewys et al.; Hammerlid et al., 1998; Murry, Riva, & Poplack, 1998).

Assessment

Early nutrition screening and assessment can help to identify and minimize nutritional problems. Nutrition screening allows for risk factors associated with dietary or nutritional problems to be discovered. It is important for data to be both subjective and objective. Once the screening has been completed and if the patient has been determined to be at high risk, a more thorough nutrition assessment should be performed by a registered dietitian or nutrition professional. A comprehensive nutrition evaluation includes detailed dietary history, physical examination, anthropometric measurements, and laboratory data (Green & Watson, 2005; Huhmann & Cunningham, 2005). The Patient-Generated Subjective Global Assessment (PG-SGA) and the Mini Nutritional Assessment include both screening and assessment components. The PG-SGA is a tool that has been studied extensively in oncology, and the tool has been reprinted in a recent article addressing nutrition needs of patients with cancer (see Gosselin, Gilliard, & Tinnen, 2008, pp. 783–784). The assessment and further management of patients with anorexia with a multidisciplinary team approach are more likely to be successful in producing better clinical outcomes.

Clinical Assessment and Measurement Tools

The following clinical assessment and measurement tools for anorexia are presented in Table 3-1.
1. PG-SGA
2. Mini Nutritional Assessment
3. Malnutrition Screening Tool

Table 3-1. Clinical Assessment and Measurement Tools for Anorexia					
Name of Tool	**Number of Items**	**Domains**	**Reliability and Validity**	**Populations**	**Clinical Utility**
Patient-Generated Subjective Global Assessment (PG-SGA)	17	Weight history Food history Symptoms Activity level Metabolic demand Physical assessment	Reliability not reported Validity not specifically reported; PG-SGA is based on SGA, a previously validated tool.	Studied in patients with gastrointestinal and urologic malignancies, outpatients, and inpatients	A proactive and standardized approach to nutritional assessment in patients with cancer In pilot studies done at Fox Chase Cancer Center, PG-SGA added less than one minute to the overall patient assessment process.
					(Continued on next page)

Name of Tool	Number of Items	Domains	Reliability and Validity	Populations	Clinical Utility
					Practical for use in general oncology populations and with clinical trial assessment of nutritional interventions
Mini Nutritional Assessment (MNA)	18	Weight history Food intake Activity Psychological distress Anthropometric measurements Practitioner completed	Reliability not reported Validity not published in the literature	Validated for use with older adult population; studied with locally advanced and/or metastatic cancer (predominantly lung, breast, and prostate cancers)	Baseline weight loss and MNA score were strongly correlated to C-reactive protein (a marker of acute phase response). Testing for serum concentration of C-reactive protein at baseline may serve as an indicator of nutritional decline.
Malnutrition Screening Tool (MST)	3	Weight history Effect of appetite Patient completed	Reliability not reported Validity: positive p = 0.4; negative p = 1.0	Outpatients receiving radiation therapy and chemotherapy	MST is easy to use and a strong predictor of nutritional status. MST can be completed by medical, nursing, dietetic, and administrative personnel.

Table 3-1. Clinical Assessment and Measurement Tools for Anorexia (Continued)

Note. Based on information from Cunningham, 2004, 2005; Isenring et al., 2006.

References

Cunningham, R.S. (2004). The anorexia-cachexia syndrome. In C.H. Yarbro, M.H. Frogge, & M. Goodman (Eds.), *Cancer symptom management* (3rd ed., pp. 137–167). Sudbury, MA: Jones and Bartlett.

Cunningham, R.S. (2005). *Measuring oncology nursing-sensitive patient outcomes: Evidence-based summary: Nutritional status.* Retrieved August 31, 2008, from http://www.ons.org/outcomes/measures/nutrition.shtml

Dewys, W.D., Begg, C., Lavin, P.T., Band, P.R., Bennett, J.M., Bertino, J.R., et al. (1980). Prognostic effect of weight loss prior to chemotherapy in cancer patients. *American Journal of Medicine, 69*(4), 491–497.

Gosselin, T.K., Gilliard, L., & Tinnen, R. (2008). Assessing the need for a dietitian in radiation oncology. *Clinical Journal of Oncology Nursing, 12*(5), 781–787.

Green, S.M., & Watson, R. (2005). Nutritional screening and assessment tools for use by nurses: Literature review. *Journal of Advanced Nursing, 50*(1), 69–83.

Hammerlid, E., Wirlad, B., Sandin, C., Mercke, C., Edström, S., Kaasa, S., et al. (1998). Malnutrition and food intake in relation to quality of life in head and neck cancer patients. *Head and Neck, 20*(6), 540–548.

Huhmann, M.B., & Cunningham, R.S. (2005). Importance of nutritional screening in treatment of cancer-related weight loss. *Lancet Oncology, 6*(5), 334–343.

Isenring, E., Cross, G., Daniels, L., Kellett, E., & Koczwara, B. (2006). Validity of the malnutrition screening tool as an effective predictor of nutritional risk in oncology outpatients receiving chemotherapy. *Supportive Care in Cancer, 14*(11), 1152–1156.

Murry, D.J., Riva, L., & Poplack, D.G. (1998). Impact of nutrition on pharmacokinetics of antineoplastic agents. *International Journal of Cancer, 78*(Suppl. 11), 48–51.

Nelson, K.A. (2000). The cancer anorexia-cachexia syndrome. *Seminars in Oncology, 27*(1), 64–68.

Tisdale, M.J. (2001). Cancer anorexia and cachexia. *Nutrition, 17*(5), 438–442.

Case Study

B.K. was a 67-year-old woman with metastatic breast cancer. Her past medical history included a diagnosis of breast cancer, infiltrating lobular carcinoma, in 2001. She underwent a lumpectomy and axillary node dissection, and two of five lymph nodes were positive. The tumor was estrogen-receptor and progesterone-receptor positive. HER2/neu testing was not routinely done at the time. She received four cycles of doxorubicin and cyclophosphamide chemotherapy and three cycles of paclitaxel. She did not receive the last cycle of paclitaxel because of peripheral neuropathy. Upon completion of her radiation therapy, she began taking tamoxifen. Her medical history also included depression, hypertension, and bipolar disorder.

B.K. transferred care to another practice in 2004 and was switched to anastrozole because of the data to support use of aromatase inhibitors in postmenopausal females. She did not take the medication routinely because of poor prescription coverage. Her husband died in the fall of 2005, but otherwise she experienced no significant events.

B.K. was admitted to the hospital in November 2007 for shortness of breath. Positron-emission tomography (PET)/computed tomography (CT) findings were consistent with lung and bone metastases. She began treatment with zoledronic acid and fulvestrant.

A PET/CT scan was repeated in February 2008 that showed worsening of her disease. Her treatment was changed to bevacizumab and *nab*-paclitaxel. Follow-up in May 2008 showed some worsening of the bone metastases but improvement of the lung metastases. Radiation therapy was begun to her left sacrum because of the metastatic disease and increased pain. She was hospitalized twice for nausea, fatigue, and generalized weakness, progressing to an inability to walk. Magnetic resonance imaging studies of the brain and spine were negative for brain metastases and cord compression. She completed her radiation therapy in late June.

B.K. was admitted to the rehabilitation unit because of deconditioning, poor appetite, and weakness. During her stay there, she made considerable progress in ambulation with a walker. One of her most difficult problems was anorexia.

Patient-Generated Subjective Global Assessment Data

The PG-SGA evaluates weight change, dietary intake changes, gastrointestinal symptoms, and activity levels. The PG-SGA includes cancer-specific symptoms and information about the patient's activity level. The patient completes a portion of the assessment, thus decreasing clinician time in data collection. The clinician reviews the patient input within the context of the patient's diagnosis, stage of cancer, estimated treatment- and tumor-associated metabolic demand, and findings from a focused physical examination and develops a score. The overall score identifies the patient as being well-nourished, moderately (or suspected of being) malnourished, or severely malnourished. B.K.'s overall score on the PG-SGA was 25, indicating that she was severely malnourished. The triage recommendation should indicate the critical need for improved symptom management and/or nutrient intervention options.

Interventions Using ONS PEP Resource on Anorexia

1. Megestrol acetate 800 mg/day (see *Recommended for Practice* section)
2. Dietary counseling (see *Likely to Be Effective* section)

Evaluation

On clinic visit follow-up, the patient had gained approximately 10 pounds in six weeks and reported improved appetite. She benefited from the aforementioned interventions as well as rehabilitation stay. The nursing staff have been working with the patient to explore assistance programs for medications, including megestrol acetate, which has been beneficial in this case.

Sandy Storer, RN
Clinical Nurse III
University of Toledo Medical Center, Cancer Center
Toledo, OH

Anorexia

2009 AUTHORS
Lynn A. Adams, RN, MS, ANP, AOCN®, and Regina S. Cunningham, PhD, RN, AOCN®
ONS STAFF: Heather Belansky, RN, MSN

2008 AUTHORS
Lynn A. Adams, RN, MS, ANP, AOCN®, Regina S. Cunningham, PhD, RN, AOCN®,
Rose Ann Caruso, RN, OCN®, Martha J. Norling, RN, OCN®, and Nancy Shepard, RN, MS, AOCN®
ONS STAFF: Heather Belansky, RN, MSN

What interventions are effective in managing anorexia in people with cancer?

Recommended for Practice

Interventions for which effectiveness has been demonstrated by strong evidence from rigorously conducted studies, meta-analyses, or systematic reviews and for which expectation of harms is small compared with the benefits

CORTICOSTEROIDS

According to 2003 clinical practice guidelines (Desport et al., 2003), corticosteroids are recommended as appetite stimulants for patients with cancer. These can include
- Dexamethasone
- Methylprednisolone
- Prednisolone.

Although the most effective type, dose, or route of corticosteroids is not established, the benefit is significant yet short in duration. Long-term use is associated with significant toxicities, such as increased anxiety, immunosuppression, hyperglycemia, muscle weakness and wasting, fat redistribution, decrease in bone density, fluid retention, easy bruising, and skin fragility (Bruera, Roca, Cedaro, Carraro, & Chacon, 1985; Yavuzsen, Davis, Walsh, LeGrand, & Lagman, 2005). Therefore, corticosteroids are reserved for those with anorexia in whom short-term benefit is desired or those with limited life expectancy (Yavuzsen et al.).

PROGESTINS

Progestins are synthetic analogs of progesterone and include both medroxyprogesterone and megestrol acetate.
- Megestrol acetate is the most widely studied of the progestinal agents for its effect on anorexia. It has demonstrated a dose-related benefit (dosages ranging from 160–1,600 mg per day) on appetite, caloric intake, body weight, and sensation of well-being when compared with placebo in clinical studies. However, information remains insufficient to define the optimal dosage (Berenstein & Ortiz, 2005; Jatoi et al., 2002; Lopez et al., 2004; Maltoni et al., 2001; Nelson, Walsh, & Hussein, 2002; Tomiska, Tomiskova, Salajka, Adam, & Vorlicek, 2003; Yavuzsen et al., 2005).

- Side effects of progestinal agents include thromboembolic phenomena, breakthrough bleeding, hyperglycemia, hypertension, peripheral edema, and adrenal suppression. Patients in clinical trials rarely needed to discontinue the drug because of adverse effects. Adverse events are thought to be dose-related, so starting low and titrating upward to clinical response is justifiable (Berenstein & Ortiz, 2005; Jatoi et al., 2002; Lopez et al., 2004; Maltoni et al., 2001; Nelson et al., 2002; Tomiska et al., 2003; Yavuzsen et al., 2005).

Likely to Be Effective

Interventions for which effectiveness has been demonstrated by supportive evidence from a single rigorously conducted controlled trial, consistent supportive evidence from well-designed controlled trials using small samples, or guidelines developed from evidence and supported by expert opinion

DIETARY COUNSELING

Individualized dietary counseling has been shown to improve nutritional intake and body weight, resulting in reduction in the incidence of anorexia and improved quality of life.
- A systematic review examined the effects of nutritional counseling and/or commercial oral liquid supplements focused on increasing food intake in seven clinical trials (N = 558) (Brown, 2002). All studies reported improved caloric intake as a result of nutritional counseling and oral supplements.
- One study demonstrated that patients with colorectal cancer who received dietary counseling maintained their nutritional intake at the end of three months more successfully than those who received nutritional supplements (Ravasco, Monteiro-Grillo, Marques-Vidal, & Camilo, 2005).

Benefits Balanced With Harms

Interventions for which clinicians and patients should weigh the beneficial and harmful effects according to individual circumstances and priorities

There are no interventions as of May 2008.

Effectiveness Not Established

Interventions for which insufficient or conflicting data or data of inadequate quality currently exist, with no clear indication of harm

CYPROHEPTADINE

Cyproheptadine is an antihistamine marketed for the treatment of various allergic problems (Kardinal et al., 1990). Two trials compared the use of cyproheptadine to placebo, monitoring the outcomes of appetite, weight, and side effects.
- One trial showed that cyproheptadine 12 mg/day for eight weeks improved both appetite scores and weight gain (Yavuzsen et al., 2005).
- One trial found that people who received cyproheptadine 24 mg/day for 12 weeks had improved appetite but no significant difference in weight gain (Kardinal et al., 1990). Considerable sedative effects resulted from cyproheptadine.

EICOSAPENTAENOIC ACID

Eicosapentaenoic acid (EPA) is an essential omega-3 fatty acid present in fish. A systematic review (Yavuzsen et al., 2005) included three studies that evaluated the efficacy of EPA in improving appetite and weight gain in patients with cancer.
- **EPA in fish oil capsules:** One small randomized controlled trial (N = 60) compared an EPA dose of 1.8 g plus 1.2 g docosahexaenoic acid in capsule form to placebo (olive oil capsules). No significant difference existed in appetite or weight outcomes between the two treatments (Bruera et al., 2003).
- **EPA in supplement form:** One study compared three treatments: EPA at a dose of 2.18 g/day in supplement form; megestrol acetate alone; and a combination of the two (Jatoi et al., 2004). An improvement in overall weight gain occurred with all three treatments. In regard to appetite, a significant improvement occurred in patients who took megestrol acetate and the combination of the two, but not in the EPA-alone arm. In a systematic review (Yavuzsen et al., 2005), an energy-dense omega-3 fatty acid–enriched supplement with an EPA dose of 2.2 g/day was compared to a control group over a period of eight weeks. The results indicated a significant correlation between EPA and weight gain.

ERYTHROPOIETIN

Erythropoietin (EPO) is theorized to help reduce weight loss by decreasing the energy consumption that can occur with anemia (Lundholm, Daneryd, Bosaeus, Koerner, & Lindholm, 2004). One systematic review (Yavuzsen et al., 2005) summarized two studies that looked at whether a combination of EPO and a cyclooxygenase-2 inhibitor with or without a nutrition program can decrease weight loss. Although preliminary results look encouraging, determining what specific effect EPO had on the outcome is difficult.

GHRELIN

- One small clinical trial (N = 7) used a dose of 5 picomoles*/kg/minute infused over 180 minutes. Improvements in meal appreciation scores and energy intake occurred in patients who received ghrelin versus those receiving saline infusions (Neary et al., 2004). *Note: A picomole is one trillionth of a mole.*
- Although no side effects were observed, the long-term effects of the use of ghrelin to improve appetite have not been established (Neary et al., 2004).

METOCLOPRAMIDE

Metoclopramide does not directly stimulate appetite but is effective for decreasing nausea and early satiety (Yavuzsen et al., 2005).

ORAL BRANCHED-CHAIN AMINO ACIDS

One small study found that daily caloric intake was significantly increased and the incidence of anorexia significantly decreased in patients with cancer who received oral branched-chain amino acids over a period of seven days as compared to placebo. Oral branched-chain amino acids are thought to reduce the level of tryptophan in the brain and thus limit anorexic symptoms (Cangiano et al., 1996).

PENTOXIFYLLINE

Pentoxifylline is approved by the U.S. Food and Drug Administration for the treatment of intermittent claudication. It can inhibit tumor necrosis factor-alpha production, reducing plasma levels of this cytokine, which is thought to be a mediator in cancer-associated anorexia and cachexia (Goldberg et al., 1995). One double-blind, placebo-controlled trial (N = 70) failed to demonstrate any benefit of pentoxifylline over placebo in terms of appetite or weight gain in the treatment of cancer-related anorexia and cachexia (Goldberg et al.).

THALIDOMIDE

Small studies indicate that thalidomide may help to reduce anorexia in patients with cancer.
- One study found that a dose of 100 mg PO at bedtime can improve nausea, appetite, caloric intake, and well-being (Bruera et al., 1999).
- The results of another study using 200 mg PO daily indicated that thalidomide may effectively attenuate loss of weight and lean muscle mass (Gordon et al., 2005).
- Side effects of thalidomide may include dizziness, drowsiness, somnolence, constipation, and increased incidence of thromboembolic events (Bruera et al., 1999; Gordon et al., 2005).

Effectiveness Unlikely

Interventions for which lack of effectiveness has been demonstrated by negative evidence from a single rigorously conducted controlled trial, consistent negative evidence from well-designed controlled trials using small samples, or guidelines developed from evidence and supported by expert opinion

CANNABINOIDS

Cannabinoids are a group of substances that are structurally related to delta-9-tetrahydrocannabinol (THC). Appetite stimulation and weight gain are recognized effects of THC. Two clinical trials investigated the use of cannabinoids for cancer-related anorexia. They found that
- Megestrol acetate was more effective in improving appetite than dronabinol in patients with advanced cancer. The combination did not confer any additional benefit (Jatoi et al., 2002).
- No difference existed between cannabis extract, THC, or placebo on appetite and quality of life in patients with advanced cancer (Strasser et al., 2006).
- Side effects of cannabinoid use include dizziness, nausea, and fatigue (Strasser et al., 2006).

HYDRAZINE SULFATE

Hydrazine sulfate is sold as a dietary supplement in the United States for the treatment of cancer and cancer-related anorexia and cachexia. However, a systematic review failed to show a significant difference in appetite or weight between patients who received hydrazine sulfate and those who received placebo (Yavuzsen et al., 2005). Initial trials using hydrazine sulfate indicated an improvement in appetite with an increase or maintenance in weight when compared to placebo. However, these findings were not corroborated in subsequent trials investigating the use of hydrazine sulfate in patients with lung or colorectal cancers. This lack of significant difference provides strong evidence against the use of hydrazine sulfate (Yavuzsen et al.).

MELATONIN

Melatonin is a hormone produced by the pineal gland and regulates leptin, a hormone that plays a role in regulating energy intake and expenditure, including the regulation of appetite and metabolism ("Melatonin," n.d.).
- Melatonin has been used at doses of 20 mg/day for a duration of 1–16 weeks. Although weight loss was observed less frequently in the melatonin groups, no differences in appetite or nutritional intake could be appreciated. Side effects of the agent include sleepiness (Yavuzsen et al., 2005).

Not Recommended for Practice

Interventions for which lack of effectiveness or harmfulness has been demonstrated by strong evidence from rigorously conducted studies, meta-analyses, or systematic reviews, or interventions where the costs, burden, or harms associated with the intervention exceed anticipated benefit

There are no interventions as of May 2008.

Definitions of the interventions are available at **www.ons.org/outcomes**.
Literature search completed through May 2008.

References

Berenstein, E.G., & Ortiz, Z. (2005). Megestrol acetate for the treatment of anorexia-cachexia syndrome. *Cochrane Database of Systematic Reviews 2005*, Issue 2. Art. No.: CD004310. DOI: 10.1002/14651858 .CD004310.pub2.

Brown, J.K. (2002). A systematic review of the evidence on symptom management of cancer-related anorexia and cachexia. *Oncology Nursing Forum, 29*(3), 517–530.

Bruera, E., Neumann, C.M., Pituskin, E., Calder, K., Ball, G., & Hanson, J. (1999). Thalidomide in patients with cachexia due to terminal cancer: Preliminary report. *Annals of Oncology, 10*(7), 857–859.

Bruera E., Roca, E., Cedaro, L., Carraro, S., & Chacon, R. (1985). Action of oral methylprednisolone in terminal cancer patients: A prospective randomized double-blind study. *Cancer Treatment Reports, 69*(7–8), 751–754.

Bruera, E., Strasser, F., Palmer, J.L., Willey, J., Calder, K., Amyotte, G., et al. (2003). Effect of fish oil on appetite and other symptoms in patients with advanced cancer and anorexia/cachexia: A double-blind, placebo-controlled study. *Journal of Clinical Oncology, 21*(1), 129–134.

Cangiano, C., Laviano, A., Meguid, M.M., Mulieri, M., Conversano, L., Preziosa, I., et al. (1996). Effects of administration of oral branched-chain amino acids on anorexia and caloric intake in cancer patients. *Journal of the National Cancer Institute, 88*(8), 550–552.

Desport, J.C., Gory-Delabaere, G., Blanc-Vincent, M.P., Bachmann, P., Beal, J., Benamouzig, R., et al. (2003). Standards, options and recommendations for the use of appetite stimulants in oncology (2000). *British Journal of Cancer, 89*(Suppl. 1), S98–S100.

Goldberg, R., Loprinzi, C., Mailliard, J., O'Fallon, J., Krook, J., Ghosh, C., et al. (1995). Pentoxifylline for treatment of cancer anorexia and cachexia? A randomized, double-blind, placebo-controlled trial. *Journal of Clinical Oncology, 13*(11), 2856–2859.

Gordon, J.N., Trebble, T.M., Ellis, R.D., Duncan, H.D., Johns, T., & Goggin, P.M. (2005). Thalidomide in the treatment of cancer cachexia: A randomised placebo controlled trial. *Gut, 54*(4), 540–545.

Jatoi, A., Rowland, K., Loprinzi, C.L., Sloan, J.A., Dakhil, S.R., MacDonald, N., et al. (2004). An eicosapen-taenoic acid supplement versus megestrol acetate versus both for patients with cancer associated wasting: A North Central Cancer Treatment Group and National Cancer Institute of Canada collaborative effort. *Journal of Clinical Oncology, 22*(12), 2469–2476.

Jatoi, A., Windschitl, H.E., Loprinzi, C.L., Sloan, J.A., Dakhil, S.R., Mailliard, J.A., et al. (2002). Dronabinol versus megestrol acetate versus combination therapy for cancer associated anorexia: A North Central Cancer Treatment Group study. *Journal of Clinical Oncology, 20*(2), 567–573.

Kardinal, C.G., Loprinzi, C.L., Schaid, D.J., Hass, A.C., Dose, A.M., Athmann, L.M., et al. (1990). A controlled trial of cyproheptadine in cancer patients with anorexia and/or cachexia. *Cancer, 65*(12), 2657–2662.

Lopez, A.P., i Figuls, M.R., Cuchi, G.U., Berenstein, E.G., Pasies, B.A., Alegre, M.B., et al. (2004). Systematic review of megestrol acetate in the treatment of anorexia-cachexia syndrome. *Journal of Pain and Symptom Management, 27*(4), 360–369.

Lundholm, K., Daneryd, P., Bosaeus, I., Koerner, U., & Lindholm, E. (2004). Palliative nutritional intervention in addition to cyclooxygenase and erythropoietin treatment for patients with malignancy disease: Effects on survival, metabolism, and function. *Cancer, 100*(9), 1967–1977.

Maltoni, M., Nanni, O., Scarpi, E., Rossi, D., Serra, P., & Amadori, D. (2001). High-dose progestins for the treatment of cancer anorexia-cachexia syndrome: A systematic review of randomised clinical trials. *Annals of Oncology, 12*(3), 289–300.

Melatonin. (n.d.). *Merriam-Webster's online dictionary.* Retrieved March 6, 2008, from http://www.merriam-webster.com/dictionary/melatonin

Neary, N.M., Small, C.J., Wren, A.M., Lee, J.L., Druce, M.R., Palmieri, C., et al. (2004). Ghrelin increases energy intake in cancer patients with impaired appetite: Acute, randomized, placebo-controlled trial. *Journal of Clinical Endocrinology and Metabolism, 89*(6), 2832–2836.

Nelson, K.A., Walsh, D., & Hussein, M. (2002). A phase II study of low-dose megestrol acetate using twice-daily dosing for anorexia in nonhormonally dependent cancer. *American Journal of Hospice and Palliative Care, 19*(3), 206–210.

Ravasco, P., Monteiro-Grillo, I., Marques-Vidal, P., & Camilo, M. (2005). Dietary counseling improves patient outcomes: A prospective, randomized, controlled trial, in colorectal cancer patients undergoing radiotherapy. *Journal of Clinical Oncology, 23*(7), 1431–1438.

Strasser, F., Luftner, D., Possinger, K., Ernst, G., Ruhstaller, T., Meissner, W., et al. (2006). Comparison of orally administered cannabis extract and delta-9-tetrahydrocannabinol in treating patients with cancer-related anorexia-cachexia syndrome: A multi-center, phase III, randomized, double-blind, placebo-controlled clinical trial from the Cannabis-In-Cachexia-Study-Group. *Journal of Clinical Oncology, 24*(21), 3394–3400.

Tomiska, M., Tomiskova, M., Salajka, F., Adam, Z., & Vorlicek, J. (2003). Palliative treatment of cancer anorexia with oral suspension of megestrol acetate. *Neoplasma, 50*(3), 227–233.

Yavuzsen, T., Davis, M.P., Walsh, D., LeGrand, S., & Lagman, R. (2005). Systematic review of the treatment of cancer-associated anorexia and weight loss. *Journal of Clinical Oncology, 23*(33), 8500–8511.

CHAPTER **4**

Anxiety

Problem

Anxiety is an emotional and/or physiologic response to known or unknown causes that can range from a normal reaction to extreme dysfunction (indicative of an anxiety disorder), affect decision making and adherence to treatment, impair functioning, and affect quality of life (American Psychiatric Association [APA], 2000; Bush & Griffin-Sobel, 2002; Noyes, Holt, & Massie, 1998; Shahrokh & Hales, 2003; Vitek, Rosenzweig, & Stollings, 2007).

According to APA's (2000) *Diagnostic and Statistical Manual of Mental Disorders,* two types of anxiety disorders can occur in patients with cancer: generalized anxiety disorder (GAD) and post-traumatic stress disorder (PTSD). GAD is characterized by at least six months of persistent and severe anxiety and worry that significantly impairs social, occupational, and other important areas of functioning. PTSD is characterized by the re-experiencing of an extremely traumatic event accompanied by symptoms of increased arousal (e.g., difficulty concentrating, hypervigilance, difficulty falling or staying asleep) and avoidance of stimuli associated with the trauma. Additionally, anxiety seen in patients with cancer is accompanied by greater autonomic hyperactivity than in people with GAD who do not have cancer (Noyes et al., 1998).

Incidence

Anxiety is one of the most common psychological responses to the cancer experience and may occur at different times throughout the cancer care trajectory (Bush, 2006; Mock et al., 1997). Although anxiety levels usually decrease over time after the initial diagnosis and treatment, 20%–30% of people with cancer continue to experience increased levels of anxiety after treatment is complete (Howard & Harvey, 1998; Maher, Mackenzie, Young, & Marks, 1996; Nordin & Glimelius, 1998). Uncontrolled anxiety can be disabling and may interfere with both treatment response and psychosocial functioning (Bush).

Assessment

Assessing for anxiety at major transition points along the cancer continuum and differentiating between normal and abnormal anxiety responses are important (Bush, 2006).

Basic anxiety can be screened for by asking "How are you feeling?" (Gobel, 2004). A detailed assessment (see Table 4-1) that includes use of an anxiety clinical measurement tool is important in assessing anxiety and measuring the impact of nursing interventions.

Table 4-1. Anxiety Assessment Guide		
Assessment	**Yes**	**No**
Physical Symptoms		
Palpitations and chest pain combined with respiratory symptoms of hyperventilation and dyspnea		
Feelings of suffocation		
Anorexia, nausea, diarrhea		
Difficulty swallowing and heartburn		
Dizziness, weakness, headaches, confusion, fine tremors		
Exhaustion		
Difficulty sleeping		
Psychosocial Symptoms		
Tense and worried		
Feeling nervous		
Irritability		
Anxious foreboding or a sense of impending doom		
Impaired communication		
Cognitive Changes		
Difficulty concentrating and maintaining attention		
Memory changes		
Behavioral Responses		
Restlessness, pacing, wringing of hands, nail biting		
Risk Factors		
History of preexisting anxiety disorder (e.g., generalized anxiety disorder, panic disorder, panic disorder with phobia, post-traumatic stress disorder)		
Underlying medical conditions that may contribute to anxiety (e.g., pain, sepsis, medications, cognitive disruptions, metabolic imbalances, hormonal imbalances)		
Note. Based on information from Bush, 2006.		

Clinical Measurement Tools

The following clinical measurement tools for anxiety are presented in Table 4-2.

1. National Comprehensive Cancer Network (NCCN) Distress Thermometer (see Figure 4-1): Although this tool does not specifically measure anxiety, it is a brief and easy-to-use tool recommended by NCCN and other experts to measure distress (Badger, 2008). As defined by NCCN (2008), *distress* is an unpleasant experience of an emotional, psychological, social, or spiritual characteristic ranging from normal feelings of vulnerability, sadness, and fears to depression, anxiety, panic, social isolation, and existential and spiritual crisis. A distress level of 4 or greater on the thermometer is considered moderate to severe distress (Vitek et al., 2007). The tool also includes a problem checklist of possible factors that contribute to distress.

2. Beck Anxiety Inventory: This tool is a self-report measure of somatic and panic symptoms of anxiety (Badger, 2008).

Table 4-2. Clinical Measurement Tools for Anxiety					
Name of Tool	Number of Items	Domains	Reliability and Validity	Populations	Clinical Utility
National Comprehensive Cancer Network Distress Thermometer	1	Emotional distress, not anxiety	Correlates highly with more comprehensive cancer screening instruments and structured interviews	Breast, prostate, gastrointestinal, gynecologic, and lung cancers	Good to very good
Beck Anxiety Inventory	21	Subjective, somatic, and panic symptoms of anxiety	Adequate reliability established; Discriminate validity reported with mental health/cancer patients	Breast, gastrointestinal, and gynecologic cancers; chronic lymphocytic leukemia	Acceptable
Hospital Anxiety and Depression Scale	14	Severity of anxiety and depression	Adequate reliability established	Breast, prostate, gastrointestinal, and testicular cancers	Short and easy to use; very good to excellent

Note. Based on information from Badger, 2008.

3. Hospital Anxiety and Depression Scale (HADS): The HADS is a self-report measure of anxiety and depression (Badger, 2008).

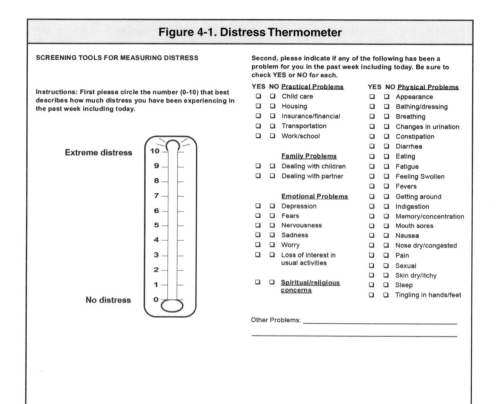

Figure 4-1. Distress Thermometer

SCREENING TOOLS FOR MEASURING DISTRESS

Instructions: First please circle the number (0-10) that best describes how much distress you have been experiencing in the past week including today.

Extreme distress 10

9

8

7

6

5

4

3

2

1

No distress 0

Second, please indicate if any of the following has been a problem for you in the past week including today. Be sure to check YES or NO for each.

YES NO **Practical Problems**
☐ ☐ Child care
☐ ☐ Housing
☐ ☐ Insurance/financial
☐ ☐ Transportation
☐ ☐ Work/school

Family Problems
☐ ☐ Dealing with children
☐ ☐ Dealing with partner

Emotional Problems
☐ ☐ Depression
☐ ☐ Fears
☐ ☐ Nervousness
☐ ☐ Sadness
☐ ☐ Worry
☐ ☐ Loss of interest in usual activities

☐ ☐ **Spiritual/religious concerns**

YES NO **Physical Problems**
☐ ☐ Appearance
☐ ☐ Bathing/dressing
☐ ☐ Breathing
☐ ☐ Changes in urination
☐ ☐ Constipation
☐ ☐ Diarrhea
☐ ☐ Eating
☐ ☐ Fatigue
☐ ☐ Feeling Swollen
☐ ☐ Fevers
☐ ☐ Getting around
☐ ☐ Indigestion
☐ ☐ Memory/concentration
☐ ☐ Mouth sores
☐ ☐ Nausea
☐ ☐ Nose dry/congested
☐ ☐ Pain
☐ ☐ Sexual
☐ ☐ Skin dry/itchy
☐ ☐ Sleep
☐ ☐ Tingling in hands/feet

Other Problems: _____
_____

References

American Psychiatric Association. (2000). *Diagnostic and statistical manual of mental disorders* (4th ed., text revision). Washington, DC: Author.

Badger, T. (2008). *Evidence-based outcomes measurement summaries—Anxiety.* Retrieved July 23, 2008, from http://www.ons.org/outcomes/measures/anxiety.shtml

Bush, N.J. (2006). Anxiety and the cancer experience. In R.M. Carroll-Johnson, L.M. Gorman, & N.J. Bush (Eds.), *Psychosocial nursing care along the cancer continuum* (2nd ed., pp. 205–221). Pittsburgh, PA: Oncology Nursing Society.

Bush, N.J., & Griffin-Sobel, J.P. (2002). Cultural dimensions of anxiety and truth telling. *Oncology Nursing Forum, 29*(5), 757–759.

Gobel, B.H. (2004). Anxiety. In C.H. Yarbro, M.H. Frogge, & M. Goodman (Eds.), *Cancer symptom management* (3rd ed., pp. 651–667). Sudbury, MA: Jones and Bartlett.

Howard, R., & Harvey, P. (1998). A longitudinal study of psychological distress in women with breast symptoms. *Journal of Health Psychology, 3*(2), 215–226.

Maher, E., Mackenzie, C., Young, T., & Marks, D. (1996). The use of the Hospital Anxiety and Depression Scale (HADS) and the EORTC QLQ-C30 questionnaires to screen for treatable unmet needs in patients attending routinely for radiotherapy. *Cancer Treatment Reviews, 22*(Suppl. A), 123–129.

Mock, V.M., Dow, K.H., Meares, C.J., Grimm, P.M., Dienemann, J.A., Haisfield-Wolfe, M.E., et al. (1997). Effects of exercise on fatigue, physical functioning, and emotional distress during radiation therapy for breast cancer. *Oncology Nursing Forum, 24*(6), 991–1000.

National Comprehensive Cancer Network. (2008). *NCCN Clinical Practice Guidelines in Oncology™: Distress management* [v.1.2008]. Retrieved August 28, 2008, from http://www.nccn.org/professionals/physician_gls/PDF/distress.pdf

Nordin, K., & Glimelius, B. (1998). Reactions to gastrointestinal cancer—Variations of mental adjustments and emotional well-being with time in patients with different prognoses. *Psycho-Oncology, 7*(5), 413–423.

Noyes, R., Holt, C.S., & Massie, M.J. (1998). Anxiety disorders. In J.C. Holland (Ed.), *Psycho-oncology* (pp. 548–563). New York: Oxford University Press.

Shahrokh, N.C., & Hales, R.E. (2003). *American psychiatric glossary.* Washington, DC: American Psychiatric Association Publishing.

Vitek, L., Rosenzweig, M.Q., & Stollings, S. (2007). Distress in patients with cancer: Definition, assessment, and suggested interventions. *Clinical Journal of Oncology Nursing, 11*(1), 413–418.

Case Study

The oncology clinical nurse specialist (CNS) educates the staff and assists with complex patient problems that arise in the clinical setting. A 67-year-old woman newly diagnosed with stage III ovarian cancer received one cycle of IV and intra-peritoneal chemotherapy prior to surgery. During the assessment, the patient rated her distress as a 6 on the distress thermometer. A distress level of 4 or greater is considered a moderate to severe distress level requiring further assessment and possibly referral and interventions.

Despite appropriate premedications, the patient experienced a mild infusion reaction during the administration of IV paclitaxel on the first day. This experience contributed to the patient's anxiety on the second day when she was to receive her intraperitoneal cisplatin. Using a multidisciplinary approach to care and applying findings cited on the Oncology Nursing Society (ONS) Putting Evidence Into Practice (PEP) resource on anxiety, the CNS discussed which interventions are most likely to reduce the patient's anxiety with the oncology pharmacist and the gyne-oncologist. As supported by the evidence on the PEP resource for interventions that are *Likely to Be Effective,* alprazolam was prescribed to help her relax before the administration of intraperitoneal cisplatin. Additionally, the alprazolam would help to prevent anticipatory nausea and vomiting, a side effect that she was at risk for developing (see the *Recommended for Practice* section of the ONS PEP resource on chemotherapy-induced nausea and vomiting).

The ONS PEP resource on anxiety lists several nonpharmacologic interventions to reduce anxiety. Evidence supports massage therapy as an intervention that is *Likely to Be Effective.* The CNS asked the patient if she was willing to try light massage as an intervention to help her relax while she received the intraperitoneal chemotherapy. Light massage could be done by either the patient's friend or by the nurse, depending on the patient's preference. The lighting in the room was dimmed, and soft music of her choice was played (an example of distraction). The patient chose to have her friend perform the light massage for 5–10 minutes as the patient received the intraperitoneal cisplatin. The friend lightly massaged the patient's back while she turned from one side to the other. This combination of evidence-based interventions—massage and pharmacologic agents—diminished the patient's anxiety tremendously. Because the same interventions were employed, the second day of the patient's chemotherapy regimen went smoothly. She reported feeling much more relaxed (distress level reported as 3) and very satisfied with the efforts to make her experience less distressing.

With each subsequent cycle of chemotherapy, the patient rated her anxiety using the distress thermometer. Using effective interventions and open communication allowed the patient to feel more in control of her care and worries and allowed her to complete four cycles of chemotherapy. The format of the ONS PEP resource on anxiety allows nurses to quickly select evidence-based interventions that will most benefit the patient. Evidence clearly supports that providing symptom management education and self-care strategies helps patients manage their anxiety. The ONS PEP Resources are vital and useful in fast-paced, busy clinical settings.

Amy H. Dolce, RN, APN, MS, AOCN®, CHPN
Oncology Clinical Nurse Specialist
Northwest Community Hospital
Arlington Heights, IL

Anxiety

2009 AUTHORS
Susan A. Swanson, RN, MS, AOCN®, and Lisa Kennedy Sheldon, PhD, APRN-BC, AOCNP®
ONS STAFF: Linda H. Eaton, MN, RN, AOCN®

2008 AUTHORS
Susan A. Swanson, RN, MS, AOCN®, Amy H. Dolce, RN, APN, MS, AOCN®, CHPN,
Kathy Marsh, RN, Julie A. Summers, RN, BSN, and Lisa Kennedy Sheldon, PhD, ARNP, AOCNP®
RESEARCH CONSULTANT: Terry A. Badger, PhD, RN, CS, FAAN
ONS STAFF: Linda H. Eaton, MN, RN, AOCN®

What interventions are effective in preventing and treating anxiety in people with cancer?

Recommended for Practice

Interventions for which effectiveness has been demonstrated by strong evidence from rigorously conducted studies, meta-analyses, or systematic reviews and for which expectation of harms is small compared with the benefits

PSYCHOEDUCATIONAL/PSYCHOSOCIAL INTERVENTIONS

Psychoeducational Interventions
- Patient-centered education materials about specific types of cancers and treatment modalities via written information or Internet sites (Hoff & Haaga, 2005; Jones et al., 2006)
- Treatment-centered orientation programs to describe the facility, staff, and contact information through individual education and written information (Katz, Irish, & Devins, 2004)
- Symptom management and self-care strategies to teach exercise and relaxation techniques and manage anxiety using audio- and/or videotapes (Deshler et al., 2006; Williams & Schreier, 2004)

Psychosocial Interventions
- Cognitive behavioral therapy (CBT) for individuals or groups to teach distraction, thought monitoring, cognitive restructuring, coping self-statements, and/or mental imagery exercises (Antoni et al., 2006; Arving et al., 2007; Kissane et al., 2003; Osborn, Demoncada, & Feuerstein, 2006)
- Individual or group sessions to counsel or provide psychotherapy in person or via telephone (Badger, Segrin, Dorros, Meek, & Lopez, 2007; Shepard et al., 2006)
- Psychosocial support group meetings offered weekly or monthly to provide anxiety management techniques, coping skills, and social support (Chujo et al., 2005; Manne et al., 2005; Miller, Chibnall, Videen, & Duckro, 2005)

Oncology nurses may provide psychoeducational/psychosocial interventions, facilitate support groups, and provide patient education and information to prevent and treat anxiety. Although the highest level of evidence also supports the use of CBT, it requires advanced educational training. However, nurses may facilitate referrals for CBT.

Likely to Be Effective

Interventions for which effectiveness has been demonstrated by supportive evidence from a single rigorously conducted controlled trial, consistent supportive evidence from well-designed controlled trials using small samples, or guidelines developed from evidence and supported by expert opinion

PHARMACOTHERAPY

Pharmacotherapy has been studied as an intervention to treat anxiety in patients with cancer (Pasquini et al., 2006). Studies over the past 20 years have examined many pharmacologic agents, including alprazolam (Holland et al., 1991; Wald, Roger, Noyes, Carroll, & Clamon, 1993), midazolam (Mentes, Unsal, Baran, Argun, & Ertunc, 2005), propofol (Mentes et al.), fluoxetine (Rasavi et al., 1996), and olanzapine (Khojainova, Santiago-Palma, Kornick, Breitbart, & Gonzales, 2002). Few studies have adequate sample sizes with patients with cancer to determine the most effective agents for decreasing anxiety. Overall, the studies combined with expert opinion (National Comprehensive Cancer Network [NCCN], 2008) show that pharmacologic agents are likely to be effective in decreasing anxiety in patients with cancer.

MEDICATIONS USED FOR ANXIETY IN PATIENTS WITH CANCER

Benzodiazepines
- Lorazepam (Ativan®, Biovail)
- Diazepam (Valium®, Roche)
- Alprazolam (Xanax®, Pfizer)

Azapirones
- Buspirone (BuSpar®, Bristol-Myers Squibb)

Antihistamines
- Hydroxyzine (Vistaril®, Pfizer)

Antidepressants
- Paroxetine (Paxil®, GlaxoSmithKline)
- Sertraline (Zoloft®, Pfizer)
- Escitalopram (Lexapro®, Forest Laboratories)
- Venlafaxine (Effexor®, Effexor XR®, Wyeth)
- Mirtazapine (Remeron®, Organon USA)

Atypical Neuroleptics
- Olanzapine (Zyprexa®, Lilly)
- Risperidone (Risperdal®, Janssen)

Other
- Propofol (Diprivan®, AstraZeneca)

A variety of tools have been used to measure response to pharmacotherapy (see ONS anxiety measurement summary at www.ons.org/outcomes).

MASSAGE THERAPY

Massage therapy involves manipulation of soft tissue areas of the body to assist in relaxation, aid in sleep, relieve muscle tension, and diminish cancer-related depression. Across studies, its most consistent effect is in reducing anxiety.
- A 2004 Cochrane Systematic Review of eight randomized controlled trials (RCTs) supported its effectiveness in decreasing anxiety in patients with cancer (Fellowes, Barnes, & Wilkinson, 2004).
- Several studies (Hernandez-Reif et al., 2005; Jane, 2005; Soden, Vincent, Craske, Lucas, & Ashley, 2004; Wilkinson et al., 2007) demonstrated significant decrease in anxiety, with the greatest reduction occurring immediately after the massage. Further studies examining the maintenance of reduced anxiety demonstrated a range from 18 hours (Jane) to 6–10 weeks (Wilkinson et al.).

Benefits Balanced With Harms

Interventions for which clinicians and patients should weigh the beneficial and harmful effects according to individual circumstances and priorities

There are no interventions as of May 2008.

Effectiveness Not Established

Interventions for which insufficient or conflicting data or data of inadequate quality currently exist, with no clear indication of harm

ART THERAPY

One quasi-experimental study demonstrated significant change in anxiety scores for patients who participated in art therapy sessions administered by a registered art therapist/counselor (Nainis et al., 2005).

COMPLEMENTARY AND ALTERNATIVE MEDICINE

Complementary and alternative medicine (CAM) comprises diverse medical practices not considered part of conventional medical treatment. Effectiveness has been proved for some CAM therapies, but few well-designed studies exist to demonstrate their efficacy in patients with cancer. The list of CAM therapies continually changes as interventions that were previously considered CAM are adopted into conventional health care and new treatments emerge (National Institutes of Health, National Center for Complementary and Alternative Medicine, 2007).
- One RCT with 181 women with breast cancer examined multiple CAM therapies for anxiety versus standard psychosocial support group meetings. CAM therapies included meditation, yoga, guided imagery, drawing, and dance therapy (Targ & Levine, 2002). Although the study demonstrated decreased anxiety in both groups, it could not determine which intervention decreased anxiety.

DISTRACTION (VIRTUAL REALITY OR MUSIC)

Two studies examined the use of distraction as a method to reduce anxiety in patients with cancer. One small RCT compared music versus simple distraction and a control group (Kwekkeboom, 2003). Another study compared patients receiving computer-simulated virtual reality (visual and auditory input) during chemotherapy versus patients in a control group (Schneider & Hood, 2007). Neither study demonstrated a statistically significant reduction in anxiety.

EXERCISE

Four studies examined the effect of exercise on anxiety in patients with cancer and demonstrated some decrease in anxiety. One RCT demonstrated significant reduction in anxiety (Badger et al., 2007). Two of the studies had very small sample sizes, which limits their significance (Burnham & Wilcox, 2002; Segar et al., 1998). One study (N = 91) was not randomized but demonstrated reduction in anxiety (Midtgaard et al., 2005).

FOOT REFLEXOLOGY

Foot reflexology is a manual technique based upon the theory that reflex areas on the feet correspond to specific glands, organs, and parts of the body. It is administered by a specially trained professional who applies pressure using his or her thumb or forefinger to stimulate the specific reflex areas (Stephenson, Swanson, Dalton, Keefe, & Engelke, 2007).
- Two studies demonstrated a significant decrease in anxiety following reflexology treatment; however, both studies had small sample sizes (Quattrin et al., 2006; Stephenson et al., 2007).

HOMEOPATHY

The effectiveness of homeopathy on anxiety levels has shown mixed and/or contradictory results in a systematic review (Pilkington, Kirkwood, Rampes, Fisher, & Richardson, 2006).

MEDITATION

Autogenic training (AT), a type of meditation, "teaches" the body to relax through controlled breathing with a resulting decrease in blood pressure and heartbeat. The goal is to achieve deep relaxation and reduce stress.
- The results of one small randomized trial demonstrated decreased anxiety in the AT group; however, the results were not statistically significant (Hidderley & Holt, 2004).

PROGRESSIVE MUSCLE RELAXATION

Progressive muscle relaxation requires participants to tense and relax different muscle groups in combination with deep breathing (Cheung, Molassiotis, & Chang, 2003).
- Three studies provided audiotapes describing the step-by-step procedure as well as written instructions. One study (Cheung et al., 2003) demonstrated reduction in the state anxiety (transitory emotional responses to stressful situations) level over a 10-week period; however, the other two studies did not demonstrate reduced anxiety (Hernandez-Reif et al., 2004; Sloman, 2002). All three studies had small sample sizes, limiting significance of the results.

REIKI

Reiki is a type of energy touch therapy requiring specialized training.
- One pilot study demonstrated statistically significant reduction in anxiety but was limited by a small sample size (Tsang, Carlson, & Olson, 2007).

RELAXATION BREATHING EXERCISE

Relaxation breathing exercise (RBE) consists of muscle relaxation exercises combined with relaxation breathing (Kim & Kim, 2005).
- In one study, the treatment group was educated by a researcher for 10 minutes and then given a 30-minute tape with specific instructions for RBE. State anxiety levels after RBE showed a significant decrease; however, the sample size was small (Kim & Kim, 2005).

THERAPEUTIC TOUCH

Therapeutic touch (TT) is an energy therapy in which specially trained practitioners, with deliberate intent, move their hands through the patient's energy field to assess and treat energy field imbalances (Shames & Keegan, 2000). The practitioners move their hands over the patient's body but do not actually touch the body.
- In one small study using mixed methods, no significant difference occurred in anxiety levels before and after TT between the intervention and control groups. Both groups expressed feelings of calmness, relaxation, security, and control (Kelly, Sullivan, Fawcett, & Samarel, 2004).

Effectiveness Unlikely

Interventions for which lack of effectiveness has been demonstrated by negative evidence from a single rigorously conducted controlled trial, consistent negative evidence from well-designed controlled trials using small samples, or guidelines developed from evidence and supported by expert opinion

There are no interventions as of May 2008.

Not Recommended for Practice

Interventions for which lack of effectiveness or harmfulness has been demonstrated by strong evidence from rigorously conducted studies, meta-analyses, or systematic reviews, or interventions where the costs, burden, or harms associated with the intervention exceed anticipated benefit

There are no interventions as of May 2008.

Expert Opinion

Low-risk interventions that are (1) consistent with sound clinical practice, (2) suggested by an expert in a peer-reviewed publication (journal or book chapter), and (3) for which limited evidence exists. An expert is an individual who has published articles in a peer-reviewed journal in the domain of interest.

Experts recommend the following interventions by the oncology team (oncologist, oncology nurse, social worker, psychologist, psychiatrist, and clergy) for distressed patients with cancer who may be experiencing anxiety (NCCN, 2008).

- Monitor and recognize the symptoms of distress.
- Assess patients for distress, including symptoms of anxiety during the initial visit, at appropriate intervals, and at vulnerable time periods (i.e., changes in disease status such as progression or recurrence, change in treatment modality, and end-of-life care).
- Use a standardized Likert-style scale of 0–10 (see ONS Outcomes Resource Area at www.ons.org/outcomes and the NCCN distress thermometer with a scale of 0 = no distress to 10 = extreme distress).
- Evaluate patients with scores ≥ 4 on the distress thermometer for overall distress and sources of distress and anxiety.
- Assess for medical causes of anxiety, including hypoxia, medications such as steroids, and hormone-secreting tumors.
- Refer patients with significant anxiety (not related to medical causes) to a social worker, psychiatrist, or psychologist for further assessment and/or treatment.
- Treat significant anxiety with psychotherapy and psychosocial interventions and/or anxiolytic and antidepressant medications.
- Provide patients and their families with information that discusses responses to a cancer diagnosis and treatment and the management of distress and anxiety.

Although evidence is insufficient to recommend specific pharmacologic agents, expert opinion and guidelines recommend psychotherapy and psychosocial interventions and/or pharmacologic agents in the management of significant anxiety.

Definitions of the interventions are available at **www.ons.org/outcomes**.
Literature search completed through May 2008.

References

Antoni, M.H., Wimberly, S.R., Lechner, S.C., Kazi, A., Sifre, T., Urcuyo, K.R., et al. (2006). Reduction of cancer-specific thought intrusions and anxiety symptoms with a stress management intervention among women undergoing treatment for breast cancer. *American Journal of Psychiatry, 163*(10), 1791–1797.

Arving, C., Sjoden, P.-O., Bergh, J., Hellbom, M., Johansson, B., Glimelius, B., et al. (2007). Individual psychosocial support for breast cancer patients: A randomized study of nurse versus psychologist interventions and standard care. *Cancer Nursing, 30*(3), E10–E19.

Badger, T., Segrin, C., Dorros, S.M., Meek, P., & Lopez, A.M. (2007). Depression and anxiety in women with breast cancer and their partners. *Nursing Research, 56*(1), 44–53.

Burnham, T.R., & Wilcox, A. (2002). Effects of exercise on physiologic and psychological variables in cancer survivors. *Medicine and Science in Sports and Exercise, 34*(12), 1863–1867.

Cheung, Y.L., Molassiotis, A., & Chang, A.M. (2003). The effect of progressive muscle relaxation training on anxiety and quality of life after stoma surgery in colorectal cancer patients. *Psycho-Oncology, 12*(3), 254–266.

Chujo, M., Mikami, I., Takashima, S., Saeki, T., Ohsumi, S., Aogi, K., et al. (2005). A feasibility study of psychosocial group intervention for breast cancer patients with first recurrence. *Supportive Care in Cancer, 13*(7), 503–514.

Deshler, A.M., Fee-Schroeder, K.C., Dowdy, J.L., Mettler, T.A., Novotny, P., Zhao, X., et al. (2006). A patient orientation program at a comprehensive cancer center. *Oncology Nursing Forum, 33*(3), 569–578.

Fellowes, D., Barnes, K., & Wilkinson, S. (2004). Aromatherapy and massage for symptom relief in patients with cancer. *Cochrane Database of Systematic Reviews* 2004, Issue 3. Art. No.: CD002287. DOI: 10.1002/14651858.CD002287.pub2.

Hernandez-Reif, M., Field, T., Ironson, G., Beutler, J., Vera, Y., Hurley, J., et al. (2005). Natural killer cells and lymphocytes increase in women with breast cancer following massage therapy. *International Journal of Neuroscience, 115*(4), 495–510.

Hernandez-Reif, M., Ironson, G., Field, T., Hurley, J., Katz, G., Diego, M., et al. (2004). Breast cancer patients have improved immune and neuroendocrine functions following massage therapy. *Journal of Psychosomatic Research, 57*(1), 45–52.

Hidderley, M., & Holt, M. (2004). A pilot randomized trial assessing the effects of autogenic training in early stage cancer patients in relation to psychological status and immune system responses. *European Journal of Oncology Nursing, 8*(1), 61–65.

Hoff, A.C., & Haaga, D.A. (2005). Effects of an education program on radiation oncology patients and families. *Journal of Psychosocial Oncology, 23*(4), 61–75.

Holland, J.C., Morrow, G., Schmale, A., Derogatis, L., Stefanek, M., Berenson, S., et al. (1991). A randomized clinical trial of alprazolam versus progressive muscle relaxation in cancer patients with anxiety and depressive symptoms. *Journal of Clinical Oncology, 9*(6), 1004–1011.

Jane, S. (2005). *Effects of full-body massage on pain intensity, anxiety, and physiologic relaxation in Taiwanese patients with metastatic bone pain: A pilot study.* Unpublished doctoral dissertation, University of Washington.

Jones, R.B., Pearson, J., Cawset, A.J., Bental, D., Barrett A., White, J., et al. (2006). Effect of different forms of information produced for cancer patients on their use of the information, social support, and anxiety: Randomised trial. *BMJ, 332*(7547), 942–948.

Katz, M.R., Irish, J.C., & Devins, G.M. (2004). Development and pilot testing of a psychoeducational intervention for oral cancer patients. *Psycho-Oncology, 13*(9), 642–653.

Kelly, A.E., Sullivan, P., Fawcett, J., & Samarel, N. (2004). Therapeutic touch, quiet time, and dialogue: Perceptions of women with breast cancer. *Oncology Nursing Forum, 31*(3), 625–631.

Khojainova, N., Santiago-Palma, J., Kornick, C., Breitbart, W., & Gonzales, G.R. (2002). Olanzapine in the management of cancer pain. *Journal of Pain and Symptom Management, 23*(4), 346–350.

Kim, S., & Kim, H. (2005). Effects of a relaxation breathing exercise on anxiety, depression, and leukocyte in hemopoietic stem cell transplantation patients. *Cancer Nursing, 28*(1), 79–83.

Kissane, D.W., Bloch, S., Smith, G.C., Miach, P., Clarke, D.M., Ikin, J., et al. (2003). Cognitive-existential group psychotherapy for women with primary breast cancer: A randomized controlled trial. *Psycho-Oncology, 12*(6), 532–546.

Kwekkeboom, K.L. (2003). Music versus distraction for procedural pain and anxiety in patients with cancer. *Oncology Nursing Forum, 30*(3), 433–440.

Manne, S.L., Ostroff, J.S., Winkel, G., Fox, K., Grana, G., Miller, E., et al. (2005). Couple-focused group intervention for women with early stage breast cancer. *Journal of Consulting and Clinical Psychology, 73*(4), 634–646.

Mentes, S.D., Unsal, D., Baran, O., Argun, G., & Ertunc, F.N. (2005). Effect of sedation with midazolam or propofol on patient's comfort during cancer chemotherapy: A prospective, randomized, double-blind study in breast cancer patients. *Journal of Chemotherapy, 17*(3), 327–333.

Midtgaard, J., Rorth, M., Stelter, R., Tveteras, A., Andersen, C., Quist, M., et al. (2005). The impact of a multidimensional exercise program on self-reported anxiety and depression in cancer patients undergoing chemotherapy: A phase II study. *Palliative and Supportive Care, 3*(3), 197–208.

Miller, D.K., Chibnall, J.T., Videen, S.D., & Duckro, P.N. (2005). Supportive-affective group experience for persons with life-threatening illness: Reducing spiritual, psychological, and death-related distress in dying patients. *Journal of Palliative Medicine, 8*(2), 333–343.

Nainis, N., Paice, J.A., Ratner, J., Wirth, J.H., Lai, J., & Shott, S. (2005). Relieving symptoms in cancer: Innovative use of art therapy. *Journal of Pain and Symptom Management, 31*(2), 162–169.

National Comprehensive Cancer Network. (2008). *NCCN Clinical Practice Guidelines in Oncology™: Distress management* [v.1.2008]. Retrieved March 6, 2008, from http://www.nccn.org/professionals/physician_gls/PDF/distress.pdf

National Institutes of Health, National Center for Complementary and Alternative Medicine. (2007, October). *What is CAM?* Retrieved March 6, 2008, from http://nccam.nih.gov/health/whatiscam

Osborn, R.L., Demoncada, A.C., & Feuerstein, M. (2006). Psychosocial interventions for depression, anxiety and quality of life in cancer survivors: Meta-analysis. *International Journal of Psychiatry in Medicine, 36*(1), 13–34.

Pasquini, M., Biondi, M., Constantini, A., Cairoli, F., Ferrarese, G., Picardi, A., et al. (2006). Detection and treatment of depressive and anxiety disorders among cancer patients: Feasibility and preliminary findings from a liaison service in an oncology division. *Depression and Anxiety, 23*(7), 441–448.

Pilkington, K., Kirkwood, G., Rampes, H., Fisher, P., & Richardson, J. (2006). Homeopathy for anxiety and anxiety disorders: A systematic review of the research. *Homeopathy, 95*(3), 151–162.

Quattrin, R., Zanini, A., Buchini, S., Turello, D., Annunziata, M.A., Vidotti, C., et al. (2006). Use of reflexology foot massage to reduce anxiety in hospitalized cancer patients in chemotherapy treatment: Methodology and outcomes. *Journal of Nursing Management, 14*(2), 96–105.

Rasavi, D., Allilaire, J.F., Smith, M., Salimpour, A., Verra, M., Desclaux, B., et al. (1996). The effect of fluoxetine on anxiety and depression symptoms in cancer patients. *Acta Psychiatria Scandinavica, 94*(3), 205–210.

Schneider, S.M., & Hood, L.E. (2007). Virtual reality: A distraction intervention for chemotherapy. *Oncology Nursing Forum, 34*(1), 39–46.

Segar, M.L., Katch, V.L., Roth, R.S., Garcia, A.W., Portner, T.I., Glickman, S.G., et al. (1998). The effect of aerobic exercise on self-esteem and depressive and anxiety symptoms among breast cancer survivors. *Oncology Nursing Forum, 25*(1), 107–113.

Shames, K.H., & Keegan, L. (2000). Touch: Connecting with the healing power. In B.M. Dossey, L. Keegan, & C.E. Guzzetta (Eds.), *Holistic nursing: A handbook for practice* (3rd ed., pp. 613–636). Gaithersburg, MD: Aspen.

Shepherd, L., Goldstein, D., Whitford, H., Thewes, B., Brummell, V., & Hicks, M. (2006). The utility of videoconferencing to provide innovative delivery of psychological treatment for rural cancer patients: Results of a pilot study. *Journal of Pain and Symptom Management, 32*(3), 453–461.

Sloman, R. (2002). Relaxation and imagery for anxiety and depression control in community patients with advanced cancer. *Cancer Nursing, 25*(6), 432–435.

Soden, K., Vincent, K., Craske, S., Lucas, C., & Ashley, S. (2004). A randomized controlled trial of aromatherapy massage in a hospice setting. *Palliative Medicine, 18*(2), 87–92.

Stephenson, N.L., Swanson, M., Dalton, J., Keefe, F.J., & Engelke, M. (2007). Partner-delivered reflexology: Effects on cancer pain and anxiety. *Oncology Nursing Forum, 34*(1), 127–132.

Targ, E.F., & Levine, E.G. (2002). The efficacy of a mind-body-spirit group for women with breast cancer: A randomized controlled trial. *General Hospital Psychiatry, 24*(4), 238–248.

Tsang, K.L., Carlson, L.E., & Olson, K. (2007). Pilot crossover trial of Reiki versus rest for treating cancer-related fatigue. *Integrative Cancer Therapies, 6*(1), 25–35.

Wald, T.G., Roger, R.G., Noyes, R., Carroll, B.T., & Clamon, G.H. (1993). Rapid relief of anxiety in cancer patients with both alprazolam and placebo. *Psychosomatics, 34*(4), 324–332.

Wilkinson, S.M., Love, S.B., Westcombe, A.M., Gambles, M.A., Burgess, C.C., Cargill, A., et al. (2007). Effectiveness of aromatherapy massage in the management of anxiety and depression in patients with cancer: A multicenter randomized controlled trial. *Journal of Clinical Oncology, 25*(5), 532–539.

Williams, S.A., & Schreier, A.M. (2004). The effect of education in managing side effects in women receiving chemotherapy for treatment of breast cancer [Online exclusive]. *Oncology Nursing Forum, 31*(1), E16–E23. Retrieved June 14, 2008, from http://ons.metapress.com/content/b366435101rv1712/fulltext.pdf

CHAPTER **5**

Caregiver Strain and Burden

Problem

Caregiver strain is the "felt difficulty in performing the caregiver role" (Archbold, Stewart, Greenlick, & Harvath, 1990, p. 376). Caregiver burden is the alterations in caregivers' emotional and physical health that can occur when care demands outweigh available resources (Given et al., 1992).

Incidence

Many individuals with cancer require care from an informal caregiver at some point in their disease process. An informal caregiver is unpaid and provides physical, emotional, or financial support to a person with cancer (Honea et al., 2008). Informal caregivers include both family members and others who are not related in the traditional sense to the person with cancer. The demands on informal caregivers have increased with the technologic advancements in cancer management and with more cancer treatments being given on an outpatient basis and at home (Ferrall, 2006).

Assessment

Caregivers experience different challenges during the diagnosis, treatment, recurrence, and survivorship phases of cancer. These challenges can significantly impact the caregiver's quality of life. A thorough assessment allows the nurse to facilitate coping by the caregiver (Ferrall, 2006). Objective measurement of caregiver burden includes obtaining information on the number of hours that care is provided and the number of tasks performed by the caregiver on behalf of the patient (Bookwala & Schulz, 2000; Gaugler et al., 2005). Subjective measurement of caregiver burden assesses the caregiver's level of emotional distress related to providing care (Given et al., 1992; Robinson, 1983; Zarit, Reever, & Bach-Peterson, 1980).

Clinical Measurement Tools

The following clinical measurement tools for caregiver strain and burden are presented in Table 5-1.
1. Caregiver Strain Index (see Figure 5-1)
2. Zarit Burden Inventory
3. Caregiver Reaction Assessment

Table 5-1. Caregiver Strain and Burden Measurement Tools					
Name of Tool	Number of Items	Domains	Reliability and Validity	Populations	Clinical Utility
Caregiver Strain Index	13	Burden related to employment, financial, physical, social, and time aspects	Adequate reliability and validity established	Caregivers of people with advanced cancer, caregivers of people with cancer pain	The scale is easily obtainable and short; however, its unidimensional nature may limit clinical applicability.
Zarit Burden Inventory	22	Burden related to health, psychological well-being, finances, social life, and relationship with impaired person	Adequate reliability and validity established	Caregivers of people at least three months following cancer diagnosis; caregivers of people with cancer receiving palliative care	The scale is commonly used in caregivers of people with cognitive impairment.
Caregiver Reaction Assessment	24	Burden related to self-esteem, lack of family support, and impact on finances, schedule, and health	Adequate reliability and validity established	Caregivers of people with a solid tumor; caregivers of people with cancer receiving home care	Lengthy but multidimensional

Note. Based on information from Sherwood & Given, 2008.

Figure 5-1. Caregiver Strain Index		
I am going to read a list of things that other people have found to be difficult. Would you tell me if any of these apply to you? (Give examples)		
	Yes = 1	No = 0
Sleep is disturbed (e.g., because _____ is in and out of bed or wanders around at night)		
It is inconvenient (e.g., because helping takes so much time or it is a long drive over to help)		
It is a physical strain (e.g., because of lifting in and out of a chair; effort or concentration is required)		
It is confining (e.g., helping restricts free time or cannot go visiting)		
There have been family adjustments (e.g., because helping has disrupted routine; there has been no privacy)		
There have been changes in personal plans (e.g., had to turn down a job; could not go on vacation)		
There have been other demands on my time (e.g., from other family members)		
There have been emotional adjustments (e.g., because of severe arguments)		
Some behavior is upsetting (e.g., because of incontinence; _____ has trouble remembering things; or _____ accuses people of taking things)		
It is upsetting to find_____ has changed so much from his/her former self (e.g., he/she is a different person than he/she used to be)		
There have been work adjustments (e.g., because of having to take time off)		
It is a financial strain		
Feeling completely overwhelmed (e.g., because of worry about _____; concerns about how you will manage)		
TOTAL SCORE (Count yes responses. Any positive answer may indicate a need for intervention in that area. A score of 7 or higher indicates a high level of stress.)		

Note. From "Validation of a Caregiver Strain Index," by B. Robinson, 1983, *Journal of Gerontology, 38*(3), p. 345. Copyright 1983 by Gerontological Society of America. Reprinted with permission.

References

Archbold, P.G., Stewart, B.J., Greenlick, M.R., & Harvath, T. (1990). Mutuality and preparedness as predictors of caregiver role strain. *Research in Nursing and Health, 13*(6), 375–384.

Bookwala, J., & Schulz, R. (2000). A comparison of primary stressors, secondary stressors, and depressive symptoms between elderly caregiving husbands and wives. *Psychology and Aging, 15*(4), 607–616.

Ferrall, S.M. (2006). Caring for the family caregiver. In R.M. Carroll-Johnson, L.M. Gorman, & N.J. Bush (Eds.), *Psychosocial nursing care along the cancer continuum* (2nd ed., pp. 603–610). Pittsburgh, PA: Oncology Nursing Society.

Gaugler, J.E., Hanna, N., Linder, J., Given, C.W., Tolbert, V., Kataria, R., et al. (2005). Cancer caregiving and subjective stress: A multi-site, multi-dimensional analysis. *Psycho-Oncology, 14*(9), 771–785.

Given, C.W., Given, B., Stommel, M., Collins, C., King, S., & Franklin, S. (1992). The Caregiver Reaction Assessment (CRA) for caregivers to persons with chronic physical and mental impairments. *Research in Nursing and Health, 15*(4), 271–283.

Holland, J.C., & Lewis, S. (2000). *The human side of cancer: Living with hope, coping with uncertainty.* New York: HarperCollins.

Honea, N.J., Brintnall, R., Given, B., Sherwood, P., Colao, D., Somers, S., et al. (2008). Putting Evidence Into Practice: Nursing assessment and interventions to reduce family caregiver strain and burden. *Clinical Journal of Oncology Nursing, 12*(3), 507–516.

Robinson, B. (1983). Validation of a caregiver strain index. *Journal of Gerontology, 38*(3), 344–348.

Sherwood, P., & Given, B. (2008). *Measuring oncology-nursing sensitive patient outcomes: Evidence-base summary.* Retrieved August 1, 2008, from http://www.ons.org/outcomes/measures/caregiver.shtml

Zarit, S., Reever, K., & Bach-Peterson, J. (1980). Relatives of the impaired elderly: Correlates of feelings of burden. *Gerontologist, 20*(6), 649–655.

Case Study

The oncology clinical nurse specialist (CNS) meets with patients' families who are struggling with caring for their loved one. A request for the CNS to meet with a family came shortly after the Oncology Nursing Society (ONS) Putting Evidence Into Practice (PEP) Resources on caregiver strain and burden were published. The caregiver was a woman caring for her husband. The cancer course for this gentleman was long, indolent, and palliative. The caregiver was well aware of the diagnosis, treatment plan, and need for symptom management. The tasks of caring for her husband were a daily challenge. They had been dealing with the disease for almost six years. She was thinking about retirement but continued to work part-time as a secretary in human resources. She verbally recognized her difficulty in asking for help from family and friends yet agreed that she felt overloaded in her role as a caregiver.

Within the CNS scope of practice and using the ONS PEP resource on caregiver strain and burden, the CNS began the meeting by merely validating the real phenomenon of caregiver strain and burden. The CNS used the Caregiver Strain Index to gather more information about the burden and strain that the caregiver was experiencing. The CNS shared with her several books and national associations that addressed the problem, including the work of ONS. Simply learning that role overload is common among people caring for the chronically ill seemed to validate and normalize her feelings.

The ONS PEP resource on caregiver strain and burden lists multicomponent interventions among those likely to be effective. The circumstances of this caregiver fit several of the specific situations highlighted on the resource. Together the CNS and the caregiver rehearsed a combination of interventions that the caregiver was willing to try in an attempt to understand and relieve the strain of caregiving, including the following.

• Educational: reading about caregiver burden and strain in *The Human Side of Cancer* (Holland & Lewis, 2000)
• Supportive: visting a local Gilda's Club; asking family to help her with specific tasks, such as mowing the lawn and purchasing a few months of housecleaning service; asking family and friends to focus their conversation on topics other than cancer
• Psychotherapy: This intervention was already in place at the time of the CNS's first meeting with the caregiver.
• Miscellaneous: encouraging the couple to engage in pleasant, positive experiences such as a tai chi class or massage

One of the interventions listed on the ONS PEP resource for which effectiveness has not been established is massage. The CNS shared with the caregiver that even though the evidence for this intervention is not sufficient to recommend its effectiveness in relieving caregiver strain and burden, it may provide a reduction in anxiety and depressive feelings. The caregiver participated in massage therapy and felt it provided an hour of respite while relieving muscle tension.

The ONS PEP resource packaged the principles for relieving caregiver strain and burden into a useable format. After a brief review of the evidence cited on the resource, the CNS had a structured framework that guided the choice of interventions—interventions that had the potential for effectiveness in the lives of two people facing life with cancer together.

Carolene B. Robinson, RN, MA, CNS, AOCN®
Oncology Clinical Nurse Specialist
Trinity Medical Center
Rock Island, IL

Caregiver Strain and Burden

2009 AUTHORS
Norissa J. Honea, PhD(c), MSN, RN, AOCN®, CCRP, and Paula R. Sherwood, PhD, RN, CNRN
ONS STAFF: Heather Belansky, RN, MSN

2007 AUTHORS
Norissa J. Honea, MSN, RN, AOCN®, Laurel L. Northouse, PhD, RN, FAAN, Ruth Ann Brintnall, PhD, RN, CHPN, Deirdre B. Colao, RN, OCN®, Susan Claire Somers, RN, BSN, OCN®, Barbara A. Given, PhD, RN, FAAN, and Paula R. Sherwood, PhD, RN, CNRN
ONS STAFF: Robi Thomas, MS, RN, AOCN®, CHPN, and Gail Mallory, PhD, RN, NEA-BC

What can nurses do to assist family caregivers of people with cancer to reduce strain and burden?

Recommended for Practice

Interventions for which effectiveness has been demonstrated by strong evidence from rigorously designed studies, meta-analyses, or systematic reviews and for which expectation of harms is small compared with the benefits

COGNITIVE BEHAVIORAL INTERVENTIONS

Cognitive behavioral interventions center on changing caregivers' perceptions of their ability to control a situation (Sorensen, Pinquart, & Duberstein, 2002). Such skills include
- Challenging negative thoughts or assumptions
- Using strategies that facilitate development of problem-solving abilities
- Focusing on time management, work overload, or emotional reactivity management
- Encouraging caregivers to re-engage in pleasant activities and positive experiences.

Cognitive behavioral interventions are recommended for practice in assisting oncology family caregivers to deal with their reactions to and assistance with patients' symptom management (Given et al., 2006). It may be most effective at reducing caregiver burden and strain for
- Caregivers who are younger than the patient
- Female caregivers.

Likely to Be Effective

Interventions for which effectiveness has been demonstrated by supportive evidence from a single rigorously conducted controlled trial, consistent supportive evidence from well-designed controlled trials using small samples, or guidelines developed from evidence and supported by expert opinion

Research in the area of caregiver burden has focused primarily on other chronic illness populations (e.g., dementia) rather than cancer populations (less than 10% of studies). Because of this, several interventions are listed as *Likely to Be Effective* rather than *Recommended for Practice* at this time.

PSYCHOEDUCATIONAL INTERVENTIONS

Psychoeducational interventions involve structured programs that provide education to caregivers delivered in either an individual (McMillan et al., 2006) or group format (Sorensen et al., 2002). Groups are commonly led by a trained leader and may include lectures, group discussions, and written materials. Content in the psychoeducational interventions may include

- The care recipient's disease process
- Information about resources and services
- Training for caregivers to respond effectively to disease- and treatment-related problems.

Support (which includes facilitating discussion of feelings about caregiving) may be part of a psychoeducational intervention, but it is secondary to the educational content (Sorensen et al., 2002).

Psychoeducational interventions are likely to be effective at reducing caregiver strain and burden, especially when they

- Occur in multiple sessions over time (McMillan et al., 2006; Sorensen et al., 2002)
- Teach problem-solving skills (McMillan et al., 2006; Sorensen et al., 2002; Toseland, Blanchard, & McCallion, 1995)
- Include patient symptom assessment and management (McMillan et al., 2006)
- Teach coping skills (Toseland et al., 1995)
- Are directed to caregivers with greater burden (Toseland et al., 1995).

PSYCHOTHERAPY INTERVENTIONS

Psychotherapy involves a therapeutic relationship between the caregiver and a trained professional in which the caregiver identifies strategies to manage his or her emotional/psychological distress. (Special training is required.) The conclusions from one meta-analysis point to psychotherapy interventions as likely to be effective in reducing caregiver burden (Sorensen et al., 2002). These may include

- Teaching caregivers to monitor their own feelings
- Helping caregivers to challenge negative thoughts that increase emotional distress
- Helping caregivers to develop problem-solving abilities by focusing on time management and role overload and managing their emotions
- Helping caregivers to engage in pleasant activities and positive experiences.

SUPPORTIVE INTERVENTIONS

Supportive interventions can be offered in an individual or group format led by either a professional or peer (McMillan et al., 2006; Sorensen et al., 2002). These interventions focus on building rapport and creating opportunities in which to discuss problems as well as successes and feelings regarding caregiving. Findings from one meta-analysis indicated that supportive interventions are likely to be effective in reducing caregiver burden (Sorensen et al.). Supportive interventions that are likely to be effective include

- Teaching caregivers problem-solving skills
- Teaching caregivers coping skills.

MULTICOMPONENT INTERVENTIONS

Multicomponent interventions use various combinations of educational, supportive, psychotherapy, respite, and miscellaneous interventions (Sorensen et al., 2002). These interventions are likely to be effective at reducing caregiver strain and burden because they use a variety of techniques to reduce burden and are able to address a variety of caregiver needs. Multicomponent interventions also have a *moderate* effect on reducing caregiver burden, whereas interventions that focus on a single therapeutic activity, such as supportive interventions (e.g., support groups) and psychoeducational interventions, have only a *small* effect on reducing burden (Martire, Lustig, Schulz, Miller, & Helgeson, 2004; Sorensen et al.).

Specific situations exist in which multicomponent interventions are more likely to reduce caregiver burden. Greater reduction in burden may be seen when the intervention is directed or offered

- To **older caregivers** rather than to younger caregivers (Sorensen et al., 2002)
- To caregivers of **older rather than younger care recipients** (Sorensen et al., 2002)
- To **female caregivers** rather than to male caregivers (Sorensen et al., 2002)
- To **caregivers who report greater subjective burden** than to caregivers with less subjective burden (Sorensen et al., 2002; Toseland et al., 1995)
- To **individual caregivers** rather than to caregivers in a group setting (McMillan et al., 2006)
- To **spouses alone or to a combination of family members** (Martire et al., 2004)
- To **both the patient and family member or to family members alone** (Martire et al., 2004)
- **When relationship issues between care recipients and caregivers are addressed** (Martire et al., 2004).

Benefits Balanced With Harms

Interventions for which clinicians and patients should weigh the beneficial and harmful effects according to individual circumstances and priorities

There are no interventions as of May 2008.

Effectiveness Not Established

Interventions for which insufficient or conflicting data or data of inadequate quality currently exist, with no clear indication of harm

DISCUSSING PSYCHOSOCIAL ISSUES

A nonrandomized, multisite trial examined a formalized intervention program, the *Family Caregiver Cancer Education Program,* which included strategies such as controlling symptoms, managing psychosocial issues, and identifying available resources. No overall improvement in caregiver burden was observed. However, the impact of caregiving on household finances and caregiver knowledge showed significant improvement, and caregivers perceived an improvement in their health (Pasacreta, Barg, Nuamah, & McCorkle, 2000). A second study explored informal short-term teaching and group support sessions aimed at self-care promotion for adult caregivers and found no significant difference in caregiver burden (Harding et al., 2004).

IDENTIFYING AVAILABLE RESOURCES AND DISCUSSING COORDINATION OF SERVICES

Three studies (Harding et al., 2004; Jepson, McCorkle, Adler, Nuamah, & Lusk, 1999; Pasacreta et al., 2000) used multicomponent interventions to examine the benefit of educational sessions on coping skills and on caregivers' ability to identify supportive resources. No significant difference was seen on outcome measures, suggesting that the interventions were not effective in reducing caregiver burden or strain. However, caregivers in one study reported feeling more confident in their ability to handle the caregiver role following the educational sessions (Pasacreta et al.).

MASSAGE

One quasi-experimental study examined the benefit of massage therapy or healing touch on caregivers of patients with cancer (Rexilius, Mundt, Erickson Megel, & Agrawal, 2002). The intervention was not effective in reducing caregiver burden or strain. However, a significant decline was observed in depression and anxiety scores of caregivers in the treatment group receiving massage therapy (Rexilius et al.).

RESPITE/ADULT DAY CARE

The benefit of respite (adult day care) was examined in a multicomponent meta-analysis (Sorensen et al., 2002). Preliminary results suggested that respite care may reduce caregiver burden and strain. However, as study populations were not limited to oncology, the benefit for caregivers of patients with cancer was not established.

TEACHING CAREGIVER SELF-CARE

One randomized trial (Jepson et al., 1999) and one nonrandomized study (Pasacreta et al., 2000) taught self-care behaviors to caregivers. One of the studies also addressed common emotional reactions to caregiving, such as depression and anger (Pasacreta et al.). No difference in caregiver strain or burden was observed in either study, but other benefits, such as increased caregiver esteem and perceived competence, were reported (Pasacreta et al.).

TEACHING PAIN MANAGEMENT

Two studies tested the impact of one-on-one pain management education on cancer caregivers' feelings of efficacy and reported subjective burden and strain. The one study (Keefe et al., 2005) showed a trend in improvement for reported levels of caregiver strain, whereas the second (Ferrell, Grant, Chan, Ahn, & Ferrell, 1995) reported that education improved caregivers' attitudes about pain management and about their ability to handle their partner's pain but led to no measurable change in caregiver strain or burden.

TEACHING SYMPTOM MANAGEMENT

One observational study (Harding et al., 2004), one nonrandomized study (Pasacreta et al., 2000), and one randomized trial (Jepson et al., 1999) investigated the benefits of using supportive interventions, including teaching symptom management in the cancer caregiving population. Two studies used multisession group interactions (Harding et al.; Pasacreta et al.), and the other used in-home and telephone educational interventions aimed at improving caregiver competency in dealing with their care recipient's symptoms. One study showed no improvement in reported caregiver burden or strain but demonstrated positive effects on other measured indicators (Pasacreta et al.). The other studies were inconclusive (Harding et al.; Jepson et al.).

Effectiveness Unlikely

Interventions for which lack of effectiveness has been demonstrated by negative evidence from a single rigorously conducted controlled trial, consistent negative evidence from well-designed controlled trials using small samples, or guidelines developed from evidence and supported by expert opinion

INTERVENTIONS DIRECTED AT IMPROVING CARE RECIPIENT COMPETENCE

A meta-analysis found no effect on caregiver burden when the intervention was directed only toward the care recipient to improve the care recipient's competence (Sorensen et al., 2002). Examples of this type of intervention include memory clinics for those with dementia and activity therapy programs designed to improve the care recipient's affect and everyday competence.

Not Recommended for Practice

Interventions for which lack of effectiveness or harmfulness has been demonstrated by strong evidence from rigorously conducted studies, meta-analyses, or systematic reviews, or interventions where the costs, burden, or harms associated with the intervention exceed anticipated benefit

There are no interventions as of May 2008.

Definitions of the interventions are available at **www.ons.org/outcomes**.
Literature search completed through May 2008.

References

Ferrell, B.R., Grant, M., Chan, J., Ahn, C., & Ferrell, B.A. (1995). The impact of cancer pain education on family caregivers of elderly patients. *Oncology Nursing Forum, 22*(8), 1211–1218.

Given, B., Given, C.W., Sikorski, A., Jeon, S., Sherwood, P., & Rahbar, M. (2006). The impact of providing symptom management assistance on caregiver reaction: Results of a randomized trial. *Journal of Pain and Symptom Management, 32*(5), 433–443.

Harding, R., Higginson, I.J., Leam, C., Donaldson, N., Pearce, A., George, R., et al. (2004). Evaluation of a short-term group intervention for informal carers of patients attending a home palliative care service. *Journal of Pain and Symptom Management, 27*(5), 396–408.

Jepson, C., McCorkle, R., Adler, D., Nuamah, I., & Lusk, E. (1999). Effects of home care on caregivers' psychosocial status. *Image: The Journal of Nursing Scholarship, 31*(2), 115–120.

Keefe, F.J., Ahles, T.A., Sutton, L., Dalton, J., Baucom, D., Pope, M.S., et al. (2005). Partner-guided cancer pain management at the end of life: A preliminary study. *Journal of Pain and Symptom Management, 29*(3), 263–272.

Martire, L.M., Lustig, A.P., Schulz, R., Miller, G.E., & Helgeson, V.S. (2004). Is it beneficial to involve a family member? A meta-analysis of psychosocial interventions for chronic illness. *Health Psychology, 23*(6), 599–611.

McMillan, S.C., Small, B.J., Weitzner, M., Schonwetter, R., Tittle, M., Moody, L., et al. (2006). Impact of coping skills intervention with family caregivers of hospice patients with cancer: A randomized clinical trial. *Cancer, 106*(1), 214–222.

Pasacreta, J.V., Barg, F., Nuamah, I., & McCorkle, R. (2000). Participant characteristics before and 4 months after attendance at a family caregiver cancer education program. *Cancer Nursing, 23*(4), 295–303.

Rexilius, S.J., Mundt, C., Erickson Megel, M., & Agrawal, S. (2002). Therapeutic effects of massage therapy and healing touch on caregivers of patients undergoing autologous hematopoietic stem cell transplant [Online exclusive]. *Oncology Nursing Forum, 29*(3), E35–E44.

Sorensen, S., Pinquart, M., & Duberstein, P. (2002). How effective are interventions with caregivers? An updated meta-analysis. *Gerontologist, 42*(3), 356–372.

Toseland, R.W., Blanchard, C.G., & McCallion, P. (1995). A problem solving intervention for caregivers of cancer patients. *Social Science and Medicine, 40*(4), 517–528.

CHAPTER 6

Chemotherapy-Induced Nausea and Vomiting

Problem

Nausea is a subjective sensation associated with the conscious recognition of the will or desire to vomit. It is accompanied by symptoms such as hyperventilation, tachycardia, and potentially vomiting. Vomiting is the oral expulsion of stomach or intestinal contents, often preceded by nausea, rapid or irregular heartbeat, dizziness, sweating, pallor, pupil dilation, and retching (de Carvalho, Martins, & dos Santos, 2007). Chemotherapy-induced nausea and vomiting (CINV), a common side effect of chemotherapy regimens, may be described as acute, delayed, anticipatory, breakthrough, or refractory (National Comprehensive Cancer Network [NCCN], 2008). Uncontrolled CINV can lead to dehydration, electrolyte imbalances, malnutrition, esophageal tears, wound dehiscence, decreased self-care and functional abilities, depression, fatigue, and withdrawal from potentially useful or curable treatment (Lohr, 2008; NCCN).

Incidence

Approximately 70%–80% of patients may experience CINV if not properly prevented, despite the advances in antiemetic therapy (Morrow et al., 1998). It is reported that approximately 50%–60% of patients receiving highly emetogenic chemotherapy experience delayed nausea and emesis (Grunberg et al., 2004). Several studies documented that nausea, in particular, remains one of patients' most feared side effects (de Boer-Dennert et al., 1997; Hickok et al., 2003). Despite many advances in the pharmacologic management of nausea and vomiting, clinicians still struggle to control this problematic symptom. Studies have documented that healthcare providers underestimate the degree to which patients experience CINV (Grunberg et al.). Failing to control nausea and vomiting often leads to anticipatory nausea and is quite difficult to overcome. CINV, if uncontrolled, can become a significant quality-of-life issue for patients.

Assessment

Assessing known risk factors for CINV and selecting appropriate interventions at the outset are paramount. Table 6-1 presents an example of a baseline assessment checklist for CINV in which more affirmative responses indicate higher risk for developing CINV. In addition to the baseline assessment, it is important to consistently assess patients for nausea and vomiting post-chemotherapy and to alter the management strategies. Ongoing assessment prior to each cycle is important to modify the intervention and plan. Items for subsequent assessment should include (a) the number of episodes of nausea and vomiting after chemotherapy and number of episodes of retching, (b) timing of CINV (within first 24 hours or thereafter), (c) ability to eat after chemotherapy, (d) oral intake, (e) antiemetics taken, and (f) other related symptom problems.

Clinical Measurement Tools

The following clinical measurement tools for CINV are presented in Table 6-2.

Table 6-1. Baseline Assessment for Chemotherapy-Induced Nausea and Vomiting (CINV)		
Assessment	Yes	No
Age < 50 years		
Female gender		
History of nausea and vomiting with pregnancy		
History of motion sickness		
One or less alcoholic beverage per day		
High anxiety level		
Previous history of CINV		
High to moderate emetogenicity of chemotherapy		
Patient expectation of nausea before therapy		
Physical examination findings documented		
Laboratory data checked		
Current medications checked		
Fluid volume status assessed		
Previous interventions assessed		
Note. Based on information from Booth et al., 2007; Wickham, 2004.		

1. Index of Nausea, Vomiting, and Retching (INVR) (see Figure 6-1)
2. Functional Living Index–Emesis
3. Common Terminology Criteria for Adverse Events (CTCAE) (National Cancer Institute Cancer Therapy Evaluation Program [NCI CTEP], 2006) (see Table 6-3)

The Multinational Association of Supportive Care in Cancer developed an antiemesis tool (MAT) in 2004. This tool measures the frequency and intensity of acute and delayed nausea and vomiting (24 hours after chemotherapy and four days after chemotherapy). MAT is a computerized tool that also has a patient outcomes score sheet documenting chemotherapy, dates of treatment, antiemetic regimens, and actions taken. Although the MAT is relatively easy to use and has shown recent evidence of validation (Molassiotis et al., 2007), it does not address the symptom distress experienced by patients with nausea or vomiting. It is available online at www.mascc.org/content/126.html.

Table 6-2. Clinical Measurement Tools for Chemotherapy-Induced Nausea and Vomiting					
Name of Tool	Number of Items	Domains	Reliability and Validity	Populations	Clinical Utility
Index of Nausea, Vomiting, and Retching	8 total: 5 for occurrence, 3 for distress	Nausea, vomiting, and retching (NVR), and the components (frequency/amount, duration, severity, distress) of each symptom	Adequate reliability and validity established	Inpatients receiving chemotherapy, outpatients receiving chemotherapy, breast cancer, medical-surgical, and obstetrics Translated in Japanese and Chinese	Easy to use Provides information about NVR, total experience, occurrence, distress, and individual symptoms 12-hour time frame
Functional Living Index–Emesis	18 total: 9 for nausea, 9 for vomiting	Effect of nausea and vomiting on physical activity, social and emotional function, and eating	Reliability and validity established	Breast cancer, lung cancer, inpatients, chemotherapy-naïve patients, radiotherapy patients Translated in Japanese	Easy to use Provides information about the effect of nausea and vomiting on functional status Correlates with quality-of-life measures

(Continued on next page)

Table 6-2. Clinical Measurement Tools for Chemotherapy-Induced Nausea and Vomiting *(Continued)*

Name of Tool	Number of Items	Domains	Reliability and Validity	Populations	Clinical Utility
Common Terminology Criteria for Adverse Events	5 category grading scales for nausea and vomiting	Nausea: oral intake Vomiting: number of episodes, IV fluid requirements	Unknown	Unknown	Clinician-friendly Often used in clinical trials and outpatient flow sheets

Note. Based on information from Decker et al., 2006; National Cancer Institute Cancer Therapy Evaluation Program, 2006; Rhodes & McDaniel, 2004.

Figure 6-1. Index of Nausea, Vomiting, and Retching (INVR)

Directions: Please mark the box in each row that most clearly corresponds to your experience. Please make *one* mark on each *line*.

I.D. Number: _____ Date: _____

Time: _____

1.	In the last 12 hours, I threw up _____ times.	7 or more	5–6	3–4	1–2	I did not throw up
2.	In the last 12 hours, from retching or dry heaves I have felt _____ distress.	no	mild	moderate	great	severe
3.	In the last 12 hours, from vomiting or throwing up, I have felt _____ distress.	severe	great	moderate	mild	no
4.	In the last 12 hours, I have felt nauseated or sick at my stomach _____.	not at all	1 hour or less	2–3 hours	4–6 hours	more than 6
5.	In the last 12 hours, from nausea/sickness at my stomach, I have felt _____ distress.	no	mild	moderate	great	severe
6.	In the last 12 hours, each time I threw up I produced a _____ amount.	very large (3 cups or more)	large (2–3 cups)	moderate (½–2 cups)	small (up to ½ cup)	I did not throw up
7.	In the last 12 hours, I have felt nauseated or sick at my stomach _____ times.	7 or more	5–6	3–4	1–2	no

(Continued on next page)

Figure 6-1. Index of Nausea, Vomiting, and Retching (INVR) *(Continued)*

8.	In the last 12 hours, I have had periods of retching or dry heaves without bringing anything up _____ times.	no	1–2	3–4	5–6	7 or more

INVR Scale

Complete *one* INVR Scale starting at 7, 8, or 9 p.m. on _____.
(date)

Choose the best hour for your schedule.
Beginning with your chosen hour, complete *one* INVR Scale every 12 hours at the *same* clock hour for six times.

Example: 7 p.m. – 7 a.m.
8 p.m. – 8 a.m.
9 p.m. – 9 a.m.

Note. Copyright 1996, Curators of Missouri, Verna A. Rhodes, RN, EdS, FAAN. Used with permission.

Table 6-3. Common Terminology Criteria for Adverse Events

Grade	Nausea	Vomiting
0	None	None
1	Able to eat	1 episode/24 hours
2	Oral intake significantly decreased	2–5 episodes/24 hours
3	No significant oral intake, requiring IV fluids	> 6 episodes/24 hours or requiring IV fluids
4	–	Requiring parenteral nutrition or intensive care

Note. Based on information from National Cancer Institute Cancer Therapy Evaluation Program, 2006.

References

Booth, C.M., Clemons, M., Dranitsaris, G., Joy, A., Young, S., Callaghan, W., et al. (2007). Chemotherapy-induced nausea and vomiting in breast cancer patients: A prospective observational study. *Journal of Supportive Oncology, 5*(8), 374–380.

de Boer-Dennert, M., de Wit, R., Schmitz, P.I., Djontono, J., v Beurden, V., Stoter, G., et al. (1997). Patient perceptions of the side-effects of chemotherapy: The influence of 5HT3 antagonists. *British Journal of Cancer, 76*(8), 1055–1061.

de Carvalho, E.C., Martins, F.T.M., & dos Santos, C.B. (2007). A pilot study of a relaxation technique for management of nausea and vomiting in patients receiving cancer chemotherapy. *Cancer Nursing, 30*(2), 163–167.

Decker, G.M., DeMeyer, E.S., & Kisko, D.L. (2006). Measuring the maintenance of daily life activities using the Functional Living Index–Emesis (FLIE) in patients receiving moderately emetogenic chemotherapy. *Journal of Supportive Oncology, 4*(1), 35–52.

Grunberg, S.M., Deuson, R.R., Mavros, P., Geling, O., Hansen, M., Cruciani, G., et al. (2004). Incidence of chemotherapy-induced nausea and emesis after modern antiemetics. *Cancer, 100*(10), 2261–2268.

Hickok, J.T., Roscoe, J.A., Morrow, G.R., King, D.K., Atkins, J.N., & Fitch, T.R. (2003). Nausea and emesis remain significant problems of chemotherapy despite prophylaxis with 5-hydroxytryptamine-3 antiemetics: A University of Rochester James P. Wilmot Cancer Center Community Hospital Clinical Oncology Program study of 360 cancer patients treated in the community. *Cancer, 97*(11), 2880–2886.

Lohr, L. (2008). Chemotherapy-induced nausea and vomiting. *Cancer Journal, 14*(2), 85–93.

Molassiotis, A., Coventry, P.A., Stricker, C.T., Clements, C., Eaby, B., Velders, L., et al. (2007). Validation and psychometric assessment of a short clinical scale to measure chemotherapy-induced nausea and vomiting: The MASCC antiemesis tool. *Journal of Pain and Symptom Management, 34*(2), 148–159.

Morrow, G.R., Roscoe, J.A., Hickok, J.T., Stern, R.M., Pierce, H.I., King, D.B., et al. (1998). Initial control of chemotherapy-induced nausea and vomiting in patient quality of life. *Oncology, 12*(Suppl. 4), 32–37.

Multinational Association of Supportive Care in Cancer. (2008). *Antiemetic guidelines.* Retrieved June 23, 2008, from http://www.mascc.org/media/Resource_centers/MASCC_Guidelines _Update.pdf

National Cancer Institute Cancer Therapy Evaluation Program. (2006). *Common terminology criteria for adverse events* (version 3.0). Bethesda, MD: National Cancer Institute. Retrieved March 14, 2008, from http://ctep.cancer.gov/protocolDevelopment/electronic_applications/ docs/ctcaev3.pdf

National Comprehensive Cancer Network. (2008). *NCCN Clinical Practice Guidelines in Oncology™: Antiemesis* [v.2.2008]. Retrieved March 14, 2008, from http://www.nccn.org/ professionals/physician_gls/PDF/antiemesis.pdf

Rhodes, V., & McDaniel, R. (2004). *Measuring oncology nursing-sensitive patient outcomes: Evidence-based-summary: Nausea and vomiting.* Retrieved August 31, 2008, from http:// www.ons.org/outcomes/measures/nausea.shtml

Wickham, R. (2004). Nausea and vomiting. In C.H. Yarbro, M.H. Frogge & M. Goodman (Eds.), *Cancer symptom management* (3rd ed., pp. 187–214). Sudbury, MA: Jones and Bartlett.

Case Study

L.B. was a 49-year-old white female with stage IB breast cancer. She underwent mastectomy and sentinel lymph node biopsy. Adjuvant chemotherapy was prescribed as dose-dense chemotherapy with ACT (doxorubicin plus cyclophosphamide and paclitaxel every two weeks for four cycles). Some of L.B.'s risk factors for CINV were young age, female gender, history of nausea with pregnancy, and anxiety. According to the Oncology Nursing Society (ONS) Putting Evidence Into Practice (PEP) resource, the antiemetics recommended for prevention of acute CINV with highly to moderately emetogenic chemotherapy are a neurokinin-1 (NK1) receptor antagonist (aprepitant 125 mg PO or fosaprepitant 115 mg

IV), a 5-hydroxytryptamine-3 (5-HT$_3$) receptor antagonist (palonosetron 0.25 mg IV on day 1, ondansetron 16–24 mg PO or 32 mg IV on day 1, dolasetron 100 mg PO or IV on day 1, or tropisetron 5 mg PO or IV on day 1), and a corticosteroid (dexamethasone 12 mg PO or IV). Women receiving doxorubicin and cyclophosphamide represent a significantly high risk for CINV; therefore, the three-drug antiemetic regimen (NK1 receptor antagonist, 5-HT$_3$ receptor antagonist, and corticosteroid) is recommended. For managing delayed CINV, aprepitant 80 mg PO for days 2 and 3 and a corticosteroid (dexamethasone 12 mg PO days 2–4) is recommended. L.B. was instructed to call the oncology nurse if her nausea or vomiting was uncontrolled.

When L.B. returned for cycle 2 of doxorubicin and cyclophosphamide, she informed the nurse that she vomited on days two and three and experienced prolonged nausea for eight days. The dexamethasone caused L.B. to be extremely nervous and unable to sleep. She said that she would rather be nauseous than experience these symptoms. For cycle 2, the patient was asked to complete the INVR scale every 12 hours at the same clock time for six times, beginning the day after chemotherapy. By writing her responses down, perhaps L.B. would be able to quantify the problem and possibly be more likely to report problems earlier.

After consulting the ONS PEP resource on CINV and L.B.'s physician, a benzodiazepine, lorazepam 0.5–2 mg PO or sublingual every four to six hours on days 1–4, was added to her antiemetic regimen.

Because the ONS PEP resource on CINV included the recommendation that structured educational intervention may be helpful, a detailed instruction sheet with verbal and written information was provided.

Nonpharmacologic interventions that are cited in the *Likely to Be Effective* section of the ONS PEP resource on CINV include
- Acupuncture
- Acupressure
- Guided imagery
- Music therapy and progressive muscle relaxation.

These interventions should be used in addition to pharmacologic intervention. A common intervention for nausea is ginger, but according to the ONS PEP resource, its effectiveness is not established. L.B. tried ginger with poor results.

L.B. also tried acupuncture two times per week from a Chinese practitioner who was a certified acupuncturist. She believed that the acupuncture helped her some.

By her fourth cycle, L.B.'s symptoms were improved but not completely resolved. According to the ONS PEP resource, dronabinol 5–10 mg every three to six hours may be added. Dronabinol was added on days 3–8 with resolution of nausea.

Laurel A. Barbour, RN, MSN, APN, AOCN®
Biotherapy Care Manager
Advocate Lutheran General Hospital
Park Ridge, IL

Chemotherapy-Induced Nausea and Vomiting

2009 AUTHORS
Patricia J. Friend, PhD, APRN, AOCN®, and Mary Pat Johnston, RN, MS, AOCN®
ONS STAFF: Linda H. Eaton, MN, RN, AOCN®

2006 AUTHORS
Janelle M. Tipton, MSN, RN, AOCN®, Roxanne W. McDaniel, PhD, RN,
Laurel A. Barbour, MSN, RN, AOCN®, Mary Pat Johnston, MS, RN, AOCN®, Patricia Starr, RN, BSN, OCN®,
Marilyn K. Kayne, BSN, RN, OCN®, and Marita L. Ripple, RN
ONS STAFF: Gail Mallory, PhD, RN, NEA-BC

What interventions are effective in preventing and treating chemotherapy-induced nausea and vomiting (CINV)?

Recommended for Practice

Interventions for which effectiveness has been demonstrated by strong evidence from rigorously designed studies, meta-analyses, or systematic reviews and for which expectation of harm is small compared to the benefits

ANTICIPATORY NAUSEA AND/OR VOMITING

Anticipatory nausea and/or vomiting is a conditioned or learned response that occurs after a negative past experience with chemotherapy in which nausea and vomiting was not controlled. Prevention is key to prevent the learned response from occurring (National Comprehensive Cancer Network [NCCN], 2008).
- Utilization of optimal treatments for acute and delayed nausea and vomiting from the initiation of chemotherapy to prevent development of anticipatory nausea and vomiting during subsequent cycles
- Behavioral therapies such as relaxation, hypnosis, guided imagery, and acupuncture may be effective in treating anticipatory nausea and vomiting (Figueroa-Moseley et al., 2007).
- Benzodiazepines
  - Alprazolam 0.5–2 mg PO three times a day, beginning the night before treatment, or
  - Lorazepam 0.5–2 mg PO the night before and the morning of treatment
(American Society of Health-System Pharmacists [ASHP], 1999; Antiemetic Subcommittee of the Multinational Association of Supportive Care in Cancer [MASCC], 2008; Gralla et al., 1999; NCCN, 2008; Polovich, White, & Kelleher, 2005)

ACUTE AND DELAYED NAUSEA AND/OR VOMITING: HIGHLY EMETOGENIC CHEMOTHERAPY

Acute nausea and/or vomiting usually occurs within a few minutes to several hours after chemotherapy administration and often resolves within the first 24 hours (NCCN, 2008). Delayed nausea and/or vomiting usually occurs more than 24 hours after chemotherapy administration. It often peaks 48–72 hours after chemotherapy and can last six to seven days (NCCN, 2006). For patients who receive multi-day emetogenic therapy, delayed nausea can last up to 10 days depending on the sequence of the regimen and the emetogenicity of the last chemotherapy agent administered. The antiemetic regimen should be based on the emetogenic potential of the chemotherapy agents. For highly emetogenic regimens, a three-drug regimen is recommended, including single doses of a 5-HT$_3$ receptor antagonist, dexamethasone, and aprepitant (or fosaprepitant) given before chemotherapy. For effective control of CINV, patients need antiemesis protection throughout the period of risk, thus antiemetic prophylaxis should be given on days 1–4 for single-day agents, and up to 10 days for multi-day emetogenic therapy.

Antiemetic regimens have shown better efficacy in controlling acute and delayed vomiting than nausea. Trials show poorer control of nausea; indeed, the prevalence of anticipatory, acute, and delayed nausea is greater than the prevalence of vomiting.

- **5-HT$_3$ receptor antagonist**
  - Palonosetron 0.25 mg IV on day 1, or
  - Granisetron 2 mg PO, or 1 mg PO twice a day, or 0.01 mg/kg (maximum 1 mg) IV on day 1, or
  - Ondansetron 16–24 mg PO or 8–32 mg IV (or oral dissolving tablet 16–24 mg, only if other routes are contraindicated) (Pectasides et al., 2007) on day 1, or
  - Dolasetron 100 mg PO or 1.8 mg/kg or 100 mg IV on day 1, or
  - Tropisetron 5 mg PO or IV on day 1 (MASCC, 2008)
- **NK1 receptor antagonist**
  - Aprepitant 125 mg PO or fosaprepitant 115 mg IV on day 1, aprepitant 80 mg PO daily on days 2–3 (MASCC, 2008; NCCN, 2008)
- **Corticosteroid**
  - Dexamethasone 12 mg PO or IV on day 1, 8 mg PO or IV once daily on days 2–4
  - Because of its interaction with the cytochrome P450 enzyme system, aprepitant can alter the metabolism of certain drugs. Specifically, when given with aprepitant, the efficacy of dexamethasone is increased. Thus, the recommendations stated previously reflect a reduced dose of dexamethasone.
  - If aprepitant or fosaprepitant is **not** given, the corticosteroid dose is dexamethasone 20 mg PO or IV on day 1, 8 mg PO or IV twice a day on days 2–4.
- **Benzodiazepine** (may or may not be given with other antiemetics because of its sedating effects)
  - Lorazepam 0.5–2 mg PO, IV, or sublingual every four to six hours on days 1–4

(ASHP, 1999; Gralla et al., 1999; MASCC, 2008; NCCN, 2008; Polovich et al., 2005)

ACUTE AND DELAYED NAUSEA AND/OR VOMITING: MODERATELY EMETOGENIC CHEMOTHERAPY

- **5-HT$_3$ receptor antagonist**
  - Palonosetron 0.25 mg IV on day 1, or
  - Granisetron 1–2 mg PO, 1 mg PO twice per day, or 1 mg IV on day 1, or
  - Ondansetron 16–24 mg PO or 8–32 mg IV (or oral dissolving table 16–24 mg, only if other routes are contraindicated [Pectasides et al., 2007]) on day 1, or
  - Dolasetron 100 mg PO or IV on day 1, or
  - Tropisetron 5 mg PO or IV on day 1 (MASCC, 2008)

- **NK1 receptor antagonist**
  - Aprepitant 125 mg PO or fosaprepitant 115 mg IV on day 1, aprepitant 80 mg PO daily on days 2–3 (MASCC, 2008; NCCN, 2008)
- **Corticosteroid**
  - Dexamethasone 12 mg PO or IV on day 1, 8 mg PO or IV once daily on days 2–4
  - Because of its interaction with the cytochrome P450 enzyme system, aprepitant can alter the metabolism of certain drugs. Specifically, when given with aprepitant, the efficacy of dexamethasone is increased. Thus, the recommendations stated previously reflect a reduced dose of dexamethasone.
  - If aprepitant or fosaprepitant is not given, the corticosteroid dose is dexamethasone 20 mg PO or IV on day 1, 8 mg PO or IV twice a day on days 2–4.
- **Benzodiazepine** (may or may not be given with other antiemetics because of its sedating effects)
  - Lorazepam 0.5–2 mg PO, IV, or sublingual every four to six hours, and

On days 2–4, consider:

- **Corticosteroid**
  - Dexamethasone 8 mg PO or IV daily, or
- **5-HT$_3$ receptor antagonist**
  - Ondansetron 8 mg PO twice daily, 16 mg PO daily, or 8 mg IV, or
  - Granisetron 1–2 mg PO daily, 1 mg PO twice daily, or 1 mg IV, or
  - Dolasetron 100 mg PO or IV daily
  - Tropisetron 5 mg PO or IV daily (MASCC, 2008)
- **Substituted benzamide**
  - Metoclopramide 0.5 mg/kg PO or IV every six hours or 20 mg PO four times daily ± diphenhydramine 25–50 mg PO or IV every four to six hours as needed

(ASHP, 1999; Gralla et al., 1999; MASCC, 2008; NCCN, 2008; Polovich et al., 2005)

ACUTE AND DELAYED NAUSEA AND/OR VOMITING: LOW EMETOGENIC CHEMOTHERAPY

No routine antiemetic prophylaxis for delayed emesis is indicated, but the following can be given to prevent acute emesis.
- **Corticosteroid**
  - Dexamethasone 12 mg PO or IV on the day of treatment, or
- **Phenothiazine**
  - Prochlorperazine 10 mg PO or IV every four to six hours, or
- **Substituted benzamide**
  - Metoclopramide 10–40 mg PO every four to six hours or 1–2 mg/kg every three to four hours ± diphenhydramine 25–50 mg PO or IV every four to six hours, or
- **Benzodiazepine** (may or may not be given with other antiemetics because of its sedating effects)
  - Lorazepam 0.5–2 mg PO or IV every four to six hours

(ASHP, 1999; Gralla et al., 1999; MASCC, 2008; NCCN, 2008; Polovich et al., 2005)

ACUTE AND DELAYED NAUSEA AND/OR VOMITING: MINIMAL EMETOGENIC CHEMOTHERAPY

No routine antiemesis prophylaxis is recommended.

BREAKTHROUGH OR REFRACTORY NAUSEA AND/OR VOMITING

Preventing is much easier than treating breakthrough or refractory nausea and/or vomiting; however, the general principle is to give an agent from a drug class not previously used. Also consider around-the-clock rather than PRN dosing. Furthermore, often the oral route will be contraindicated (if breakthrough emesis is a problem), so parenteral and rectal routes are preferred (NCCN, 2008).

- **Corticosteroids**
  - Dexamethasone 12 mg PO or IV daily, if not previously given, or
- **5-HT$_3$ receptor antagonist**
  - Granisetron 1–2 mg PO daily, 1 mg PO twice daily, or 1 mg IV, or
  - Ondansetron 16 mg PO or 8 mg IV daily, or
  - Dolasetron 100 mg PO or IV daily, or
  - Tropisetron 5 mg PO or IV on day 1
- **Phenothiazine**
  - Prochlorperazine 25 mg suppository every 12 hours, or 10 mg PO or IV every four to six hours, or
- **Substituted benzamide**
  - Metoclopramide 10–40 mg PO every four to six hours or 1–2 mg/kg IV every three to four hours ± diphenhydramine 25–50 mg PO or IV every four to six hours, or
- **Butyrophenones**
  - Haloperidol 1–2 mg PO every four to six hours or 1–3 mg IV every four to six hours, or
- **Benzodiazepine**
  - Lorazepam 0.5–2 mg PO every four to six hours, or
- **Cannabinoid**
  - Dronabinol 5–10 mg PO every three to six hours, or
  - Nabilone 1–2 mg PO twice daily
- **Olanzapine:** 2.5–5 mg PO twice daily as needed
- **Promethazine:** 12.5–25 mg PO or IV every four hours as needed

(ASHP, 1999; Gralla et al., 1999; MASCC, 2008; NCCN, 2008; Polovich et al., 2005)

Likely to Be Effective

Interventions for which effectiveness has been demonstrated by supportive evidence from a single rigorously conducted controlled trial, consistent supportive evidence from well-designed controlled trials using small samples, or guidelines developed from evidence and supported by expert opinion

Nonpharmacologic interventions are to be used in conjunction with pharmacologic interventions.

Provide referral to appropriate practitioners as needed.

ACUPRESSURE

- Three small randomized controlled trials (RCTs) found limited evidence that P6 acupressure reduced CINV compared to no intervention. The studies demonstrated decreases in severity, frequency, and duration of nausea and vomiting after chemotherapy in postoperative patients with gastric cancer receiving their first cycle of cisplatin and 5-fluorouracil, and in patients with other mixed cancer types (Dibble, Chapman, Mack, & Shih, 2000; Klein & Griffiths, 2004; Shin, Kim, Shin, & Juon, 2004). In a recent study, acupressure significantly decreased the nausea and vomiting experience and nausea, vomiting, and retching occurrence and distress after chemotherapy (doxorubicin-containing regimen) for breast cancer (Molassiotis, Helin, Dabbour, & Hummerston, 2007).

- One multicenter, longitudinal RCT of 160 women beginning second- and third-cycle adjuvant chemotherapy (cyclophosphamide, methotrexate, 5-fluorouracil) for breast cancer concluded that acupressure at P6 significantly reduced the frequency of vomiting and intensity of nausea following chemotherapy over time when compared to placebo at P13 or usual care (Dibble et al., 2007).

ACUPUNCTURE

- Two systematic reviews concluded that acupuncture can provide a statistically reliable and clinically significant reduction in nausea and vomiting (Collins & Thomas, 2004; Mayer, 2000). This benefit, when compared to pharmacotherapy alone, also was observed in one RCT with high-dose myeloablative chemotherapy using electroacupuncture (Shen et al., 2000). In a more recent systematic review, acupuncture reduced acute vomiting but not nausea severity (Klein & Griffiths, 2004). Study populations: Patients with mixed cancer types experiencing refractory emesis after first-cycle doxorubicin.
- One small, prospective trial found that electroacupuncture decreased overall nausea and severity of vomiting in patients with breast cancer with refractory emesis. Most of the patients indicated that electroacupuncture was an acceptable procedure and helpful in managing refractory emesis. The study was not controlled, 42% of eligible patients declined participation, and placebo effect may have been a factor, as 8 of 27 participants had previous experiences with acupuncture (Choo, 2006).

ACUPUNCTURE, ACUPRESSURE, AND ACUSTIMULATION

- One small, randomized crossover pilot with hematology and gastroenterology patients receiving highly to moderately emetogenic chemotherapy found no difference between combined acupuncture and acupressure at the P6 point and the sham point. There was no control for the acupressure group. The sham group reported a low incidence of nausea and vomiting. The short distance between the acupoints and needle depth were potential variables. However, half of the participants reported an irradiating feeling, a sign of effective acupuncture (Melchart, Ihbe-Heffinger, Leps, von Schilling, & Linde, 2006).
- A Cochrane review (11 trials, N = 1,247) concluded that overall, acupuncture-point stimulation of all methods combined reduced the incidence of acute vomiting but not acute or delayed nausea severity compared to control. By modality, stimulation with needles reduced the proportion of acute vomiting but not acute nausea severity. Electroacupuncture reduced the proportion of acute vomiting, but manual acupuncture did not. Acupressure reduced mean acute nausea severity. Noninvasive electrostimulation showed no benefit for any outcome. All trials used concomitant pharmacologic antiemetics, and all, except electroacupuncture trials, used state-of-the-art antiemetics. Demonstrated effects are most profound for acute vomiting (Ezzo, Streitberger, & Schneider, 2006).

GUIDED IMAGERY, MUSIC THERAPY, AND PROGRESSIVE MUSCLE RELAXATION

- A systematic review, a meta-analysis, and five RCTs found that guided imagery, music therapy, and progressive muscle relaxation reduce nausea, vomiting, and/or retching. The adjuvant behavioral techniques are useful complements to antiemetics. Many of the strategies may be helpful interventions for the prevention and treatment of anticipatory nausea and vomiting. In many studies, at least two interventions were used together (e.g., guided imagery with music therapy) (Arakawa, 1997; Ezzone, Baker, Rosselet, & Terepka, 1998; King, 1997; Luebbert, Dahme, & Hasenbring, 2001; Miller & Kearney, 2004; Molassiotis, Yung, Yam, Chan, & Mok, 2002; Sahler, Hunter, & Liesveld, 2003; Troesch, Rodehaver, Delaney, & Yanes, 1993).
- Study populations: Patients with mixed cancer types; women with breast cancer receiving doxorubicin and cyclophosphamide; bone marrow transplant (BMT) recipients; and patients receiving cisplatin-based chemotherapy, some of whom were chemotherapy naïve.

PSYCHOEDUCATIONAL SUPPORT AND INFORMATION

- Two studies of nursing interventions with increased support and education and standard antiemetics resulted in the reduction of nausea and improvement in well-being in women receiving cisplatin-based chemotherapy for ovarian cancer and in women receiving chemotherapy for breast cancer. Verbal, written, and audiotaped information was effective in improving symptoms (Borjeson, Hursti, Tishelman, Peterson, & Steineck, 2002; Williams & Schreier, 2004). Further study should be conducted to evaluate the interventions and characterize the methods.

Benefits Balanced With Harms

Interventions for which clinicians and patients should weigh the beneficial and harmful effects according to individual circumstances and priorities

Nonpharmacologic interventions are to be used in conjunction with pharmacologic interventions.

Provide referral to appropriate practitioners as needed.

VIRTUAL REALITY

- A single, small study using a virtual reality intervention with outpatients during chemotherapy showed some preliminary evidence for reducing emesis three to five days after chemotherapy. Nausea was not measured. Motion sickness, however, is a potential side effect (Oyama, Kaneda, Katsumata, Akechi, & Ohsuga, 2000).
- Study populations: Patients with mixed cancer diagnoses, but primarily women with breast and ovarian cancers

Effectiveness Not Established

Interventions for which insufficient data or data of inadequate quality currently exist, with no clear indication of harm

PHARMACOLOGIC INTERVENTIONS

Several pharmacologic studies have been completed that evaluate using suggested drugs in alternative routes or different dosing regimens; however, insufficient data exist at this point to recommend any practice changes. Some of the alternative regimens studied are

- Olanzapine for prevention of CINV with highly and moderately emetogenic chemotherapy. Navari et al. (2007) studied a higher dose of olanzapine (10 mg PO) up front and through days 2–4 and eliminated the use of dexamethasone after day 1. This was a small trial with some limitations.
- Mirtazapine (a noradrenergic antidepressant) was evaluated for its ability to treat nausea and insomnia in depressed patients with cancer (Kim et al., 2008), but its effectiveness was not established.
- Other studies have looked at different dosing schedules of antiemetics, such as skipping day 2 antiemetics (Lajolo & del Giglio, 2007) and repeated doses of palonosetron (Einhorn et al., 2007). The Lajolo and del Giglio study hypothesized that delayed CINV may be improved by skipping day 2 antiemetics, thereby preventing the accumulation of 5-HT_3 at the presynaptic level in the gastrointestinal tract; however, this was a small, nonrandomized study that warrants further investigation. Similarly, Einhorn et al. administered a longer-acting 5-HT_3 receptor antagonist (palonosetron) at multiple time points for a multiday cisplatin regimen. Concern about the higher binding affinity and longer half-life of this agent has prevented its repeated use in patients receiving multi-day regimens but who might benefit from its superior efficacy.
- Gurpide et al. (2007) performed a pharmacokinetic study to evaluate the bioavailability of subcutaneous granisetron and determined it to be similar to the IV route.
- Bleicher et al. (2008) reported the results of two small, institution-based pilot trials on lorazepam, diphenhydramine, and haloperidol (ABH) transdermal gel, demonstrating a decrease in the severity of delayed CINV after application of ABH gel. Further study is needed.

NONPHARMACOLOGIC INTERVENTIONS ARE TO BE USED IN CONJUNCTION WITH PHARMACOLOGIC INTERVENTIONS.

Provide referral to appropriate practitioners as needed.

Acustimulation With a Wristband Device

- Two studies were positive but not conclusive for use of wristbands in CINV (Roscoe, Morrow, Matteson, Bushunow, & Tian, 2002; Treish et al., 2003). Two studies have shown no significant differences for the acustimulation group (Roscoe et al., 2003, 2005). In both studies, most of the subjects were female patients with breast cancer, and the acustimulation intervention was not effective as an adjunct to antiemetics in this population. Further study is needed to evaluate this intervention in other populations, including males, and with other malignancies. In a recent systematic review, no benefit was found for this outcome (Collins & Thomas, 2004).
- Study populations: Women with breast cancer receiving their second course of chemotherapy (doxorubicin-based); chemotherapy-naïve patients with mixed cancers receiving cisplatin or doxorubicin; and patients with mixed cancers receiving moderately high to highly emetogenic chemotherapy (Roscoe et al., 2002, 2003, 2005; Treish et al., 2003)

Chinese Herbal Medicine

In one double-blinded, placebo-controlled RCT, Chinese herbal medicine (CHM) reduced nausea in patients receiving adjuvant chemotherapy for early-stage breast and colon cancers. The study was terminated early because it was difficult to recruit patients to a placebo-controlled study where CHM is widely accepted (Mok et al., 2007).

- Two Cochrane reviews summarized current evidence on the use of CHM in the management of CINV. These reviews included RCTs assessing the effect of herbal medicines on chemotherapy-related side effects, quality of life, and objective measures of immune function in patients with colorectal cancer and RCTs comparing chemotherapy with or without Chinese herbs in women with breast cancer. The studies were of low quality, with methodologic limitations and no strong demonstration of benefit (Tiaxaing, Munro, & Guanjian, 2005; Zhang, Liu, Ji, He, & Tripathy, 2007).

Exercise

- One RCT suggested that moderate aerobic activity may be beneficial as an adjunct to antiemetic therapy in controlling CINV and in promoting physical well-being (Winningham & MacVicar, 1988). Study population: Women with breast cancer receiving chemotherapy (not doxorubicin) who had received at least three treatments prior to the study (Winningham & MacVicar).
- One prospective, exploratory study of patients receiving chemotherapy for adjuvant treatment or advanced disease (N = 54) found that a multidimensional, structured, supervised exercise program decreased the symptoms following chemotherapy. Ten of 12 symptoms were reduced, including nausea and vomiting, with the exercise program. Patients with evidence of disease scored symptoms higher than patients without evidence of disease. Patients responded positively to the intervention regardless of participation in a high- or low-intensity exercise program (Andersen et al., 2006).

Ginger

- In a small study on the effectiveness of ginger on various types of nausea and vomiting, not enough evidence was found to support the effectiveness of ginger in treating CINV for 40 patients with leukemia (Ernst & Pittler, 2000). In another small study with 40 patients being treated for gynecologic cancer, ginger was compared to placebo and metoclopramide. Ginger was not found to be effective in treating acute nausea and was not significantly different than metoclopramide in treating delayed nausea (Manusirivithaya et al., 2004).
- Study populations: Patients with leukemia; patients with gynecologic cancer receiving cisplatin

Hypnosis

- A small, nonrandomized study examined hypnosis as an intervention in patients affected by anticipatory CINV. Fourteen of 16 patients experienced a major response, showing a complete remission of anticipatory nausea and vomiting following hypnotherapy intervention. The responses were achieved primarily in patients with breast and ovarian cancers who had received at least four cycles of chemotherapy combined with a 5-HT$_3$ receptor antagonist who developed nausea and vomiting within the first six hours prior to receiving chemotherapy (drugs included cisplatin, carboplatin, cyclophosphamide, dacarbazine, doxorubicin, and epirubicin) (Marchioro et al., 2000).
- A systematic review summarized six RCTs (five with children) that involved a hypnosis intervention to relieve CINV. The study evaluating effectiveness of hypnosis for CINV in adult BMT recipients had no significant findings (Richardson et al., 2007).

Massage and Aromatherapy
A systematic review of the use of massage and aromatherapy for symptom relief in patients with cancer identified two small RCTs (N = 34, N = 87) where nausea was assessed in autologous BMT recipients and hospital inpatients (Fellowes, Barnes, & Wilkinson, 2004). The massage groups experienced a significant decrease in nausea following the first massage (Ahles et al., 1999) and a significant reduction in nausea following massage overall (Cassileth & Vickers, 2004; Grealish, Lomasney, & Whiteman, 2000).

Massage
One prospective RCT of women with breast cancer (prior to third chemotherapy cycle) found that massage significantly reduced nausea. However, the raw data were not reported, only the percentage improved (Billhult, Bergbom, & Stener-Victorin, 2007).

Progressive Muscle Relaxation
- A pilot study found that progressive muscle relaxation (PMR) decreased physiologic conditions (e.g., vital signs) and muscle reactions (e.g., forearm, leg, forehead, and eye tension) and demonstrated a statistically significant reduction in the intensity of nausea and vomiting. The PMR intervention was tensing and releasing muscle groups and control of respirations, combined in an environment of reduced artificial lighting, adequate music, and no interruptions (de Carvalho, Martins, & dos Santos, 2007).
- Study populations: Hematology patients receiving chemotherapy and experiencing nausea and vomiting (de Carvalho et al., 2007)

Yoga
One small RCT found that yoga reduced the frequency and intensity of nausea and the intensity of anticipatory nausea and vomiting in chemotherapy-naïve women with early-stage breast cancer. The vomiting severity was mild to moderate in both groups. The nausea severity was mild to moderate in the yoga group but moderate to severe in the control group (Raghavendra et al., 2007).

Expert Opinion

Low-risk interventions that are (1) consistent with sound clinical practice, (2) suggested by an expert in a peer-reviewed publication (journal or book chapter), and (3) for which limited evidence exists. An expert is an individual with peer-reviewed journal publications in the domain of interest.

Consensus exists recognizing the growing evidence that the following interventions may be effective in the prevention and management of CINV (ASHP, 1999; Gralla et al., 1999; MASCC, 2008; NCCN, 2008; Polovich et al., 2005).
- Prevention of nausea and vomiting is the goal.
- Oral and IV antiemetics have equivalent effectiveness.
- The period of expected CINV should be covered with appropriate antiemetics (anticipatory, acute, and delayed period for at least four days or longer if using a multi-day regimen).
- The lowest efficacious dose of the antiemetics should be used.
- Clinicians should base selection of antiemetics on the emetic potential of the chemotherapy agent(s), as well as patient risk factors.
- Healthcare providers need to consider the many potential causes of nausea and emesis in patients with cancer that may be contributing factors.

Limited evidence exists, but experts recommend the following dietary interventions in patients receiving chemotherapy to minimize nausea and vomiting (Polovich et al., 2005).
- Eat a small amount of food prior to treatment, as receiving chemotherapy on an empty stomach has been linked to the development of severe emesis (Booth et al., 2007).
- Eat smaller, more frequent meals.
- Reduce food aromas and other stimuli with strong odors.
- Avoid foods that are spicy, fatty, and highly salty.
- Take antiemetics prior to meals so that the effect is present during and after meals.
- Repeat previous measures, and consume foods that minimize nausea and that are "comfort foods."

Definitions of the interventions are available at **www.ons.org/outcomes**.
Literature search completed through May 2008.

References

Ahles, T.A., Tope, D.M., Pinkson, B., Walch, S., Hann, D., Whedon, M., et al. (1999). Massage therapy for patients undergoing autologous bone marrow transplantation. *Journal of Pain and Symptom Management, 18*(3), 157–163.

American Society of Health-System Pharmacists. (1999). ASHP therapeutic guidelines on the pharmacologic management of nausea and vomiting in adult and pediatric patients receiving chemotherapy or radiation therapy or undergoing surgery. *American Journal of Health-System Pharmacy, 56*(8), 729–764.

Andersen, C., Adamsen, L., Moeller, T., Midtgaard, J., Quist, M., Tveteraas, A., et al. (2006). The effect of a multidimensional exercise programme on symptoms and side-effects in cancer patients undergoing chemotherapy—The use of semi-structured diaries. *European Journal of Oncology Nursing, 10*(4), 247–262.

Antiemetic Subcommittee of the Multinational Association of Supportive Care in Cancer. (2006). Prevention of chemotherapy- and radiotherapy-induced emesis: Results of the 2004 Perugia International Antiemetic Consensus Conference. *Annals of Oncology, 17*(1), 20–28.

Arakawa, S. (1997). Relaxation to reduce nausea, vomiting, and anxiety induced by chemotherapy in Japanese patients. *Cancer Nursing, 20*(5), 342–349.

Billhult, A., Bergbom, I., & Stener-Victorin, E. (2007). Massage relieves nausea in women with breast cancer who are undergoing chemotherapy. *Journal of Alternative and Complementary Medicine, 13*(1), 53–57.

Bleicher, J., Bhaskara, A., Huyck, T., Constantino, S., Bardia, A., Loprinzi, C.L., et al. (2008). Lorazepam, diphenhydramine, and haloperidol gel for rescue from chemotherapy-induced nausea and vomiting: Results of two pilot trials. *Journal of Supportive Oncology, 6*(1), 27–32.

Booth, C.M., Clemons, M., Dranitsaris, G., Joy, A., Young, S., Callaghan, W., et al. (2007). Chemotherapy-induced nausea and vomiting in breast cancer patients: A prospective observational study. *Journal of Supportive Oncology, 5*(8), 374–380.

Borjeson, S., Hursti, T.J., Tishelman, C., Peterson, C., & Steineck, G. (2002). Treatment of nausea and emesis during cancer chemotherapy: Discrepancies between antiemetic effect and well-being. *Journal of Pain and Symptom Management, 24*(3), 345–358.

Cassileth, B.R., & Vickers, A.J. (2004). Massage therapy for symptom control: Outcome study at a major cancer center. *Journal of Pain and Symptom Management, 28*(3), 244–249.

Choo, S.P., Kong, K.H., Lim, W.T., Gao, F., Chua, K., & Leong, S.S. (2006). Electroacupuncture for refractory acute emesis caused by chemotherapy. *Journal of Alternative and Complementary Medicine, 12*(10), 963–969.

Collins, K.B., & Thomas, D.J. (2004). Acupuncture and acupressure for the management of chemotherapy-induced nausea and vomiting. *Journal of the American Academy of Nurse Practitioners, 16*(2), 76–80.

de Carvalho, E.C., Martins, F.T.M., & dos Santos, C.B. (2007). A pilot study of a relaxation technique for management of nausea and vomiting in patients receiving cancer chemotherapy. *Cancer Nursing, 30*(2), 163–167.

Dibble, S.L., Chapman, J., Mack, K.A., & Shih, A. (2000). Acupressure for nausea: Results of a pilot study. *Oncology Nursing Forum, 27*(1), 41–47.

Dibble, S.L., Luce, J., Cooper, B.A., Israel, J., Cohen, M., Nussey, B., et al. (2007). Acupressure for chemotherapy-induced nausea and vomiting: A randomized clinical trial. *Oncology Nursing Forum, 34*(4), 813–820.

Einhorn, L.H., Brames, M.J., Dreicer, R., Nichols, C.R., Cullen, M.T., Jr., & Bubalo, J. (2007). Palonosetron plus dexamethasone for prevention of chemotherapy-induced nausea and vomiting in patients receiving multiple-day cisplatin chemotherapy for germ cell cancer. *Supportive Care in Cancer, 15*(11), 1293–1300.

Ernst, E., & Pittler, M.H. (2000). Efficacy of ginger for nausea and vomiting: A systematic review of randomized clinical trials. *British Journal of Anaesthesia, 84*(3), 367–371.

Ezzo, J., Streitberger, K., & Schneider, A. (2006). Cochrane systematic reviews examine p6 acupuncture-point stimulation for nausea and vomiting. *Journal of Alternative and Complementary Medicine, 12*(5), 489–495.

Ezzone, S., Baker, C., Rosselet, R., & Terepka, E. (1998). Music as an adjunct to antiemetic therapy. *Oncology Nursing Forum, 25*(9), 1551–1556.

Fellowes, D., Barnes, K., & Wilkinson, S. (2004). Aromatherapy and massage for symptom relief in patients with cancer. *Cochrane Database of Systematic Reviews* 2004, Issue 3. Art. No.: CD002287. DOI: 10.1002/14651858.CD002287.pub2.

Figueroa-Moseley, C., Jean-Pierre, P., Roscoe, J.A., Ryan, J.L., Kohli, S., Palesh, O.G., et al. (2007). Behavioral interventions in treating anticipatory nausea and vomiting. *Journal of the National Comprehensive Cancer Network, 5*(1), 44–50.

Gralla, R.J., Osoba, D., Kris, M.G., Kirkbride, P., Hesketh, P.J., Chinnery, L.W., et al. (1999). Recommendations for the use of antiemetics: Evidence-based, clinical practice guidelines. *Journal of Clinical Oncology, 17*(9), 2971–2994.

Grealish, L., Lomasney, A., & Whiteman, B. (2000). Foot massage: A nursing intervention to modify the distressing symptoms of pain and nausea in patients hospitalized with cancer. *Cancer Nursing, 23*(3), 237–243.

Gurpide, A., Sadaba, B., Martin-Algarra, S., Azanza, J.R., Lopez-Picazo, J.M., Campanero, M.A., et al. (2007). Randomized crossover pharmacokinetic evaluation of subcutaneous versus intravenous granisetron in cancer patients treated with platinum-based chemotherapy. *Oncologist, 12*(9), 1151–1155.

Kim, S.W., Shin, I.S., Kim, J.M., Kim, Y.C., Kim, K.S., Kim, K.M., et al. (2008). Effectiveness of mirtazapine for nausea and insomnia in cancer patients with depression. *Psychiatry and Clinical Neurosciences, 62*(1), 75–83.

King, C.R. (1997). Nonpharmacologic management of chemotherapy-induced nausea and vomiting. *Oncology Nursing Forum, 24*(Suppl. 7), 41–48.

Klein, J., & Griffiths, P. (2004). Acupressure for nausea and vomiting in cancer patients receiving chemotherapy. *British Journal of Community Nursing, 9*(9), 383–387.

Lajolo, P.P., & del Giglio, A. (2007). Skipping day 2 antiemetic medications may improve chemotherapy-induced delayed nausea and vomiting control: Results of two pilot phase II trials. *Supportive Care in Cancer, 15*(3), 343–346.

Luebbert, K., Dahme, B., & Hasenbring, M. (2001). The effectiveness of relaxation training in reducing treatment-related symptoms and improving emotional adjustment in acute non-surgical cancer treatment: A meta-analytical review. *Psycho-Oncology, 10*(6), 490–502.

Manusirivithaya, S., Sripramote, M., Tangjitgamol, S., Sheanakul, C., Leelahakorn, S., Thavaramara, T., et al. (2004). Antiemetic effect of ginger in gynecologic oncology patients receiving cisplatin. *International Journal of Gynecologic Cancer, 14*(6), 1063–1069.

Marchioro, G., Azzarello, G., Viviani, F., Barbato, F., Pavanetto, M., Rosetti, F., et al. (2000). Hypnosis in the treatment of anticipatory nausea and vomiting in patients receiving cancer chemotherapy. *Oncology, 59*(2), 100–104.

Mayer, D.J. (2000). Acupuncture: An evidence-based review of the clinical literature. *Annual Review of Medicine, 51,* 49–63.

Melchart, D., Ihbe-Heffinger, A., Leps, B., von Schilling, C., & Linde, K. (2006). Acupuncture and acupressure for the prevention of chemotherapy-induced nausea—A randomised cross-over pilot study. *Supportive Care in Cancer, 14*(8), 878–882.

Miller, M., & Kearney, N. (2004). Chemotherapy-related nausea and vomiting—Past reflections, present practice and future management. *European Journal of Cancer Care, 13*(1), 71–81.

Mok, T.S., Yeo, W., Johnson, P.J., Hui, P., Ho, W.M., Lam, K.C., et al. (2007). A double-blind placebo-controlled randomized study of Chinese herbal medicine as complementary therapy for reduction of chemotherapy-induced toxicity. *Annals of Oncology, 18*(4), 768–774.

Molassiotis, A., Helin, A.M., Dabbour, R., & Hummerston, S. (2007). The effects of P6 acupressure in the prophylaxis of chemotherapy-related nausea and vomiting in breast cancer patients. *Complementary Therapies in Medicine, 15*(1), 3–12.

Molassiotis, A., Yung, H.P., Yam, B.M., Chan, F.Y., & Mok, T.S. (2002). The effectiveness of progressive muscle relaxation training in managing chemotherapy-induced nausea and vomiting in Chinese breast cancer patients: A randomised controlled trial. *Supportive Care in Cancer, 10*(3), 237–246.

Multinational Association of Supportive Care in Cancer. (2008). *Antiemetic guidelines.* Retrieved June 23, 2008, from http://www.mascc.org/media/Resource_centers/MASCC_Guidelines_Update.pdf

National Comprehensive Cancer Network. (2008). *NCCN Clinical Practice Guidelines in Oncology™: Antiemesis* [v.3.2008]. Retrieved March 14, 2008, from http://www.nccn.org/professionals/physician_gls/PDF/antiemesis.pdf

Navari, R.M., Einhorn, L.H., Loehrer, P.J., Sr., Passik, S.D., Vinson, J., McClean, J., et al. (2007). A phase II trial of olanzapine, dexamethasone, and palonosetron for the prevention of chemotherapy-induced nausea and vomiting: A Hoosier Oncology Group study. *Supportive Care in Cancer, 15*(11), 1285–1291.

Oyama, H., Kaneda, M., Katsumata, N., Akechi, T., & Ohsuga, M. (2000). Using the bedside wellness system during chemotherapy decreases fatigue and emesis in cancer patients. *Journal of Medical Systems, 24*(3), 173–182.

Pectasides, D., Dafni, U., Aravantinos, G., Timotheadou, E., Skarlos, D.V., Pavlidis, N., et al. (2007). A randomized trial to compare the efficacy and safety of antiemetic treatment with ondansetron and ondansetron zydis in patients with breast cancer treated with high-dose epirubicin. *Anticancer Research, 27*(6C), 4411–4417.

Polovich, M., White, J.M., & Kelleher, L.O. (Eds.). (2005). *Chemotherapy and biotherapy guidelines and recommendations for practice* (2nd ed.). Pittsburgh, PA: Oncology Nursing Society.

Raghavendra, R.M., Nagarathna, R., Nagendra, H.R., Gopinath, K.S., Srinath, B.S., Ravi, B.D., et al. (2007). Effects of an integrated yoga programme on chemotherapy-induced nausea and emesis in breast cancer patients. *European Journal of Cancer Care, 16*(6), 462–474.

Richardson, J., Smith, J.E., McCall, G., Richardson, A., Pilkington, K., & Kirsch, I. (2007). Hypnosis for nausea and vomiting in cancer chemotherapy: A systematic review of the research evidence. *European Journal of Cancer Care, 16*(5), 402–412.

Roscoe, J.A., Matteson, S.E., Morrow, G.R., Hickok, J.T., Bushunow, P., Griggs, J., et al. (2005). Acustimulation wrist bands are not effective for the control of chemotherapy-induced nausea in women with breast cancer. *Journal of Pain and Symptom Management, 29*(4), 376–384.

Roscoe, J.A., Morrow, G.R., Hickok, J.T., Bushunow, P., Pierce, I., Flynn, P.J., et al. (2003). The efficacy of acupressure and acustimulation wrist bands for the relief of chemotherapy-induced nausea and vomiting: A University of Rochester Cancer Center Community Clinical Oncology Program multicenter study. *Journal of Pain and Symptom Management, 22*(2), 731–740.

Roscoe, J.A., Morrow, G.R., Matteson, S., Bushunow, P., & Tian, L. (2002). Acustimulation wristbands for the relief of chemotherapy-induced nausea. *Alternative Therapies, 8*(4), 56–63.

Sahler, O.J.Z., Hunter, B.C., & Liesveld, J.L. (2003). The effect of using music therapy with relaxation imagery in the management of patients undergoing bone marrow transplantation: A pilot feasibility study. *Alternative Therapies, 9*(6), 70–74.

Shen, J., Wenger, N., Glaspy, J., Hays, R.D., Albert, P.S., Choi, C., et al. (2000). Electroacupuncture for control of myeloablative chemotherapy-induced emesis: A randomized controlled trial. *JAMA, 284*(21), 2755–2761.

Shin, Y.H., Kim, T.I., Shin, M.S., & Juon, H. (2004). Effect of acupressure on nausea and vomiting during chemotherapy cycle for Korean postoperative stomach cancer patients. *Cancer Nursing, 27*(4), 267–274.

Taixiang, W., Munro, A.J., & Guanjian, L. (2005). Chinese medical herbs for chemotherapy side effects in colorectal cancer patients. *Cochrane Database of Systematic Reviews* 2005, Issue 1. Art. No.: CD004540. DOI: 10.1002/14651858.CD004540.pub2.

Treish, I., Shord, S., Valgus, J., Harvey, D., Nagy, J., Stegal, J., et al. (2003). Randomized double-blind study of the Reliefband as an adjunct to standard antiemetics in patients receiving moderately-high to highly emetogenic chemotherapy. *Supportive Care in Cancer, 11*(8), 516–521.

Troesch, L.M., Rodehaver, C.B., Delaney, E.A., & Yanes, B. (1993). The influence of guided imagery on chemotherapy-related nausea and vomiting. *Oncology Nursing Forum, 20*(8), 1179–1185.

Williams, S.A., & Schreier, A.M. (2004). The effect of education in managing side effects in women receiving chemotherapy for treatment of breast cancer [Online exclusive]. *Oncology Nursing Forum, 31*(1), E16–E23. Retrieved March 2005 from http://ons.metapress.com/content/b366435101rv1712/fulltext.pdf

Winningham, M.L., & MacVicar, M.G. (1988). The effect of aerobic exercise on patient reports of nausea. *Oncology Nursing Forum, 15*(4), 447–450.

Zhang, M., Liu, X., Li, J., He, L., & Tripathy, D. (2007). Chinese medicinal herbs to treat the side-effects of chemotherapy in breast cancer patients. *Cochrane Database of Systematic Reviews* 2007, Issue 2. Art. No.: CD004921. DOI: 10.1002/14651858.CD004921.pub2.

CHAPTER 7

Constipation

Problem

Constipation is defined as a decrease in the passage of formed stool characterized by stools that are hard and difficult to pass. Patients have fewer than two to three stools per week and may strain to have a bowel movement. Constipation can be accompanied by abdominal pain, nausea and vomiting, abdominal distention, loss of appetite, headache, and dry, hard, formed stools (Cope, 2001; Petticrew, Rodgers, & Booth, 2001; Tamayo & Diaz-Zuluaga, 2004; Thompson, Boyd-Carson, Trainor, & Boyd, 2003).

Incidence

The prevalence of constipation is difficult to determine in patients with cancer. In the palliative care population, constipation has been reported as high as 40%–64% (McMillan, 2002; McMillan & Weitzner, 2000; Weitzner, Moody, & McMillan, 1997). Constipation in hospitalized patients with cancer receiving treatment varies but can approach 70%–100% (McMillan & Tittle, 1995; McMillan & Williams, 1989; Tittle & McMillan, 1994). Constipation can affect many patients with cancer at different points in the care continuum, related to specific treatment such as surgery or chemotherapy, or because of other concurrent medications, diet, mobility, and the palliative care setting.

Assessment

Constipation is a common clinical problem that is very amenable to nursing intervention. Constipation often goes unrecognized and can be untreated or undertreated in patients with cancer in a variety of oncology settings. Failure to anticipate and adequately treat constipation can cause unnecessary discomfort that can affect quality of life. Constipation can be one of the most sensitive nursing-sensitive patient outcomes if assessment and intervention are planned early.

One of the problems with patient report of constipation is that many patients are attuned to self-management of constipation and may not think to mention it to their healthcare provider. Directed questions need to be asked specifically about bowel function. Constipation will continue to be a poorly understood and managed problem in patients with cancer unless healthcare professionals do a complete assessment and understand the origins of the problem. Figure 7-1 provides risk assessment questions

Figure 7-1. Constipation Risk Assessment Scale

Circle risk factors in table and total

GENDER:

Male	1
Female	2

MOBILITY:

Independently mobile	0
Dependent on walking aids/assistance from others	1
Restricted to bed/chair	2
Spinal cord injury/spinal cord compression	3

FIBRE INTAKE:

5 pieces fruit/veg or more consumed daily	0
3 or 4 pieces fruit/veg consumed daily	1
2 pieces fruit/veg or less consumed daily	2

Bran products consumed daily	Yes	0
	No	2

FLUID INTAKE:

10 cups/glasses or more consumed daily	0
6 to 9 cups/glasses consumed daily	1
5 cups/glasses or less consumed daily	2

PERSONAL BELIEFS:

Does patient believe they are prone to constipation?   Yes/No _____

Has laxatives ever been used for constipation?   Yes/No _____

_____

Current bowel habit: _____

SECTION SUB TOTAL [ ]

_____

WARD PATIENTS ONLY:
Does patient have difficulty evacuating bowels in hospital toilets?

No	0
Yes	2

PATIENTS REQUIRING COMMODE/BEDPAN:
Does patient anticipate problems using a commode or bedpan?

No/Not applicable	0
Yes	2

SECTION SUB TOTAL [ ]

(Continued on next page)

Figure 7-1. Constipation Risk Assessment Scale *(Continued)*

Conditions which increase risk of constipation.

From medical notes, patient history and blood results, assess presence of the following:

PHYSIOLOGICAL CONDITIONS
Metabolic disorders:
Hypokalaemia/uraemia/lead poisoning   2
Pelvic conditions:
Hysterectomy/ovarian tumour/uterine prolapse/pregnancy   3
Neuromuscular disorders:
Parkinson's Disease/Multiple Sclerosis/Systemic Sclerosis/Hirschsprung's Disease/
Cerebrovascular Accident/Spina Bifida/Rheumatoid Arthritis/cerebral tumour   3
Endocrine disorders:
Diabetes Mellitus/hypothyroidism/ hypopituitarism/hypercalcaemia   3
Colorectal/abdominal disorders:
Irritable Bowel Syndrome/Crohn's disease/Diverticulitis/Ulcerative Colitis/colorectal
tumour/anorectal stricture/anorectal fissure/anorectal prolapse/haemorrhoids/hernias   3

PSYCHOLOGICAL CONDITIONS
Psychiatric illness:
Depression/Anorexia Nervosa/Bulimia Nervosa   2
Learning disabilities or dementia
(as evidenced by lack of understanding of speech or situations)   2

SECTION SUB TOTAL ☐

Medications which increase risk of constipation.

Is patient presently taking any of the following medications on a regular basis?

Antiemetics	2	**Analgesics:**		
Calcium channel blockers	2	Non-opioid analgesia	3	
Iron supplements	2	OR continuous opioid therapy	5	

Anticholinergic containing medication:

Anticonvulsants	2	**Cytotoxic chemotherapy:**	
Antidepressants	2	Cytotoxic chemotherapy	3
Antiparkinson drugs	2	OR Vinca alkaloid agents	5
Antispasmodics	2		

SECTION SUB TOTAL ☐

Low risk for constipation: score ≤10
Medium risk for constipation: score 11-15   **TOTAL SCORE** ☐
High risk for constipation: score ≥16

that may assist in beginning the baseline assessment. By performing the assessment at diagnosis and prior to therapy initiation, the goal of preventing constipation may be possible by assessing risk factors. Follow-up evaluations are also necessary to monitor the effect of treatment of constipation.

Clinical Measurement Tools

The following clinical measurement tools are presented in Table 7-1.
1. Constipation Assessment Scale (CAS) (see Table 7-2)
2. Common Terminology Criteria for Adverse Events (CTCAE) (National Cancer Institute Cancer Therapy Evaluation Program, 2006)
3. Modified CAS

Table 7-1. Clinical Measurement Tools					
Name of Tool	Number of Items	Domains	Reliability and Validity	Populations	Clinical Utility
Constipation Assessment Scale (CAS)	8	Subjectively reported symptoms: abdominal distention or bloating, change in the amount of gas passed rectally, less frequent bowel movements, oozing liquid stool, rectal fullness or pressure, rectal pain with bowel movements, small volume of stool, inability to pass stool	Reliability and content validity established	Studied in outpatients receiving radiation therapy to gastrointestinal or head/neck areas, and patients receiving opioids versus vinca alkaloids	Simple and easy to use. Takes about 2 minutes to complete.
Common Terminology Criteria for Adverse Events	One-item graded scale	Symptoms Use of stool softeners and laxatives Dietary modification Use of manual evacuation or enemas	Unknown	Patients with a variety of malignancies	Commonly used practice; does not assess symptomatology

(Continued on next page)

Table 7-1. Clinical Measurement Tools *(Continued)*					
Name of Tool	Number of Items	Domains	Reliability and Validity	Populations	Clinical Utility
CAS (Pediatric)	8	Subjectively reported symptoms	Reliability and validity established	Pediatric patients with cancer who are on opioids or vinca alkaloids	The scale was modified from the adult version for use with children. The language was changed to include terms such as "poop."

Note. Based on information from McMillan, 2007; National Cancer Institute Cancer Therapy Evaluation Program, 2006; Woolery et al., 2006.

Table 7-2. Constipation Assessment Scale*			
Item	No Problem	Some Problem	Severe Problem
Abdominal distention or bloating	0	1	2
Change in amount of gas passed rectally	0	1	2
Less frequent bowel movements	0	1	2
Oozing liquid stool	0	1	2
Rectal fullness or pressure	0	1	2
Rectal pain with bowel movement	0	1	2
Small stool size	0	1	2
Urge but inability to pass stool	0	1	2

*Patients are instructed to circle the appropriate number to indicate whether, during the past three days, they have had no problem, some problem, or a severe problem with each item.

Note. Copyright by Susan C. McMillan, PhD, ARNP, FAAN. Used with permission.

References

Cope, D.G. (2001). Management of chemotherapy-induced diarrhea and constipation. *Nursing Clinics of North America, 36*(4), 695–707.

McMillan, S.C. (2002). Presence and severity of constipation in hospice patients with advanced cancer. *American Journal of Hospice and Palliative Care, 19*(6), 426–430.

McMillan, S.C. (2007). *Measuring oncology nursing-sensitive patient outcomes: Evidence-based summary: Constipation.* Retrieved August 31, 2008, from http://www.ons.org/outcomes/measures/constipation.shtml

McMillan, S.C., & Tittle, M. (1995). A descriptive study of the management of pain and pain-related side effects in a cancer center and a hospice. *Hospice Journal, 10*(1), 89–108.

McMillan, S.C., & Weitzner, M.A. (2000). How problematic are various aspects of quality of life in patients with cancer at the end of life? *Oncology Nursing Forum, 27*(5), 817–823.

McMillan, S.C., & Williams, F.A. (1989). Validity and reliability of the Constipation Assessment Scale. *Cancer Nursing, 12*(3), 183–188.

National Cancer Institute Cancer Therapy Evaluation Program. (2006). *Common terminology criteria for adverse events* (version 3.0). Bethesda, MD: National Cancer Institute. Retrieved August 31, 2008, from http://ctep.cancer.gov/protocolDevelopment/electronic_applications/docs/ctcaev3.pdf

Petticrew, M., Rodgers, M., & Booth, A. (2001). Effectiveness of laxatives in adults. *Quality in Health Care, 10*(4), 268–273.

Tamayo, A.C., & Diaz-Zuluaga, P.A. (2004). Management of opioid-induced bowel dysfunction in cancer patients. *Supportive Care in Cancer, 12*(9), 613–618.

Thompson, M.J., Boyd-Carson, W., Trainor, B., & Boyd, K. (2003). Management of constipation. *Nursing Standard, 18*(14–16), 41–42.

Tittle, M., & McMillan, S.C. (1994). Pain and pain-related side effects in an ICU and on a surgical unit. *American Journal of Critical Care, 3*(1), 25–30.

Weitzner, M.A., Moody, L.N., & McMillan, S.C. (1997). Symptom management issues in hospice care. *American Journal of Hospice and Palliative Care, 14*(4), 190–195.

Woolery, M., Carroll, E., Fenn, E., Wieland, H., Jarosinksi, P., Corey, B., et al. (2006). A constipation assessment scale for use in pediatric oncology. *Journal of Pediatric Oncology Nursing, 23*(2), 65–74.

Case Study

M.R. was a 73-year-old man with a history of multiple myeloma diagnosed in 2005. He was treated successfully with thalidomide and dexamethasone for one year. During that time, he experienced some problems with constipation related to the thalidomide; however, he was able to maintain regular bowel movements at least every other day by taking two tablets of senna plus 100 mg docusate sodium twice a day. Prior to treatment, he reported that he had a bowel movement every day after his morning coffee. He ate a salad for dinner every night and had a banana with breakfast, but otherwise he was a "meat and potatoes" man.

In December 2006, M.R. developed back pain and was diagnosed with disease progression in his lumbar spine. He was started on opiates for pain management. In addition, he completed a course of palliative radiation therapy to his lumbar spine followed by kyphoplasty. In March 2007, bortezomib was added to M.R.'s treatment regimen and his long-acting oxycodone was increased to 40 mg PO BID with 5–10 mg immediate-release oxycodone every four hours as needed. The nurse recommended that he increase his senna to three to four tablets PO BID and continue his docusate sodium 100 mg PO BID. He also was instructed to take 30 ml of milk of magnesia at bedtime if he went two days without a bowel movement and was given a prescription for lactulose 30 ml PO BID as needed if the aforementioned regimen did not work.

In May 2007, M.R. presented to the outpatient medical oncology clinic with a 10-pound weight loss over two months, poor appetite, and no bowel movement for five days. Using the CAS, he was noted to have severe problems with less than normal bowel movements and some problems with the urge to defecate but an inability to pass stool. He did not report any abdominal bloating or an inability to pass gas.

M.R. was more reticent than usual. His wife reported that he was very depressed and sat in his recliner most of the day. Further assessment by the nurse revealed that his appetite was poor and he was only drinking a cup of coffee in the morning and at lunch and a glass of water with dinner (approximately 24 oz/day). His last bowel movement was hard, brown, and painful to pass. No blood was noted in the stool. In addition, he refused to take the lactulose because of the sweet taste. On examination, the patient was cachectic, and his abdomen was slightly distended but soft, with positive bowel sounds in all quadrants. His right upper quadrant was dull to percussion, and his right and left lower quadrants were tympanic. His electrolytes were all within normal limits.

The nurse identified three major contributors to constipation for this patient: medications associated with constipation (oxycodone, thalidomide, and bortezomib), poor oral intake of fluids and fiber, and decreased mobility. In collaboration with the oncology clinical specialist and M.R. and his wife, the nurse determined that based on his oral intake, a soft bowel movement every three days was a reasonable goal for M.R., and a plan was developed to achieve this. Guided by M.R.'s individual needs and risk factors and recommendations from the Oncology Nursing Society Putting Evidence Into Practice resource on constipation, the following changes were made to his bowel regimen and treatment plan.

- Increase the stimulant laxative and stool softener (docusate sodium to 100 mg PO TID and senna to two tablets PO TID); see *Likely to Be Effective* and *Expert Opinion* for opioid-induced constipation: stimulant laxatives plus stool softener.
- Add an osmotic laxative: Replace lactulose with one packet of MiraLax® (polyethylene glycol 3350) per day; see *Likely to Be Effective* for refractory constipation in adults.
- Provide a dietary consult with the goal of increasing fluid intake, especially warm liquids, and adding nutritional supplements; see *Expert Opinion* for constipation in adults.

Other strategies that were considered included changing the opiate to methadone or fentanyl (see *Likely to Be Effective* for opioid-induced constipation: opioid rotation) and adding metoclopramide four times a day (see *Expert Opinion* for constipation in adults, pharmacologic interventions); however, M.R.'s care team decided to reserve these options if the changes stated previously failed.

Patient education reinforcing the rationale for each element of the bowel regimen was provided to M.R. and his wife (see *Expert Opinion* for constipation in adults). The patient was not very receptive but agreed to try the first three interventions to start. He agreed to physical therapy once he was feeling better. The patient was successfully maintained on the bowel regimen until he was transitioned to hospice in October 2007.

Hannah F. Lyons, RN, MSN, AOCN®, BC
Oncology Clinical Nurse Specialist
Inpatient Oncology/Hematology
Massachusetts General Hospital
Boston, MA

Constipation

2009 AUTHORS
Annette Kay Bisanz, RN, BSN, MPH, and Myra J. Woolery, MN, RN, CPON®
ONS STAFF: Linda H. Eaton, MN, RN, AOCN®

2007 AUTHORS
Annette Kay Bisanz, RN, BSN, MPH, Myra J. Woolery, MN, RN, CPON®, Hannah F. Lyons, MSN, RN, BC,
AOCN®, Lindsay Gaido, MSN, RN, Mary Yenulevich, BSN, RN, OCN®, and Stephanie Fulton, MSIS
ONS STAFF: Linda H. Eaton, MN, RN, AOCN®

What interventions are effective for preventing and treating constipation in people with cancer?

Recommended for Practice

Interventions for which effectiveness has been demonstrated by strong evidence from rigorously designed studies, meta-analyses, or systematic reviews and for which expectation of harm is small compared with the benefits

No interventions are recommended as of May 2008.

Likely to Be Effective

Interventions for which effectiveness has been demonstrated by supportive evidence from a single rigorously conducted controlled trial, consistent supportive evidence from well-designed controlled trials using small samples, or guidelines developed from evidence and supported by expert opinion

CONSTIPATION IN ADULTS

Polyethylene: Polyethylene Glycol With or Without Electrolytes

Although a lack of evidence exists in the oncology population, a high level of evidence was found in the non-oncology population regarding the safety and efficacy of polyethylene glycol (PEG) with or without electrolytes (Attar et al., 1999; Brandt et al., 2005; DiPalma, Cleveland, McGowan, & Herrera, 2006; Frizelle & Barclay, 2005; Petticrew, Rodgers, & Booth, 2001; Ramkumar & Rao, 2005). **Caution:** Do not administer electrolytes when kidney function is compromised.

Opioid-Induced Constipation: Prophylactic Regimen

A proactive approach, including initiation of a prophylactic regimen, is needed to prevent constipation when taking opioids (McNicol et al., 2003; Miaskowski et al., 2005; National Comprehensive Cancer Network [NCCN], 2009). However, not enough evidence exists to identify the most effective regimen (see *Expert Opinion* section).

Opioid-Induced Constipation: Opioid Rotation

Research has demonstrated that some opioids have less constipating effect than others, and rotating opioids would decrease the associated side effects (McNicol et al., 2003; Miaskowski et al., 2005; NCCN, 2009; Radbruch, Sabatwski, Loick, Kulbe, & Casper, 2000).

- Switching opioids from sustained-release oral morphine to transdermal fentanyl patches may decrease constipation (Ahmedzai & Brooks, 1997; Allan et al., 2001; McNicol et al., 2003; Miaskowski et al., 2005; Radbruch et al., 2000).
- Switching opioids to methadone may result in a reduction in laxative use (McNicol et al., 2003; Miaskowski et al., 2005).

Refractory Constipation in Adults

NCCN recommends the use of PEG as a treatment alternative for patients with cancer with persistent constipation (NCCN, 2009). Standard-dose PEG with electrolytes in the United States is known as Golytely® (Braintree Laboratories) and Colyte® (Schwarz Pharma). Low-dose PEG, referred to as PEG 3350, is available without electrolytes in the United States and is marketed as MiraLAX® (Schering-Plough). Stimulant or osmotic laxatives are effective in improving bowel function in patients with cancer with persistent constipation and/or at the end of life, and some patients may need both types of laxatives to achieve optimal results (Agra et al., 1998; Chessman, 2008; DiPalma, Cleveland, McGowan, & Herrera, 2007a, 2007b; NCCN, 2009; Wirz & Klaschik, 2005).

Benefits Balanced With Harms

Interventions for which clinicians and patients should weigh the beneficial and harmful effects according to individual circumstances and priorities

OPIOID-INDUCED CONSTIPATION: NALOXONE

Naloxone is an opioid receptor antagonist. Both oral and enteral routes have shown mixed results for managing opioid-induced constipation, potentially causing adverse reactions, including loss of analgesia and withdrawal symptoms (Choi & Billings, 2002; Friedman & Dello Buono, 2001; McNicol et al., 2003; Meissner, Schmidt, Hartmann, Kath, & Reinhart, 2000; Miaskowski et al., 2005; Thomas, 2007b; Tofil, Benner, Faro, & Winkler, 2006).

Effectiveness Not Established

Interventions for which insufficient or conflicting data or data of inadequate quality currently exist, with no clear indication of harm

PHARMACOLOGIC INTERVENTIONS FOR CONSTIPATION IN ADULTS

These interventions are based on high-level evidence in non-oncology populations and need to be studied in the oncology population.

Bulk Laxatives (Psyllium)

Psyllium is recommended for patients with good functional status, including the ability to tolerate adequate fluids for the prevention and treatment of constipation (Frizelle & Barclay, 2005; Petticrew et al., 2001; Ramkumar & Rao, 2005). Most bulk laxatives need to be taken with at least 200–300 ml of water (Miaskowski et al., 2005). Psyllium should be avoided in patients who do not have adequate physical activity or fluid intake and/or who have severe constipation, as it may worsen manifestations of constipation (Petticrew et al.). Psyllium administered in large amounts has been associated with increased flatulence, abdominal distention and bloating, mechanical obstruction of the esophagus and colon, and anaphylactic reactions (Brandt et al., 2005; Frizelle & Barclay).

Osmotic Laxatives (Sorbitol, Lactulose)

Osmotic laxatives such as sorbitol or lactulose are associated with significant improvements in stool consistency, fecal impaction, and other symptoms of chronic constipation, such as straining of stool (Brandt et al., 2005; Petticrew et al., 2001). Adverse effects include abdominal cramping, flatulence, bowel distention, an unpleasant sweet taste, and diarrhea. In many cases, osmotic laxatives were no better than other laxatives such as senna (Agra et al., 1998; Kot & Pettit-Young, 1992). Lactulose often is used in combination with a stimulant laxative in constipation that is difficult to treat (Brandt et al.; Kot & Pettit-Young; Lederle, Busch, Mattox, West, & Aske, 1990).

PHARMACOLOGIC INTERVENTION IN PEDIATRIC PATIENTS WITH CHRONIC CONSTIPATION

This intervention is based on high-level evidence in non-oncology populations and needs to be studied in the oncology population.

PEG 3350

Although studies have not been conducted in the oncology population, PEG 3350 has been found to be safe, effective, and well-tolerated in pediatric patients (Arora & Srinivasan, 2005; Baker et al., 2006; Bell & Wall, 2004; Hardikar, Cranswick, & Heine, 2007; Kinservik & Friedhoff, 2004; Loening-Baucke & Pashankar, 2006).

Mineral Oil and Magnesium Hydroxide, Lactulose, and Sorbitol

Research has demonstrated these agents are safe and effective medications for children (Baker et al., 2006). **Caution:** Do not administer oral mineral oil if potential for aspiration exists (Zanetti, Marchiori, Gasparetto, Escuissato, & Souza, 2007).

INTERVENTIONS FOR CONSTIPATION IN ADULTS AND PEDIATRIC PATIENTS WHERE DATA ARE INSUFFICIENT

The effectiveness of the interventions described below has not been established because they are based on studies that are inadequately powered, have limited sample sizes, or have flaws in study design or in study procedures. The majority of the research is in non-oncology patients who have chronic constipation. Further study using randomized controlled trials is needed.

Pharmacologic Interventions (Adults)

- Laxatives
  - Bulk-forming laxatives
    * Methylcellulose (Brandt et al., 2005; Frizelle & Barclay, 2005; Newey & Goetzi, 1949; Ramkumar & Rao, 2005)
  - Lubricants
    * Glycerin suppositories (Frizelle & Barclay, 2005; Tofil et al., 2006)
    * Mineral oil (Brandt et al., 2005)

- Osmotic laxatives (saline)
  * Magnesium salts (Frizelle & Barclay, 2005; Ghoshal, 2007)
  * Magnesium hydroxide (Phillips' Milk of Magnesia®, Bayer Consumer Care) (Brandt et al., 2005; Ramkumar & Rao, 2005)
- Stimulant laxatives
  * Bisacodyl (Frizelle & Barclay, 2005; Kienzle-Horn et al., 2006, 2007)
  * Senna (Brandt et al., 2005; Frizelle & Barclay, 2005; Hawley & Byeon, 2008)
- Non-bulk-forming fiber laxatives (Petticrew et al., 2001)
- Stool softeners: Systematic reviews of the chronic constipation population found insufficient data to make a recommendation, and the consensus was that stool softeners are minimally effective in improving symptoms of constipation (Brandt et al., 2005; Frizelle & Barclay, 2005; Ramkumar & Rao, 2005).
  * Docusate sodium and docusate calcium (Frizelle & Barclay, 2005; Hurdon, Viola, & Schroder, 2000)
- Colchicine (Thomas, 2007a)
- Lubiprostone (Thomas, 2007a)
- Misoprostol (Ramkumar & Rao, 2005; Thomas, 2007a)
- Prokinetic agent: Erythromycin (Ramkumar & Rao, 2005)
- Enemas: Phosphate enema and sodium citrate enema (Frizelle & Barclay, 2005; Mendoza, Legido, Rubio, & Gisbert, 2007)

Caution: Water/electrolyte imbalances are usually minimal; however, imbalances may be severe in patients < 5 or > 65 years old (Thomas, 2007a) and in patients with chronic renal failure, diseases altering intestinal motility (Hsu & Wu, 2008; Mendoza et al., 2007), and tumor lysis syndrome, bowel obstruction, and small intestinal disorders (Hsu & Wu, 2008).

- Partially hydrolysed guar gum (Sutton, Dumbleton, & Allway, 2007)
- Peripheral opioid antagonists
  - Alvimopan was approved by the U.S. Food and Drug Administration (FDA) in May 2008 for use after partial large or small bowel resection surgery (Becker, Galandi, & Blum, 2007; Choi & Billings, 2002; Neary & Delaney, 2005; Taguchi et al., 2001; Thomas, 2007a; Thomas et al., 2008; Webster et al., 2008).
  - Methylnaltrexone was FDA approved in April 2008 for refractory opioid-induced constipation in patients with advanced illness who are receiving palliative care (Becker et al., 2007; Choi & Billings, 2002; Foss, 2001; Friedman & Dello Buono, 2001; McNicol, Boyce, Schumann, & Carr, 2008; Portenoy et al., 2008; Shivoa, Rim, Friedman, & Jahdi, 2007; Thomas, 2007a; Thomas et al., 2008; Yuan & Israel, 2006).

Nonpharmacologic Interventions (Adults)

- Activity/increased mobility (Bennett & Cresswell, 2003; Frizelle & Barclay, 2005; Richmond & Wright, 2004)
- Aromatherapy, massage therapy, and aromatherapy massage (Fellowes, Barnes, & Wilkinson, 2004)
- Biofeedback: Many studies excluded patients with cancer. Of the studies found, the data were inadequate to support its efficacy in treating chronic constipation (Brandt et al., 2005; Coulter et al., 2002; Frizelle & Barclay, 2005; Ghoshal, 2007).

- Dietary fiber: A relatively large body of mixed-quality evidence indicates positive effects of dietary fiber on bowel function in oncology and non-oncology populations (Griffenberg, Morris, Atkinson, & Levenback, 1997; Muller-Lissner, 1988; Richmond & Wright, 2004). *Note:* Fiber is not recommended in patients with inadequate fluid intake, such as patients with advanced disease (McEligot et al., 2002; NCCN, 2009; Sutton et al., 2007).
- Fresh baker's yeast (Wenk et al., 2000)
- Herbal supplements (Brandt et al., 2005)

Pharmacologic Interventions (Pediatrics)
- Stimulant laxatives (Bell & Wall, 2004; Rubin, 2004)
- Enemas in children: Phosphate soda, saline, or mineral oil enemas (Baker et al., 2006; Bell & Wall, 2004); see enema caution under adult section.

Nonpharmacologic Interventions (Pediatrics)
- Biofeedback: The evidence supporting the use of biofeedback in children is inconsistent and primarily relates to defecation disorders (Brazzelli & Griffiths, 2006; Coulter et al., 2002; Rubin, 2004).
- Dietary fiber (Bell & Wall, 2004; Rubin, 2004)
- Soy milk in children who are lactose intolerant (Iacono et al., 1998)

Effectiveness Unlikely

Interventions for which lack of effectiveness has been demonstrated by negative evidence from a single rigorously conducted controlled trial, consistent negative evidence from well-designed controlled trials using small samples, or guidelines developed from evidence and supported by expert opinion

There are no interventions as of May 2008.

Not Recommended for Practice

Interventions for which lack of effectiveness or harmfulness has been demonstrated by strong evidence from rigorously conducted studies, meta-analyses, or systematic reviews, or interventions where the costs, burden, or harms associated with the intervention exceed anticipated benefit

- Cisapride: A prokinetic drug that is known to increase gastrointestinal motility (Ramkumar & Rao, 2005). **Caution:** Restricted access exists in some countries because of adverse cardiac effects. Cisapride was taken off the market in the United States in 2000 by the FDA (Coggrave, Wiesel, & Norton, 2006).
- Dantron™ (Hexal Pharma): This drug has not been approved by the FDA for use in the United States because it has been associated with rodent cancer (Bennett & Cresswell, 2003).
- Enemas
  - Infants: Not recommended in infants younger than 12 months (Bell & Wall, 2004)
  - Children: Soap suds, tap water, and magnesium enemas are contraindicated because of the potential toxicity and side effects (Baker et al., 2006).

- Nalmefene: Limited studies of the efficacy of oral nalmefene in humans are available because of its propensity to reverse analgesia or to induce withdrawal (Choi & Billings, 2002).
- Naltrexone: A lipid soluble drug that crosses the blood-brain barrier and may negatively affect the analgesic effects of opioids (Choi & Billings, 2002). It has been associated with dose-related elevations in serum transaminase levels, resulting in the discontinuation of the drug (Choi & Billings). (*Note:* This is different from methylnaltrexone.)
- Tegaserod: The effectiveness of tegaserod, a 5-HT$_4$ agonist, in patients with cancer has not been established because this population was excluded from published premarketing studies; however, it was found to be effective in non-oncology patients (Brandt et al., 2005; Johanson, 2004; Kamm et al., 2005). **Caution:** Tegaserod was taken off the market in April 2007 by the FDA because of adverse cardiovascular effects. In July 2007, the FDA approved restricted use of this drug only (FDA, 2007).

Expert Opinion

Low-risk interventions that are (1) consistent with sound clinical practice, (2) suggested by an expert in a peer-reviewed publication (journal or book chapter), and (3) for which limited evidence exists. An expert is an individual with peer-reviewed journal publications in the domain of interest.

Although randomized controlled trials are lacking, experts agree that routine bowel care is an important element of care for prevention and management of constipation. In fact, it would be regarded as unethical to withhold basic bowel care as one arm of a research study in order to validate the benefit of such care.

SPECIAL NOTE: MYELOSUPPRESSED PATIENTS

Avoid rectal agents and/or manipulation (i.e., rectal examinations, suppositories, enemas) in myelosuppressed patients. These actions can lead to development of bleeding, anal fissures, or abscesses. In addition, avoid manipulation of the stoma of neutropenic patients (National Cancer Institute [NCI], 2006).

GENERAL CONSTIPATION (BOTH ADULT AND PEDIATRIC)

Prevention

- Take preventive measures in anticipation of constipation for those receiving medications, such as vincristine or other chemotherapies, that slow colonic transit times (Cope, 2001; Harris & Jackson, 1977).

Assessment

- Perform a thorough history and physical examination in evaluation of constipation before determining the treatment plan, including assessment of individual risk factors (Baker et al., 2006; Bisanz, 2005; Brandt et al., 2005; Coggrave et al., 2006; Cope, 2001; Klaschik, Nauck, & Ostgathe, 2003; Mancini & Bruera, 1998; NCCN, 2009; NCI, 2006; Richmond & Wright, 2004).
- Obtain a nutritional consult (Bisanz, 2005).
- Consider in-depth diagnostic workup for constipation *after* patient fails initial treatment (Bisanz, 2005; Brandt et al., 2005).

Interventions

- Teach the patient about bowel function (Baker et al., 2006; Bisanz, 2005).
- Provide a comfortable, quiet, private environment for defecating (Folden, 2002; NCI, 2006; Smith, 2001).
- Provide a toilet, bedside commode, and any necessary assistive devices. Avoid the use of a bedpan when possible (Folden, 2002; NCI, 2006).
- Minimize the use of constipating medications when possible (Bisanz, 2005; NCCN, 2009).
- Involve the patient in development of a bowel regimen (Bisanz, 2005).
- Encourage the intake of warm or hot liquids (Consortium for Spinal Cord Medicine, 1998; NCI, 2006).
- Castor oil: Not recommended secondary to severe cramping (Mancini & Bruera, 1998)

OPIOID-INDUCED CONSTIPATION

Stimulant Laxatives Plus Stool Softener

This combination is recommended when initiating opioid therapy (Bisanz, 2005; Kalso, Edwards, Moore, & McQuay, 2004; Miaskowski et al., 2005; NCCN, 2009; NCI, 2006; Robinson et al., 2000). A useful bowel regimen includes docusate sodium (100–300 mg/day) along with senna (two to six tablets twice a day) (Miaskowski et al.; NCI). Bulk laxatives are not recommended for opioid-induced constipation because of the risk of bowel impaction in poorly hydrated patients (Miaskowski et al.).

- The laxative dose should be individually titrated for effectiveness according to bowel function, not opioid dosing (Bennett & Cresswell, 2003; Meissner et al., 2000; Miaskowski et al., 2005; Tamayo & Diaz-Zuluaga, 2004).

CONSTIPATION IN ADULTS

Pharmacologic Interventions

- Prokinetic medication (i.e., metoclopramide) should be reserved for use in individuals with severe constipation and those resistant to bowel programs (Consortium for Spinal Cord Medicine, 1998; Mancini & Bruera, 1998; NCCN, 2009). **Caution:** Avoid in patients with large abdominal tumors or bowel obstruction (Bisanz, 2005; NCCN, 2009).
- Oral mineral oil is effective for hard stool but should not be used for routine prevention of constipation because it may interfere with absorption of some nutrients (Bisanz, 2005; Mancini & Bruera, 1998).
- PEG 4000 (Szodja, Mulder, & Felt-Bersma, 2007): PEG 4000 tastes better than PEG 3350, implying better patient compliance and effectiveness of treatment in patients with chronic constipation.
- Expert opinion supports the use of a stimulant laxative plus a stool softener in preventing and managing constipation in patients at the end of life (NCCN, 2009).

Nonpharmacologic Interventions

- Recommended fluid intake per day is eight 8-oz glasses in adults (Bisanz, 2005; NCCN, 2009; Richmond & Wright, 2004).
- Treat high and low impactions differently (Bisanz, 2005).
  - High impactions: These are comfortably relieved with low-volume (< 300 ml) milk and molasses enemas up to four times per day along with an oral laxative (Bisanz, 2005). (For enema recipe, see definition table at www.ons.org/outcomes.)

- Low impactions: Oil-retention enemas soften hard stool. In nonmyelosuppressed patients, stool can be disimpacted manually followed by enemas of choice (Bisanz, 2005).

Individualized Bowel Management Program

- After three days without a bowel movement, initiate a bowel management program (Bisanz, 2005; NCI, 2006).
- A good program includes fluids, fiber, and a decrease in constipating medications or provisio of medications to offset constipating side effects of medications (Bisanz, 2005; Cope, 2001; NCCN, 2009; NCI, 2006).

CONSTIPATION IN PEDIATRIC PATIENTS

Pharmacologic Interventions

- Children
  - Senna and bisacodyl (stimulant laxatives) can be useful (Baker et al., 2007).
  - PEG and milk of magnesia are effective in long-term treatment in children (Loening-Baucke & Pashankar, 2006).
  - Disimpaction can be achieved with either oral or rectal medications, including enemas in age-appropriate children (Baker et al., 2006).
- Infants
  - Lactulose and sorbitol (osmotic laxatives) can be used as stool softeners (Baker et al., 2006).
  - Mineral oil and stimulant laxatives are not recommended (Baker et al., 2006).
  - Rectal disimpaction can be achieved with glycerin suppositories (Baker et al., 2006).

For specifics, see the detailed ONS PEP resource on constipation at www.ons.org/outcomes.

Nonpharmacologic Interventions

- A balanced diet containing whole grains, fruits, and vegetables is recommended as part of the treatment of constipation (Baker et al., 2006; NCCN, 2007)
- Infants
  - Juices that contain sorbitol, such as prune, pear, and apple juices, can decrease constipation (Baker et al., 2006).
  - Barley malt extract and corn syrup can be used as stool softeners (Baker et al., 2006).

Definitions of the interventions are available at **www.ons.org/outcomes**.
Literature search completed through May 2008.

References

Agra, Y., Sacristan, A., Gonzalez, M., Ferrari, M., Portugues, A., & Calvo, M.J. (1998). Efficacy of senna versus lactulose in terminal cancer patients treated with opioids. *Journal of Pain and Symptom Management, 15*(1), 1–7.

Ahmedzai, S., & Brooks, D. (1997). Transdermal fentanyl versus sustained-release oral morphine in cancer pain: Preference, efficacy, and quality of life. The TTS-Fentanyl Comparative Trial Group. *Journal of Pain and Symptom Management, 13*(5), 254–261.

Allan, L., Hays, H., Jensen, N.H., de Waroux, B.L., Bolt, M., Donald, R., et al. (2001). Randomised cross-over trial of transdermal fentanyl and sustained release oral morphine for treating chronic non-cancer pain. *BMJ, 322*(7295), 1154–1158.

Arora, R., & Srinivasan, R. (2005). Is polyethylene glycol safe and effective for chronic constipation in children? *Archives of Disease in Childhood, 90*(6), 643–646.

Attar, A., Lemann, M., Ferguson, A., Halphen, M., Boutron, M.C., Flourie, B., et al. (1999). Comparison of a low dose polyethylene glycol electrolyte solution with lactulose for treatment of chronic constipation. *Gut, 44*(2), 226–230.

Baker, S.S., Liptak, G.S., Colletti, R.B., Croffie, J.M., Di Lorenzo, C., Ector, W., et al. (2006). Clinical practice guideline. Evaluation and treatment of constipation in infants and children: Recommendations of the North American Society for Pediatric Gastroenterology, Hepatology, and Nutrition. *Journal of Pediatric Gastroenterology and Nutrition, 43*(3), e1–e13.

Becker, G., Galandi, D., & Blum, H.E. (2007). Peripherally acting opioid antagonists in the treatment of opiate-related constipation. A systematic review. *Journal of Pain and Symptom Management, 34*(5), 547–565.

Bell, E.A., & Wall, G.C. (2004). Pediatric constipation therapy using guidelines and polyethylene glycol 3350. *Annals of Pharmacotherapy, 38*(4), 686–693.

Bennett, M., & Cresswell, H. (2003). Factors influencing constipation in advanced cancer patients: A prospective study of opioid dose, dantron dose and physical functioning. *Palliative Medicine, 17*(5), 418–422.

Bisanz, A. (2005). Bowel management in patients with cancer. In J.A. Ajani (Ed.), *Gastrointestinal cancer* (pp. 313–345). New York: Springer.

Brandt, L.J., Prather, C.M., Quigley, E.M., Schiller, L.R., Schoenfeld, P., & Talley, N.J. (2005). Systematic review on the management of chronic constipation in North America. *American Journal of Gastroenterology, 100*(Suppl. 1), S5–S21.

Brazzelli, M., & Griffiths, P. (2006). Behavioural and cognitive interventions with or without other treatments for the management of faecal incontinence in children. *Cochrane Database of Systematic Reviews* 2006, Issue 2. Art. No.: CD002240. DOI: 10.1002/14651858.CD002240.pub3.

Chessman, A. (2008). Daily polyethylene glycol over 6 months was effective for chronic constipation. *Evidence-Based Medicine, 13*(1), 20.

Choi, Y.S., & Billings, J.A. (2002). Opioid antagonists: A review of their role in palliative care, focusing on use in opioid-related constipation. *Journal of Pain and Symptom Management, 24*(1), 71–90.

Coggrave, M., Wiesel, P.H., & Norton, C. (2006). Management of faecal incontinence and constipation in adults with central neurological diseases. *Cochrane Database of Systematic Reviews* 2006, Issue 2. Art. No.: CD002115. DOI: 10.1002/14651858.CD002115.pub3.

Consortium for Spinal Cord Medicine. (1998). *Neurogenic bowel management in adults with spinal cord injury.* Washington, DC: Paralyzed Veterans of America.

Cope, D.G. (2001). Management of chemotherapy-induced diarrhea and constipation. *Nursing Clinics of North America, 36*(4), 695–707.

Coulter, I.D., Favreau, J.T., Hardy, M.L., Morton, S.C., Roth, E.A., & Shekelle, P. (2002). Biofeedback interventions for gastrointestinal conditions: A systematic review. *Alternative Therapies in Health and Medicine, 8*(3), 76–83.

DiPalma, J.A., Cleveland, M.B., McGowan, J., & Herrera, J.L. (2006). An open-labeled study of chronic polyethylene glycol laxative use in chronic constipation. *Alimentary Pharmacology and Therapeutics, 25*(6), 703–708.

DiPalma, J.A., Cleveland, M.B., McGowan, J., & Herrera, J.L. (2007a). A comparison of polyethylene glycol laxative and placebo relief of constipation from constipating medications. *Southern Medical Journal, 100*(11), 1085–1090.

DiPalma, J.A., Cleveland, M.B., McGowan, J., & Herrera, J.L. (2007b). A randomized, multi-centered, placebo-controlled trial of polyethylene glycol laxative for chronic treatment of chronic constipation. *American Journal of Gastroenterology, 102*(7), 1436–1441.

Fellowes, D., Barnes, K., & Wilkinson, S. (2004). Aromatherapy and massage for symptom relief in patients with cancer. *Cochrane Database of Systematic Reviews* 2004, Issue 3. Art. No.: CD002287. DOI: 10.1002/14651858.CD002287.pub2.

Folden, S.L. (2002). Current issues. Practice guidelines for the management of constipation in adults. *Rehabilitation Nursing, 27*(5), 169–175.

Foss, J.F. (2001). A review of the potential role of methylnaltrexone in opioid bowel dysfunction. *American Journal of Surgery, 182*(Suppl. 5A), 19S–26S.

Friedman, J.D., & Dello Buono, F.A. (2001). Opioid antagonists in the treatment of opioid-induced constipation and pruritus. *Annals of Pharmacotherapy, 35*(1), 85–91.

Frizelle, F., & Barclay, M. (2005, December). Constipation in adults. *Clinical Evidence, 2005*(14), 557–566.

Ghoshal, U.C. (2007). Review of pathogenesis and management of constipation. *Topical Gastroenterology, 28*(3), 91–95.

Griffenberg, L., Morris, M., Atkinson, N., & Levenback, C. (1997). The effect of dietary fiber on bowel function following radical hysterectomy: A randomized trial. *Gynecologic Oncology, 66*(3), 417–424.

Hardikar, W., Cranswick, N., & Heine, R.F. (2007). Macrogol 3350 plus electrolytes for chronic constipation in children: A single-centre, open-label study. *Journal of Paediatrics and Child Health, 43*(7–8), 527–531.

Harris, A.C., & Jackson, J.M. (1977). Lactulose in vincristine-induced constipation. *Medical Journal of Australia, 2*(17), 573–574.

Hawley, P.H., & Byeon, J.J. (2008). A comparison of sennosides-based bowel protocols with and without docusate in hospitalized patients with cancer. *Journal of Palliative Medicine, 11*(4), 575–581.

Hsu, H.L., & Wu, M.-S. (2008). Extreme hyperphosphatemia and hypocalcemic coma associated with phosphate enema. *Internal Medicine, 47*(7), 643–646.

Hurdon, V., Viola, R., & Schroder, C. (2000). How useful is docusate in patients at risk for constipation? A systematic review of the evidence in the chronically ill. *Journal of Pain and Symptom Management, 19*(2), 130–136.

Iacono, G., Cavataio, F., Montalto, G., Florena, A., Tumminello, M., Soresi, M., et al. (1998). Intolerance of cow's milk and chronic constipation in children. *New England Journal of Medicine, 339*(16), 1100–1104.

Johanson, J.F. (2004). Review article: Tegaserod for chronic constipation. *Alimentary Pharmacology and Therapeutics, 20*(Suppl. 7), 20–24.

Kalso, E., Edwards, J.E., Moore, R.A., & McQuay, H.J. (2004). Opioids in chronic non-cancer pain: Systematic review of efficacy and safety. *Pain, 112*(3), 372–380.

Kamm, M.A., Muller-Lissner, S., Talley, N.J., Tack, J., Boeckxstaens, G., Minushkin, O.N., et al. (2005). Tegaserod for the treatment of chronic constipation: A randomized, double-blind, placebo-controlled multinational study. *American Journal of Gastroenterology, 100*(2), 362–372.

Kienzle-Horn, S., Vix, J.M., Schuijt, C., Peil, H., Jordan, C.C., & Kamm, M.A. (2006). Efficacy and safety of bisacodyl in acute treatment of constipation: A double-blind, randomized, placebo-controlled study. *Aliment Pharmacology and Therapeutics, 23*(10), 1479–1488.

Kienzle-Horn, S., Vix, J.M., Schuijt, C., Peil, H., Jordan, C.C., & Kamm, M.A. (2007). Comparison of bisacodyl and sodium picosulfate in the treatment of chronic constipation. *Current Medical Research and Opinion, 23*(4), 691–699.

Kinservik, M.A., & Friedhoff, M.M. (2004). The efficacy and safety of polyethylene glycol 3350 in the treatment of constipation in children. *Pediatric Nursing, 30*(3), 232–237.

Klaschik, E., Nauck, F., & Ostgathe, C. (2003). Constipation—Modern laxative therapy. *Supportive Care in Cancer, 11*(11), 679–685.

Kot, T.V., & Pettit-Young, N.A. (1992). Lactulose in the management of constipation: A current review. *Annals of Pharmacotherapy, 26*(10), 1277–1282.

Lederle, F.A., Busch, D.L., Mattox, K.M., West, M.J., & Aske, D.M. (1990). Cost-effective treatment of constipation in the elderly: A randomized double-blind comparison of sorbitol and lactulose. *American Journal of Medicine, 89*(5), 597–601.

Loening-Baucke, V., & Pashankar, D.S. (2006). A randomized, prospective, comparison study of polyethylene glycol 3350 without electrolytes and milk of magnesia for children with constipation and fecal incontinence. *Pediatrics, 118*(20), 528–535.

Mancini, I., & Bruera, E. (1998). Constipation in advanced cancer patients. *Supportive Care in Cancer, 6*(4), 356–364.

McEligot, A.J., Gilpin, E.A., Rock, C.L., Newman, V., Hollenbach, K.A., Thomson, C.A., et al. (2002). Research and professional briefs. High dietary fiber consumption is not associated with gastrointestinal discomfort in a diet intervention trial. *Journal of the American Dietetic Association, 102*(4), 549–551.

McNicol, E., Horowicz-Mehler, N., Fisk, R.A., Bennett, K., Gialeli-Goudas, M., Chew, P.W., et al. (2003). Management of opioid side effects in cancer-related and chronic noncancer pain: A systematic review. *Journal of Pain, 4*(5), 231–256.

McNicol, E.D., Boyce, D., Schumann, R., & Carr, D.B. (2008). Mu-opioid antagonists for opioid-induced bowel dysfunction. *Cochrane Database of Systematic Reviews* 2008, Issue 2. Art. No.: CD006332. DOI: 10.1002/14651858.CD006332.pub2.

Meissner, W., Schmidt, U., Hartmann, M., Kath, R., & Reinhart, K. (2000). Oral naloxone reverses opioid-associated constipation. *Pain, 84*(1), 105–109.

Mendoza, J., Legido, J., Rubio, S., & Gisbert, J.S.P. (2007). Systematic review: The adverse effects of sodium phosphate enema. *Alimentary Pharmacology and Therapeutics, 26*(1), 9–20.

Miaskowski, C., Cleary, J., Burney, R., Coyne, P., Finley, R., Foster, R., et al. (2005). *Guideline for the management of cancer pain in adults and children. APS clinical practice guidelines* [Series No. 3]. Glenview, IL: American Pain Society.

Muller-Lissner, S.A. (1988). Effect of wheat bran on weight of stool and gastrointestinal transit time: A meta analysis. *BMJ, 296*(6622), 615–617.

National Cancer Institute. (2006, April). *Gastrointestinal complications (PDQ®)* [Health professional version]. Retrieved November 17, 2006, from http://www.cancer.gov/cancertopics/pdq/supportivecare/gastrointestinalcomplications/healthprofessional

National Comprehensive Cancer Network. (2007). *NCCN Clinical Practice Guidelines in Oncology™: Pediatric cancer pain* [v.1.2007]. Retrieved May 12, 2007, from http://www.nccn.org/professionals/physician_gls/PDF/pediatric_pain.pdf

National Comprehensive Cancer Network. (2009). *NCCN Clinical Practice Guidelines in Oncology™: Palliative care* [v.1.2009]. Retrieved December 6, 2008, from http://www.nccn.org/professionals/physician_gls/PDF/palliative.pdf

Neary, P., & Delaney, C.P. (2005). Alvimopan. *Expert Opinion on Investigational Drugs, 14*(4), 479–488.

Newey, J.A., & Goetzi, F.R. (1949). Methyl cellulose therapy in chronic constipation with a brief summary of the etiology of this condition. *Permanente Foundation Medical Bulletin, 7*(2), 67–78.

Petticrew, M., Rodgers, M., & Booth, A. (2001). Effectiveness of laxatives in adults. *Quality in Health Care, 10*(4), 268–273.

Portenoy, R.K., Thomas, J., Moehl Boatwright, M.L., Tran, D., Galasso, F.L., Stambler, N., et al. (2008). Subcutaneous methylnaltrexone for the treatment of opioid-induced constipation in patients with advanced illness: A double-blind, randomized, parallel group, dose-ranging study. *Journal of Pain and Symptom Management, 5*(5), 458–468.

Radbruch, L., Sabatwski, R., Loick, G., Kulbe, C., & Casper, M. (2000). Constipation and the use of laxatives: A comparison between transdermal fentanyl and oral morphine. *Palliative Medicine, 13*(2), 111–119.

Ramkumar, D., & Rao, S.S. (2005). Efficacy and safety of traditional medical therapies for chronic constipation: Systematic review. *American Journal of Gastroenterology, 100*(4), 936–971.

Richmond, J.P., & Wright, M.E. (2004). Review of the literature on constipation to enable development of a constipation risk assessment scale. *Clinical Effectiveness in Nursing, 8*(1), 11–25.

Robinson, C.B., Fritch, M., Hullett, L., Petersen, M.A., Sikkema, S., Theuninck, L., et al. (2000). Development of a protocol to prevent opioid-induced constipation in patients with cancer: A research utilization project. *Clinical Journal of Oncology Nursing, 4*(2), 79–84.

Rubin, G. (2004, June). Constipation in children. *Clinical Evidence, 2004*(11), 385–390.

Shiova, L., Rim, F., Friedman, D., & Jahdi, M. (2007). A review of methylnaltrexone, a peripheral opioid receptor antagonist, and its role in opioid-induced constipation. *Palliative and Supportive Care, 5*(2), 161–166.

Smith, S. (2001). Evidence-based management of constipation in the oncology patient. *European Journal of Oncology Nursing, 5*(1), 18–25.

Sutton, D., Dumbleton, S., & Allway, C. (2007). Can increased dietary fiber reduce laxative requirement in peritoneal dialysis patients? *Journal of Renal Care, 33*(4), 177–178.

Szodja, M.M., Mulder, C.J., & Felt-Bersma, R.J. (2007). Differences in taste between two polyethylene glycol preparations. *Journal of Gastrointestinal and Liver Diseases, 16*(4), 379–381.

Taguchi, A., Sharma, N., Saleem, R.M., Sessler, D.I., Carpenter, R.L., Seyedsadr, M., et al. (2001). Selective postoperative inhibition of gastrointestinal opioid receptors. *New England Journal of Medicine, 345*(13), 935–940.

Tamayo, A.C., & Diaz-Zuluaga, P.A. (2004). Management of opioid-induced bowel dysfunction in cancer patients. *Supportive Care in Cancer, 12*(9), 613–618.

Thomas, J. (2007a). Cancer-related constipation. *Current Oncology Reports, 9*(4), 278–284.

Thomas, J. (2007b). Opioid-induced bowel dysfunction. *Journal of Pain and Symptom Management, 35*(1), 103–113.

Thomas, J., Karver, S., Cooney, G.A., Chamberlain, B.H., Watt, C.K., Slatkin, N.E., et al. (2008). Methylnaltrexone for opioid induced constipation in advanced illness. *New England Journal of Medicine,* 358(22), 2332–2343.

Tofil, N.M., Benner, K.W., Faro, S.J., & Winkler, M.K. (2006). The use of enteral naloxone to treat opioid-induced constipation in a pediatric intensive care unit. *Pediatric Critical Care Medicine, 7*(3), 252–254.

U.S. Food and Drug Administration. (2007). *FDA public health advisory: Tegaserod maleate (marketed as Zelnorm).* Retrieved March 30, 2007, from http://www.fda.gov/cder/drug/advisory/tegaserod.htm

Webster, L., Jansen, J.P., Peppin, J., Lasko, B., Iriving, G., Morlion, B., et al. (2008). Alvimopan, a peripherally acting mu-opioid receptor (PAM-OR) antagonist for the treatment of opioid-induced bowel dysfunction: Results from a randomized, double-blind, placebo controlled, dose-finding study in subjects taking opioids for chronic non-cancer pain. *Pain, 137*(2), 428–440.

Wenk, R., Bertolino, M., Ochoa, J., Cullen, C., Bertucelli, N., & Bruera, E. (2000). Laxative effects of fresh baker's yeast. *Journal of Pain and Symptom Management, 19*(3), 163–164.

Wirz, S., & Klaschik, E. (2005). Management of constipation in palliative care patients undergoing opioid therapy: Is polyethylene glycol an option? *American Journal of Hospice and Palliative Medicine, 22*(5), 375–381.

Yuan, C.S., & Israel, R.J. (2006). Methylnaltrexone, a novel peripheral opioid receptor antagonist for the treatment of opioid side effects. *Expert Opinion on Investigational Drugs, 15*(5), 541–552.

Zanetti, G., Marchiori, E., Gasparetto, T.D., Escuissato, D.L., & Souza, A.S. (2007). Lipoid pneumonia in children following aspiration of mineral oil used in the treatment of constipation: High resolution CT findings in 17 patients. *Pediatric Radiology, 37*(11), 1135–1139.

CHAPTER 8

Depression

Problem

According to the American Psychiatric Association's (APA's) *Diagnostic and Statistical Manual of Mental Disorders*, symptoms indicative of a depression diagnosis include depressed mood, markedly diminished interest or pleasure in activities that formerly were enjoyed, behavioral disturbances in eating and sleeping, social withdrawal, loss of energy, feelings of worthlessness or excessive guilt, diminished ability to think or concentrate, and recurrent thoughts of death or suicide. These symptoms are present much of the time for more than two weeks (APA, 2000). Depressive symptoms are present in several psychiatric disorders common to patients with cancer, including major depressive disorder, adjustment disorder, and depression secondary to a medical condition. Depressive symptoms also can be present in the absence of a psychiatric disorder (Pirl, 2004).

Incidence

The incidence of depression in people with cancer is significantly higher than in the general population (Holland, 2002). At least 25% of people diagnosed with cancer experience depression (Martin & Jackson, 2000).

Assessment

The two levels of assessment for depression are screening and diagnostic. Screening is a brief process to establish the presence and intensity of the problem. The U.S. Preventive Services Task Force (2002) recommends that primary care clinicians routinely screen adult and older adult clients for depression. Screening can be done by asking a question such as "Are you depressed most of the day nearly every day?" (Barsevick & Much, 2004). Because some individuals may not admit to feeling depressed, clinicians should not rely solely on one screening question but should do a more detailed assessment (see Table 8-1) that includes use of a clinical measurement tool. The diagnosis of clinical depression is made by a trained professional through the evaluation of specific symptoms or behaviors.

Table 8-1. Depression Assessment Guide		
Assessment	Yes	No
Physical Symptoms		
• Changes in appetite, weight, sleep, and psychomotor activity		
• Decreased energy		
Psychosocial Symptoms		
• Feelings of worthlessness or guilt		
• Recurrent thoughts of death or suicidal ideation, plans, or attempts		
Cognitive Changes		
• Difficulty thinking, concentrating, or making decisions		
• Flat affect		
Risk and Contributing Factors		
• Medications		
• Family history		
• Medical conditions (e.g., endocrine disorders, cardiovascular conditions, neurologic conditions, immune disorders)		
• History of substance abuse		
Note. Based on information from Albright & Valente, 2006; Dahlin, 2006.		

Clinical Measurement Tools

The following self-report clinical measurement tools (see Table 8-2) can help busy clinicians identify people with cancer who may be at risk for clinical depression and need further evaluation by a trained professional (Valente & Saunders, 2005).
1. Hospital Anxiety and Depression Scale
2. Beck Depression Inventory
3. Zung Self-Rating Depression Scale (ZSDS) (see Figure 8-1)

References

Albright, A.V., & Valente, S.M. (2006). Depression and suicide. In R.M. Carroll-Johnson, L.M. Gorman, & N.J. Bush (Eds.), *Psychosocial nursing care along the cancer continuum* (2nd ed., pp. 241–260). Pittsburgh, PA: Oncology Nursing Society.

American Psychiatric Association. (2000). *Diagnostic and statistical manual of mental disorders* (4th ed., text revision). Washington, DC: Author.

Badger, T. (2005). *Measuring oncology-nursing sensitive patient outcomes: Evidence-based summary.* Retrieved March 4, 2008, from http://www.ons.org/outcomes/measures/pdf/DepressionOverview.pdf

Barsevick, A.M., & Much, J.K. (2004). Depression. In C.H. Yarbro, M.H. Frogge, & M. Goodman (Eds.), *Cancer symptom management* (3rd ed., pp. 668–692). Sudbury, MA: Jones and Bartlett.

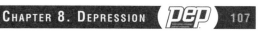

Table 8-2. Clinical Measurement Tools for Depression

Name of Tool	Number of Items	Domains	Reliability and Validity	Populations	Clinical Utility
Hospital Anxiety and Depression Scale	14 (7 items for each subscale)	Severity of depression and anxiety	Adequate reliability and validity established	Mixed cancer diagnoses, breast cancer	Easy to use Short
Beck Depression Inventory	21 (long form) 13 (short form)	Behavioral, cognitive, and somatic components of depression; focuses on negative attitudes of the patient toward self	Adequate reliability established; construct and criterion validity supported	Breast, lymphoma, head and neck, prostate	Two to five minutes to complete Easy to use
Zung Self-Rating Depression Scale	20	Frequency of symptoms and depression	Adequate reliability established; adequate construct and criterion validity supported	Mixed cancer diagnoses	Easy to use

Note. Based on information from Badger, 2005.

Figure 8-1. Zung Self-Rating Depression Scale

	None or a Little of the Time	Some of the Time	Good Part of the Time	Most or All of the Time
1. I feel down-hearted and sad	1	2	3	4
2. Morning is when I feel the best	1	2	3	4
3. I have crying spells or feel like it	1	2	3	4
4. I have trouble sleeping through the night	1	2	3	4
5. I eat as much as I used to	1	2	3	4
6. I still enjoy sex	1	2	3	4
7. I notice that I am losing weight	1	2	3	4

(Continued on next page)

Figure 8-1. Zung Self-Rating Depression Scale *(Continued)*				
	None or a Little of the Time	Some of the Time	Good Part of the Time	Most or All of the Time
8. I have trouble with constipation	1	2	3	4
9. My heart beats faster than usual	1	2	3	4
10. I get tired for no reason	1	2	3	4
11. My mind is as clear as it used to be	1	2	3	4
12. I find it easy to do the things I used to	1	2	3	4
13. I am restless and can't keep still	1	2	3	4
14. I feel hopeful about the future	1	2	3	4
15. I am more irritable than usual	1	2	3	4
16. I find it easy to make decisions	1	2	3	4
17. I feel that I am useful and needed	1	2	3	4
18. My life is pretty full	1	2	3	4
19. I feel that others would be better off if I were dead	1	2	3	4
20. I still enjoy the things I used to do	1	2	3	4

Key for Scoring the Zung Self-Rating Depression Scale

Raw Score

Total SDS Index = _____ × 100

Maximum Score of 80

SDS Index	Equivalent Clinical Global Impression
Below 50	= Within normal range, no psychopathology
50–59	= Presence of minimal to mild depression
60–69	= Presence of moderate to marked depression
70 & over	= Presence of severe to most extreme depression

Note. From "A Self-Rating Depression Scale," by W.K. Zung, 1965, *Archives of General Psychiatry, 12,* 65–66. Copyright 1965 by American Medical Association. Reprinted with permission.

Dahlin, C. (2006). Depression. In D. Camp-Sorrell & R.A. Hawkins (Eds.), *Clinical manual for the oncology advanced practice nurse* (2nd ed., pp. 1119–1125). Pittsburgh, PA: Oncology Nursing Society.

Holland, J.C. (2002). History of psycho-oncology: Overcoming attitudinal and conceptual barriers. *Psychosomatic Medicine, 64*(2), 206–221.

Martin, A.C., & Jackson, K.C. (2000). Depression in palliative care patients. *Journal of Pharmaceutical Care in Pain and Symptom Control, 7*(4), 71–89.

Pirl, W.F. (2004). Evidence report on the occurrence, assessment, and treatment of depression in cancer patients. *Journal of the National Cancer Institute Monographs, 2004*(32), 32–39.

U.S. Preventive Services Task Force. (2002). *Screening for depression.* Retrieved August 20, 2008, from http://www.ahrq.gov/clinic/uspstf/uspsdepr.htm

Valente, S.M., & Saunders, J. (2005). Screening for depression and suicide: Self-report instruments that work. *Journal of Psychosocial Nursing and Mental Health Services, 43*(11), 22–31, 46–47.

Case Study

J.D. was a 44-year-old male who was diagnosed with multiple myeloma three years ago. He was married and had a teenage daughter and a son in elementary school. Before his diagnosis, he owned a successful lawn care company but later had to sell the company. His wife worked, and he was receiving Social Security disability insurance. His health insurance coverage was Medicaid, and he had a monthly spenddown. J.D. quit smoking soon after he was diagnosed. He had used alcohol socially in the past, but his wife stated that he had been drinking beer every night recently. His current treatment plan included PO daily thalidomide and weekly IV bortezomib maintenance.

J.D. and his wife had recently separated but were back together. They both admitted that he had anger issues. In fact, on the way to the office visit, he became enraged at another driver and almost ran him off the road. His wife stated that J.D. spent most of his time in a chair in the living room, often sleeping during the day, and then was unable to sleep at night. He rarely helped with household chores or child care. J.D. admitted that he did very little but said that he loved his wife and children. He said that he was very angry about having an "old man's disease" and that he often felt anxious, overwhelmed, and depressed.

After first assessing J.D.'s risk for harm to himself or others (he denied any suicidal ideality or thoughts of harming others), the nurse reviewed the interventions listed on the Oncology Nursing Society (ONS) Putting Evidence Into Practice (PEP) resource on depression. His score for depression on the ZSDS was 66.

Recommended for Practice

As recommended on the ONS PEP resource on depression, the nurse should discuss counseling and/or antidepressant medication with the patient. The nurse also should assess the patient and family members for depression and depression symptoms at every visit as well as their understanding of depression. Verbal and written information on depression in patients with cancer and treatment options should be offered.

Likely to Be Effective

Interventions found likely to be effective include offering a referral for relaxation therapy. This includes progressive muscle relaxation, guided imagery, and combination therapy with both progressive muscle relaxation and guided imagery.

Effectiveness Not Established

Complementary and alternative therapy has been characterized as effectiveness not established. This includes the interventions of massage therapy and hypnotherapy.

Initial Visit

J.D. declined counseling and psychotherapy at the time but promised to reconsider his decision in the future. He also declined referral for relaxation therapy. He agreed to pharmacologic intervention. Zoloft® (sertraline, Pfizer Inc.) 50 mg PO daily was prescribed for depression, and Ativan® (lorazepam, Biovail Corp.) 0.5 mg PO was prescribed up to three times daily PRN for anxiety for short-term use. The nurse practitioner worked with J.D. and his wife to set reasonable daily activity goals, and J.D. agreed to physical therapy referral for reconditioning if he was not successful on his own. A follow-up appointment was scheduled for one month.

One-Month Follow-Up

At his one-month follow-up appointment, both J.D. and his wife expressed that they had seen some improvement in his anxiety, anger, and depression. He had increased his daily activity but not on a consistent basis. His Zoloft was increased to 100 mg PO daily, and his Ativan was continued for one more month. A follow-up appointment was made for one month. His ZSDS score for depression was 62.

Two-Month Follow-Up

At the return appointment, J.D. and his wife voiced much improvement in his anxiety, anger, and depression. His level of daily activity and family involvement had increased, and he was now getting the children up for school on a daily basis. Zoloft was continued at 100 mg daily, and J.D. will be weaned off the PRN Ativan. For the time being, J.D. preferred to continue with monthly follow-ups. His ZSDS score for depression was 54.

Kristi Bowser, NPC, AOCNP®
Oncology Nurse Practitioner, Gynecologic Oncology
University of Toledo Medical Center
Toledo, OH

Depression

2009 AUTHORS
Caryl D. Fulcher, RN, MSN, CNS-BC, and Terry A. Badger, PhD, PMHCNS-BC, FAAN
ONS STAFF: Heather Belansky, RN, MSN

2007 AUTHORS
Terry A. Badger, PhD, RN, CS, FAAN, Caryl D. Fulcher, MSN, RN, CNS-BC,
Ashley K. Gunter, RN, BSN, OCN®, Joyce A. Marrs, MS, APRN,BC, AOCNP®, and Jill M. Reese, RN, BSN, OCN®
ONS STAFF: Robi Thomas, MS, RN, AOCN®, CHPN

What can nurses do to assist people with cancer who also have depression or depressive symptoms?

Recommended for Practice

Interventions for which effectiveness has been demonstrated by strong evidence from rigorously designed studies, meta-analyses, or systematic reviews and for which expectation of harms is small compared with the benefits

PSYCHOEDUCATIONAL/PSYCHOSOCIAL INTERVENTIONS

Psychoeducational/psychosocial interventions include
- Cognitive behavioral therapy
- Patient education and information
- Counseling/psychotherapy
- Behavioral therapy
- Social support.

With the exception of patient education and information and social support, these psychoeducational and psychosocial interventions require advanced education and training.

Evidence at the highest level (Antoni et al., 2001; Barsevick, Sweeney, Haney, & Chung, 2002; Bennett & Badger, 2005; Given et al., 2004; Manne et al., 2007; Newell, Sanson-Fisher, & Savolainem, 2002; Osborn, Demoncada, & Feuerstein, 2006; Pirl, 2004; Scheier et al., 2005; Uitterhoeve et al., 2004; Vilela et al., 2006; Williams & Dale, 2006) supports the benefit of psychoeducational/psychosocial interventions in the management of depressive symptoms during and following cancer treatment in patients with different types of cancer. Although considerable variability exists in the frequency and duration of the interventions, the majority of studies support that such interventions are effective for reducing depressive symptoms; fewer studies support that such interventions are effective for a diagnosis of depression (Williams & Dale). Of the psychosocial interventions studied, the strongest evidence is for cognitive behavioral therapy. Effectiveness was found for both individual and group interventions. However, in one study of highly distressed, recurrent-disease patients, a peer-delivered telephone intervention to provide support was well accepted but produced no benefit on depressive symptoms (Gotay et al., 2007). More research is needed to systematically examine the intervention dosage (frequency, duration) required for effectiveness among the different types of psychoeducational/psychosocial interventions for diverse cancer subpopulations.

PHARMACOLOGIC INTERVENTIONS

Antidepressant Medications

Several treatment studies of depression in patients with cancer support using tricyclic antidepressants (TCAs), selective serotonin reuptake inhibitors (SSRIs), mianserin*, and others (Goodnick & Hernandez, 2000; Ly, Chidgey, Addington-Hall, & Hotopf, 2002; Pirl, 2004; Rodin et al., 2007; Schwartz, Lander, & Chochinov, 2002). No differences were found in the effectiveness between TCAs and SSRIs; however, the lower incidence of side effects in SSRIs makes them preferable in patients with cancer. In older patients with cancer, the anticholinergic effects of TCAs are particularly problematic, and their use for treatment of depression has diminished. SSRIs should be started at lower doses in older patients and titrated more slowly (Winell & Roth, 2005). Although no studies have specifically examined the newer serotonin-norepinephrine reuptake inhibitor duloxetine in patients with depression and cancer, its similarity to venlafaxine makes it likely to be similarly effective. One study found that pretreatment of patients with malignant melanoma with paroxetine significantly decreased the development of major depression in patients receiving interferon and decreased the likelihood that interferon would have to be discontinued because of severe depression (Musselman et al., 2001).

Clinical practice guidelines also support the benefit of medication interventions and concur that no evidence exists that a particular antidepressant is superior to another, but rather selection should be based on side effects and patient needs (National Comprehensive Cancer Network [NCCN], 2006; National Health and Medical Research Council, 2003; Qaseem et al., 2008). The clinical practice guidelines also state that patients with cancer may respond to a lower dose of TCAs and recommend medications with short half-lives in patients with hepatic or renal dysfunction. Palliative care guidelines also derived evidence from patients with cancer (Qaseem et al.) and support use of TCAs or SSRIs; other guidelines exist for the treatment of depression, and although they are not specific to patients with cancer and depression, they provide useful information on antidepressant selection, dose adjustment, and monitoring (American Psychiatric Association [APA], 2000; Ministry of Health, Singapore, 2004).

Antidepressant Medications Used in Patients With Cancer

SSRIs
- Fluoxetine (Prozac®, Eli Lilly & Co.)
- Fluvoxamine
- Sertraline (Zoloft®, Pfizer)
- Paroxetine (Paxil®, GlaxoSmithKline)
- Citalopram (Celexa®, Forest Laboratories)
- Escitalopram (Lexapro®, Forest Laboratories)

TCAs
- Amitriptyline
- Imipramine (Tofranil®, Tyco Healthcare)
- Desipramine (Norpramin®, Sanofi-Aventis)
- Nortriptyline (Pamelor®, Tyco Healthcare)
- Doxepin (Sinequan®, Pfizer)

Serotonin-Norepinephrine Reuptake Inhibitors
- Venlafaxine (Effexor®, Wyeth)
- Desvenlafaxine (Pristiq®, Wyeth)
- Duloxetine (Cymbalta®, Eli Lilly & Co.)

Other Antidepressants
- Mirtazapine (Remeron®, Organon USA)
- Bupropion (Wellbutrin®, GlaxoSmithKline)
- Trazodone (Desyrel®, Bristol-Myers Squibb)
- Mianserin*

Likely to Be Effective

Interventions for which effectiveness has been demonstrated by supportive evidence from a single rigorously conducted controlled trial, consistent supportive evidence from well-designed controlled trials using small samples, or guidelines developed from evidence and supported by expert opinion

METHYLPHENIDATE (RITALIN®)

The benefit of this central nervous system stimulant in patients with advanced cancer and associated depression is discussed in one phase II study (Homsi et al., 2001) and one systematic review (Rozans, Dreisbach, Lertora, & Kahn, 2002). It is used most often in advanced cancer and palliative situations because of its rapid onset of action and low record of side effects. Doses range from 10–40 mg daily. In a review of nine studies, it was concluded that methylphenidate is useful in treating depression in a variety of malignancies, with > 80% of patients responding favorably and < 20% reporting side effects (Rozans et al.). Methylphenidate also is used to address opioid-induced somnolence, to augment opioid effects, and to improve cognitive functioning in patients with cancer. These benefits may contribute to mood improvement (Rozans et al.).

COMPLEMENTARY/ALTERNATIVE THERAPY

Relaxation Therapy
This includes techniques that focus on inducing a relaxed physical and mental state, such as progressive muscle relaxation with or without guided imagery, hypnosis, and autogenic training (Luebbert, Dahme, & Hasenbring, 2001). Relaxation training was found to have a significant impact on reducing cancer treatment–related side effects, including depression. Another small study assigned patients to one of four treatment conditions: progressive muscle relaxation, guided imagery, both progressive muscle relaxation and guided imagery, or a control group with no treatment (Sloman, 2002). Those in the three treatment conditions showed a reduction in depression three weeks after the initial session; no one treatment proved to be superior.

Benefits Balanced With Harms

Interventions for which clinicians and patients should weigh the beneficial and harmful effects according to individual circumstances and priorities

There are no interventions as of May 2008.

Effectiveness Not Established

Interventions for which insufficient or conflicting data or data of inadequate quality currently exist, with no clear indication of harm

COMPLEMENTARY/ALTERNATIVE THERAPY

Exercise

The impact of a multidimensional exercise program on self-reported anxiety and depression was examined in a voluntary sample of men and (predominantly) women undergoing chemotherapy (Berglund et al., 2007). A moderate but significant reduction in depression scores was demonstrated from baseline to six weeks, but depression was already low at baseline, and the self-referred sample and lack of control group contribute to limited ability to generalize. Another study retrospectively analyzed physical function, fatigue, and mood in a small sample of adult patients with cancer, most of whom had completed treatment (Hanna, Avila, Meteer, Nicholas, & Kaminsky, 2008). Exercise and educational sessions were evaluated at baseline and after the completion of 16 exercise sessions, and all three outcomes demonstrated improvement. Although promising, the study's limitations do not allow practice recommendation; thus, effectiveness is not established for exercise programs as an intervention for depression in people with cancer.

Hypnotherapy

This intervention is a behavioral therapy using hypnosis to induce heightened concentration, receptivity, and relaxation. One systematic review reported the results of 27 studies conducted between 1974 and 2003 using hypnotherapy for symptom relief in terminally ill adult patients with cancer (Rajasekaran, Edmonds, & Higginson, 2005). Of the studies reported, only one was a randomized controlled trial. In this study, a statistically significant reduction in depression and anxiety scores was demonstrated in patients who were assigned hypnotherapy compared with the standard group (Rajasekaran et al.). It should be noted that although few adverse effects were reported overall, some patients reported that they were unable to enter a deep trance or were frightened by the treatment (Rajasekaran et al.).

Massage Therapy

This therapy involves manipulation of soft tissue areas of the body and is offered to assist in relaxation, aid in sleep, and relieve muscle tension and pain (Cassileth & Vickers, 2004). Approximately one in three studies that were included in a systematic review (Fellowes, Barnes, & Wilkinson, 2004) found a beneficial effect on cancer-related depression. The most consistent effect on symptom relief in patients with cancer was reduction in anxiety following intervention (Fellowes et al.).

Three studies evaluated the effect of massage therapy. One group conducted a randomized study with female participants with breast cancer who were at least three months post-treatment (Hernandez-Reif et al., 2004). They received massage three times weekly for five weeks, and their depressed mood decreased, both pre- and post-session and first-last days. The other group conducted a nonrandomized study looking at symptom relief from massage therapy (Cassileth & Vickers, 2004). Self-reported symptom scores were reduced by approximately 50%; those reporting depression demonstrated 48.9% improvement in their scores. Scoring was done 2–48 hours after massage, so the scores reflect immediate rather than long-term effect. In a third study of aromatherapy, 42 patients with advanced cancer received weekly massages with lavender, with an inert oil, or no intervention. A statistically significant reduction in depression scores was observed in the inert oil massage group; however, study limitations do not allow widespread generalizability, making effectiveness not established (Soden, Vincent, Craske, Lucas, & Ashley, 2004).

Special Considerations

Other complementary methods such as taking St. John's wort or other nutritional and herbal supplements and practicing yoga, acupuncture, aromatherapy, and meditation have not been studied specifically in the setting of patients with cancer and depression. Some of these interventions may benefit quality of life or even mood; however, they should not be generalized to depression.

Effectiveness Unlikely

Interventions for which lack of effectiveness has been demonstrated by negative evidence from a single rigorously conducted controlled trial, consistent negative evidence from well-designed controlled trials using small samples, or guidelines developed from evidence and supported by expert opinion

There are no interventions as of May 2008.

Not Recommended for Practice

Interventions for which lack of effectiveness or harmfulness has been demonstrated by strong evidence from rigorously conducted studies, meta-analyses, or systematic reviews, or interventions where the costs, burden, or harms associated with the intervention exceed anticipated benefit

There are no interventions as of May 2008.

Expert Opinion

Low-risk interventions that are (1) consistent with sound clinical practice, (2) suggested by an expert in a peer-reviewed publication (journal or book chapter), and (3) for which limited evidence exists. An expert is an individual who has published articles in a peer-reviewed journal in the domain of interest.

Experts recommend the following interventions for patients experiencing depressive symptoms and/or depression during and following cancer treatment (NCCN, 2006; Sadock & Sadock, 2003; Sharpe et al., 2004).
- Assess patients and family members for depression and depressive symptoms at every encounter.
  - When evaluating depressed patients with cancer, include consideration of medical, endocrine, and neurologic problems. Also evaluate losses secondary to cancer, the patients' experience of cancer deaths, and their understanding of their current medical illness, including prognosis (Miller & Massie, 2006).

- Assess patients' and families' understanding of depression and its role in cancer recovery, as well as the meaning of depression to patients and their families.
- Provide education to patients and their families about depression and its management.

Although no evidence exists on the combination of antidepressant medication plus psycho-educational/psychosocial therapy in patients with cancer and depression, expert opinion and clinical practice guidelines for treatment of depression recommend combined therapy for severe and chronic depression, finding it more effective than either alone (APA, 2000; Miller & Massie, 2006; Ministry of Health, Singapore, 2004).

* This drug has not been approved by the U.S. Food and Drug Administration for use in the United States.

Definitions of the interventions are available at **www.ons.org/outcomes**.
Literature search completed through May 2008.

References

American Psychiatric Association. (2000, April). *Practice guideline for the treatment of patients with major depressive disorder* (2nd ed.). Retrieved November 10, 2006, from http://www.psychiatryonline.com/pracGuide/pracGuideChapToc_7.aspx

Antoni, M.H., Lehman, J.M., Kilbourn, K.M., Boyers, A.E., Culver, J.L., Alferi, S.M., et al. (2001). Cognitive-behavioral stress management intervention decreases the prevalence of depression and enhances benefit finding among women under treatment for early-stage breast cancer. *Health Psychology, 20*(1), 20–32.

Barsevick, A.M., Sweeney, C., Haney, E., & Chung, E. (2002). A systematic qualitative analysis of psychoeducational interventions for depression in patients with cancer. *Oncology Nursing Forum, 29*(1), 73–84.

Bennett, G., & Badger, T.A. (2005). Depression in men with prostate cancer. *Oncology Nursing Forum, 32*(3), 545–556.

Berglund, G., Petersson, L.-M, Eriksson, K.C., Wallenius, I., Roshanai, A., Nordin, K.M., et al. (2007). "Between Men": A psychosocial rehabilitation programme for men with prostate cancer. *Acta Oncologica, 46*(1), 83–89.

Cassileth, B.R., & Vickers, A.J. (2004). Massage therapy for symptom control: Outcome study at a major cancer center. *Journal of Pain and Symptom Management, 28*(3), 244–249.

Fellowes, D., Barnes, K., & Wilkinson, S. (2004). Aromatherapy and massage for symptom relief in patients with cancer. *Cochrane Database of Systematic Reviews* 2004, Issue 3. Art. No.: CD002287. DOI: 10.1002/14651858.CD002287.pub3.

Given, C., Given, B., Rahbar, M., Jean, S., McCorkle, R., & Cimprich, B. (2004). Does a symptom management intervention affect depression among cancer patients: Results from a clinical trial. *Psycho-Oncology, 13*(11), 818–830.

Goodnick, P.J., & Hernandez, M. (2000). Treatment of depression in comorbid medical illness. *Expert Opinion on Pharmacotherapy, 1*(7), 1367–1384.

Gotay, C.C., Moinpour, C.M., Unger, J.M., Jiang, C.S., Coleman, D., Martino, S., et al. (2007). Impact of a peer-delivered telephone intervention for women experiencing a breast cancer recurrence. *Journal of Clinical Oncology, 25*(15), 2093–2098.

Hanna, L.R., Avila, P.F., Meteer, J.D., Nicholas, D.R., & Kaminsky, L.A. (2008). The effects of a comprehensive exercise program on physical function, fatigue, and mood in patients with various types of cancer. *Oncology Nursing Forum, 35*(3), 461–469.

Hernandez-Reif, M., Ironson, G., Field, T., Hurley, J., Katz, G., Diego, M., et al. (2004). Breast cancer patients have improved immune and neuroendocrine functions following massage therapy. *Journal of Psychosomatic Research, 57*(1), 45–52.

Homsi, J., Nelson, K.A., Sarhill, N., Rybicki, L., LeGrand, S.B., Davis, M.P., et al. (2001). A phase II study of methylphenidate for depression in advanced cancer. *American Journal of Hospice and Palliative Care, 18*(6), 403–407.

Luebbert, K., Dahme, B., & Hasenbring, M. (2001). The effectiveness of relaxation training in reducing treatment related symptoms and improving emotional adjustment in acute and non-surgical cancer treatment: A meta-analytical review. *Psycho-Oncology, 10*(6), 490–502.

Ly, K.L., Chidgey, J., Addington-Hall, J., & Hotopf, M. (2002). Depression in palliative care: A systematic review. Part 2: Treatment. *Palliative Medicine, 16*(4), 279–284.

Manne, S.L., Rubin, S., Edelson, M., Rosenblum, N., Bergman, C., Hernandez, E., et al. (2007). Coping and communication-enhancing intervention versus supportive counseling for women diagnosed with gynecological cancers. *Journal of Consulting and Clinical Psychology, 75*(4), 615–628.

Miller, K., & Massie, M.J. (2006). Depression and anxiety. *Cancer Journal, 12*(5), 388–397.

Ministry of Health, Singapore. (2004). *Clinical practice guidelines: Depression.* Retrieved November 10, 2006, from http://www.moh.gov.sg/mohcorp/publications.aspx?id=16352

Musselman, D.L., Lawson, D.H., Gumnick, J.F., Manatunga, A.K., Penna, S., Goodkin, R.S., et al. (2001). Paroxetine for the prevention of depression induced by high-dose interferon alfa. *New England Journal of Medicine, 344*(13), 961–966.

National Comprehensive Cancer Network. (2006). *NCCN Clinical Practice Guidelines in Oncology™: Distress management* [v. 1.2007]. Retrieved November 10, 2006, from http://www.nccn.org/professionals/physician_gls/PDF/distress.pdf

National Health and Medical Research Council (Australia). (2003). *Clinical practice guidelines for the psychosocial care of adults with cancer.* Retrieved November 10, 2006, from http://www.nhmrc.gov.au/publications/synopses/cp90syn.htm

Newell, S.A., Sanson-Fisher, R.W., & Savolainen, N.J. (2002). Systematic review of psychological therapies for cancer patients: Overview and recommendations for future research. *Journal of the National Cancer Institute, 94*(8), 558–584.

Osborn, R.L., Demoncada, A.C., & Feuerstein, M. (2006). Psychosocial interventions for depression, anxiety, and quality of life in cancer survivors: Meta-analyses. *International Journal of Psychiatry in Medicine, 36*(1), 13–34.

Pirl, W.F. (2004). Evidence report on the occurrence, assessment, and treatment of depression in cancer patients. *Journal of the National Cancer Institute Monographs, 2004*(32), 32–39.

Qaseem, A., Snow, V., Shekelle, P., Casey, D.E., Cross, J.R., & Owens, D.K. (2008). Evidence-based interventions to improve the palliative care of pain, dyspnea, and depression at the end of life: A clinical practice guideline from the American College of Physicians. *Annals of Internal Medicine, 148*(2), 141–146.

Rajasekaran, M., Edmonds, P.M., & Higginson, I.L. (2005). Systematic review of hypnotherapy for treating symptoms in terminally ill adult cancer patients. *Palliative Medicine, 19*(5), 418–426.

Rodin, G., Lloyd, N., Katz, M., Green, E., Mackay, J.A., & Wong, R.K.S. (2007). The treatment of depression in cancer patients: A systematic review. *Supportive Care in Cancer, 15*(2), 123–136.

Rozans, M., Dreisbach, A., Lertora, J.J., & Kahn, M.J. (2002). Palliative uses of methylphenidate in patients with cancer: A review. *Journal of Clinical Oncology, 20*(1), 335–339.

Sadock, B.J., & Sadock, V.A. (2003). *Kaplan & Sadock's synopsis of psychiatry: Behavioral sciences/clinical psychiatry* (9th ed.). Philadelphia: Lippincott Williams & Wilkins.

Scheier, M.F., Helgeson, V.S., Schulz, R., Colvin, S., Berga, S., Bridges, M.W., et al. (2005). Interventions to enhance physical and psychological functioning among younger women who are ending nonhormonal adjuvant treatment for early-stage breast cancer. *Journal of Clinical Oncology, 23*(19), 4298–4311.

Schwartz, L., Lander, M., & Chochinov, H.M. (2002). Current management of depression in cancer patients. *Oncology, 16*(8), 1102–1115.

Sharpe, M., Strong, V., Allen, K., Rush, R., Maguire, P., House, A., et al. (2004). Management of major depression in outpatients attending a centre: A preliminary evaluation of a multicomponent cancer nurse-delivered intervention. *British Journal of Cancer, 90*(2), 310–313.

Sloman, R. (2002). Relaxation and imagery for anxiety and depression control in community patients with advanced cancer. *Cancer Nursing, 25*(6), 432–435.

Soden, K., Vincent, K., Craske, S., Lucas, C., & Ashley, S. (2004). A randomized controlled trial of aromatherapy massage in a hospice setting. *Palliative Medicine, 18*(2), 87–92.

Uitterhoeve, R.J., Vernooy, M., Litjens, M., Potting, K., Bensing, J., De Mulderf, P., et al. (2004). Psychosocial interventions for patients with advanced cancer—A systematic review of the literature. *British Journal of Cancer, 91*(6), 1050–1062.

Vilela, L.D., Nicolau, B., Mahmud, S., Edgar, L., Hier, M., Black, M., et al. (2006). Comparison of psychosocial outcomes in head and neck cancer patients receiving a coping strategies intervention and control subjects receiving no intervention. *Journal of Otolaryngology, 35*(2), 88–96.

Williams, S., & Dale, J. (2006). The effectiveness of treatment for depression/depressive symptoms in adults with cancer: A systematic review. *British Journal of Cancer, 94*(3), 372–390.

Winell, J., & Roth, A. (2005). Psychiatric assessment and symptom management in elderly cancer patients. *Oncology, 19*(11), 1479–1507.

CHAPTER **9**

Diarrhea

Problem

Diarrhea is an abnormal increase in stool liquidity and stool frequency (≥ to four to six stools per day over baseline), with or without nocturnal bowel movements, and may be accompanied by abdominal cramping (Eastern Cooperative Oncology Group, 2007; National Cancer Institute Cancer Therapy Evaluation Program [NCI CTEP], 2006; Sabol & Carlson, 2007; World Health Organization, n.d.).

Incidence

In patients receiving chemotherapy, the incidence of diarrhea can approach 50%–80% (Engelking, 2000). It is a potential complication with a number of chemotherapy agents and can be particularly problematic in patients with colorectal cancer and other gastrointestinal malignancies. Diarrhea can be an underrecognized cause of symptom distress and can affect quality of life. If not managed properly, it can also become life threatening in specific subsets of patients (Engelking, 2004).

Agents such as the fluoropyrimidines and irinotecan are often the most common inducers of diarrhea. In recent years, the epidermal growth factor receptor inhibitors have emerged as newer agents that also cause diarrhea. Cancer-related diarrhea can be experienced by patients with carcinoid tumors (up to 80%), and vasoactive intestinal polypeptide tumors (known as VIPomas), a type of neuroendocrine tumor (> 30%). Diarrhea also may be a complication of bone marrow transplantation and radiation therapy, especially with abdomino-pelvic fields. It also is a common symptom seen in patients with partial bowel obstructions and can be a cardinal symptom of impaction attributable to constipation, especially related to medications such as opioids (see Chapter 7).

Assessment

Diarrhea is both a sign and a symptom, as it has objective and subjective components. A baseline assessment of bowel function is critical, as patients who have had abdomino-pelvic surgery, other abdominal comorbidities, or primary and/or metastatic disease of the abdomino-pelvic areas may have a baseline function that includes several bowel movements per day or movements that are soft, semi-formed, or liquid. This becomes extremely relevant when measuring and reporting changes from baseline after therapy has been started. Quantifying the degree of diarrhea is important, versus just reporting whether it was present or absent (Saltz, 2003). Nurses are in a position to anticipate the risk of diarrhea in association with malignancy and treatment, and in frequent contact with patients, evaluate the onset and severity of the occurrence. Figure 9-1 provides an assessment tool for baseline and ongoing assessments of diarrhea.

Figure 9-1. Assessment of Diarrhea

Patient History
- Type of cancer and extent of disease
- Past and current therapy (surgery, radiation, chemotherapy)
- History of other surgery/bowel-related problems
- Dietary and fluid habits (especially recent changes)
- Medications (prescriptions and over-the-counter/vitamins/herbals)
- Previous laxative or enema use
- Alcohol use

Baseline Bowel Habits (normal/usual bowel habits prior to cancer treatment)
- Frequency
- Usual quantity
- Consistency (need to know whether abnormal or not), including diameter, if formed
- Color (need to know whether abnormal or not)
- Odor
- History of presence of blood, undigested food, medications

Patient Definition of Diarrhea Assessed (current bowel function: frequency, quantity, character, odor)
- Associated pain, cramping, nausea
- Presence of blood, undigested food, medications
- Occurrence of fecal incontinence or urgency
- Number of stools at night
- Timing of onset of symptoms

Physical Examination Assessments
- Patient weight
- Hydration status

Abdominal Examination
- Auscultation of bowel sounds
- Percussion and palpation of abdominal quadrants

Rectal Examination (for evaluation of the following)
- Impaction
- Fissures, hemorrhoids
- Skin integrity
- Sphincter integrity
- Examination of stool

Pertinent Laboratory Data (i.e., complete blood count, electrolytes, occult blood and other stool evaluations)

Pertinent Radiologic Examinations (i.e., CT abdomen/pelvis, abdominal films, abdominal ultrasound)

Note. Based on information from Engelking, 2004; Gwede, 2003; Viele, 2003.

Clinical Measurement Tools

A summary of the following clinical measurement tools for diarrhea is presented in Table 9-1.
1. Diarrhea Assessment Scale
2. Common Terminology Criteria for Adverse Events (CTCAE) for diarrhea (NCI CTEP, 2006) (see Table 9-2)

Table 9-1. Summary of Clinical Measurement Tools for Diarrhea					
Name of Tool	Number of Items	Domains	Reliability and Validity	Populations	Clinical Utility
Diarrhea Assessment Scale	4	Stool consistency Frequency Urgency Abdominal discomfort	Reliability and validity established in one study Adequate reliability also was found in an unpublished study of quality of life.	Studied in patients receiving pelvic radiation therapy for prostate cancer versus healthy adults, and in those receiving definitive radiotherapy	Used in Radiation Therapy Oncology Group trials
Common Terminology Criteria for Adverse Events	Grading scale	Subjective report of increase in stool numbers, associated symptoms, and need for intervention Differentiates criteria for patients with colostomies	Unknown	Unknown	Primarily used for documenting adverse events in clinical trials of chemotherapy drugs Focuses primarily on number of stools rather than associated symptoms
Note. Based on information from Chambers & McMillan, 2004; National Cancer Institute Cancer Therapy Evaluation Program, 2006; Steele, in press.					

Table 9-2. Common Terminology Criteria for Adverse Events Grading Scale for Diarrhea With or Without Colostomy

Grade	Criteria
1	Increase of < 4 stools per day over baseline; mild increase in ostomy output compared to baseline
2	Increase of 4–6 stools per day over baseline; IV fluids indicated < 24 hours; moderate increase in ostomy output compared to baseline; not interfering with ADL
3	Increase of ≥ 7 stools per day over baseline; incontinence; IV fluids ≥ 24 hours; hospitalization; severe increase in ostomy output compared to baseline; interfering with ADL
4	Life-threatening consequences (e.g., hemodynamic collapse)
5	Death

ADL—activities of daily living

Note. Based on information from National Cancer Institute Cancer Therapy Evaluation Program, 2006.

References

Chambers, K.K., & McMillan, S.C. (2004). Measuring bowel elimination. In M. Frank-Stromborg & S.J. Olsen (Eds.), *Instruments for clinical health-care research* (3rd ed., pp. 487–497). Sudbury, MA: Jones and Bartlett.

Eastern Cooperative Oncology Group. (2007, June). *ECOG common toxicity criteria.* Retrieved November 15, 2007, from http://www.ecog.org/general/ctc.pdf

Engelking, C. (2000). Cancer treatment-related diarrhea: Challenges and barriers to clinical practice. *Oncology Nursing Updates, 5*(2), 1–16.

Engelking, C. (2004). Diarrhea. In C.H. Yarbro, M.H. Frogge, & M. Goodman (Eds.), *Cancer symptom management* (3rd ed., pp. 528–557). Sudbury, MA: Jones and Bartlett.

Gwede, C.K. (2003). Overview of radiation- and chemoradiation-induced diarrhea. *Seminars in Oncology Nursing, 19*(4, Suppl. 3), 6–10.

National Cancer Institute Cancer Therapy Evaluation Program. (2006). *Common terminology criteria for adverse events* (version 3.0). Bethesda, MD: National Cancer Institute. Retrieved November 13, 2007, from http://ctep.cancer.gov/protocolDevelopment/electronic_applications/docs/ctcaev3.pdf

Sabol, V.K., & Carlson, K.K. (2007). Diarrhea—Applying research to bedside practice. *AACN Advanced Critical Care, 18*(1), 32–44.

Saltz, L. (2003). Understanding and managing chemotherapy-induced diarrhea. *Journal of Supportive Oncology, 1*(1), 35–46.

Steele, S.E. (in press). *Measuring oncology nursing-sensitive patient outcomes: Evidence-based summary: Diarrhea.* Pittsburgh, PA: Oncology Nursing Society.

Viele, C.S. (2003). Overview of chemotherapy-induced diarrhea. *Seminars in Oncology Nursing, 19*(4, Suppl. 3), 2–5.

World Health Organization. (n.d.). *WHO toxicity criteria by grade.* Retrieved November 15, 2007, from http://www.fda.gov/cder/cancer/toxicityframe.htm

Case Study

History of Present Illness

S.L. was a 60-year-old male with stage IV colorectal cancer. He was being treated with irinotecan, 5-fluorouracil, and leucovorin. One week after his treatment, he presented to the emergency room complaining of diarrhea and exhaustion.

History

When questioned further, S.L. revealed that he had been having six to eight large, liquid-to-watery stools per day for the past two days. He also stated that his urine was dark in color and that although he was thirsty, he was afraid to drink too much because the fear of having more diarrhea. He also stated that he felt dizzy when standing up too quickly and had been having headaches. He denied any recent antibiotic use.

S.L.'s patient record showed that he was instructed to begin high-dose loperamide with the onset of diarrhea. When questioned how he was taking the loperamide, he replied that he took "two capsules initially and then one capsule every two hours." He stated he was told that he should not take this amount for more than 48 hours, and because his diarrhea was not getting any better, he thought he should get checked (see the *Recommended for Practice* section of the Oncology Nursing Society [ONS] Putting Evidence Into Practice [PEP] resource on diarrhea).

Physical Examination

A physical examination finding was that S.L. was orthostatic, with a lying blood pressure of 130/80 and a standing blood pressure of 100/65. His temperature was 98.8°F. His weight was 187 lbs, down 3 lbs from the documented weight of 190 lbs when he received his chemotherapy one week ago. Mucous membranes appeared dry.

Provisional Diagnosis

S.L. was diagnosed as having CTCAE grade 3 chemotherapy-induced diarrhea resulting in dehydration and electrolyte imbalances. Infectious cause was included in the differential.

Lab Work

White blood cell count = 4.1 K/cmm
Hemoglobin = 11.5 g/dl
Hematocrit = 37.2%
Platelet count = 125 K/cmm
Absolute neutrophil count = 2.38 g/dl

Sodium = 145 mmol/L
Potassium = 3.4 mmol/L
Creatinine = 1.1 mg/dl
Blood urea nitrogen = 28 mg/dl

Treatment

S.L. refused admission to the hospital for personal family reasons and lived locally; therefore, he agreed to the following outpatient treatment.

- One liter of IV normal saline over two hours
- Potassium chloride powder 40 mEq orally once and repeated at bedtime (powder ordered rather than tablets because of concern of poor gut absorption of tablets secondary to diarrhea)
- Stool sent to lab to test for blood and infectious causes (see *Expert Opinion* section of ONS PEP resource)
- Camphorated tincture of opium (0.4 mg/ml morphine): 1 tsp (5 ml) in water every three to four hours until diarrhea resolved (see *Expert Opinion* section of ONS PEP resource)
- Dietary intake counseling (see *Expert Opinion* section of ONS PEP resource)
  - General diet strategies: 8–10 servings (8 oz each) of liquid daily; drink liquids at room temperature; eat small, frequent meals (5–6 daily).
  - Avoid foods that exacerbate diarrhea: foods high in insoluble fiber (e.g., raw fruits and vegetables, whole grains, nuts, popcorn); greasy, fried, high-fat foods; foods containing lactose; large quantities of hyperosmotic liquids (e.g., fruit juice, sweetened fruit drinks); caffeinated beverages; alcohol.
  - Choose food that bulk stools: applesauce, oatmeal, bananas, cooked carrots, rice, white toast, canned or cooked fruit without skin, skinned turkey or chicken, fish.
  - Choose foods that replenish electrolytes: bananas, peach or apricot nectar, oranges, potatoes.

S.L. returned to primary care the next day for follow-up. His electrolytes returned to normal, and his number of stools per day reduced to three (CTCAE grade 1). He had a scheduled appointment in five days with the oncology fellow and was instructed to return to the emergency room if he did not continue to improve.

Arlene B. Davis, RN, MSN, AOCN®
Oncology Clinical Nurse Specialist
North Florida/South Georgia Veterans Health System
Gainesville, FL

Kourtney LaPlant, PharmD
Oncology Pharmacy Specialist
North Florida/South Georgia Veterans Health System
Gainesville, FL

Diarrhea

2009 AUTHORS
Paula Muehlbauer, RN, MSN, OCN®, and Deborah Thorpe, PhD, APRN, AOCNS®, ACHPN
ONS STAFF: Heather Belansky, RN, MSN

2008 AUTHORS
Paula Muehlbauer, RN, MSN, OCN®, Deborah Thorpe, PhD, APRN, AOCNS®, ACHPN, Arlene B. Davis,
RN, MSN, AOCN®, Rachael Christine Drabot, MPH, CNSD, RD, Elizabeth S. Kiker, RN, OCN®,
and Barbara L. Rawlings, RN, BSN
ONS STAFF: Kristen Baileys, RN, MSN, CRNP, AOCNP®

What interventions are effective for minimizing and treating diarrhea in adults with cancer receiving chemotherapy or radiation?

Chemotherapy = standard chemotherapy
The available scientific evidence does not address biologic therapies, targeted therapies, growth factors, and kinase inhibitors.

Radiation therapy = pelvic and abdominal radiation

Recommended for Practice

Interventions for which effectiveness has been demonstrated by strong evidence from rigorously conducted studies, meta-analyses, or systematic reviews and for which expectation of harms is small compared with the benefits

TREATMENT INTERVENTIONS FOR CHEMOTHERAPY-INDUCED DIARRHEA (CID)

- **Loperamide** (4 mg initial dose followed by 2 mg every four hours orally) is recommended as the standard first-line therapy for CID (Benson et al., 2004).
- **High-dose loperamide** (2 mg every two hours orally) has been shown to be moderately effective in the control of CID associated with irinotecan (Benson et al., 2004).
- **Somatostatin analog** (octreotide acetate) at a standard dose of 100–150 mcg three times daily via the subcutaneous (SC) route is recommended for second-line treatment of loperamide-refractory CID. Loperamide dosing was defined as loperamide 4 mg initially and then 2 mg every 6 hours for 48 hours (Benson et al., 2004; Zidan et al., 2001).

TREATMENT INTERVENTIONS FOR RADIATION-INDUCED DIARRHEA

- **Oral opiates,** including loperamide and diphenoxylate, are effective in the majority of patients with mild symptoms and are the standard therapy (Benson et al., 2004).

Likely to Be Effective

Interventions for which effectiveness has been demonstrated by supportive evidence from a single rigorously conducted controlled trial, consistent supportive evidence from well-designed controlled trials using small samples, or guidelines developed from evidence and supported by expert opinion

TREATMENT INTERVENTIONS FOR CHEMOTHERAPY-INDUCED DIARRHEA

- **Octreotide/IM long-acting** (Sandostatin LAR® Depot, Novartis Pharmaceuticals Corp.) for loperamide-refractory diarrhea: No specific recommendations can be made regarding a dose of 30 or 40 mg (Rosenoff et al., 2006).

PREVENTION OF RADIATION-INDUCED DIARRHEA

- **Probiotic supplementation** has been researched in the prevention of radiation-induced diarrhea because of the high risk for diarrhea among patients undergoing radiation therapy to the lower abdomen and/or pelvis (Marteau, de Vrese, Cellier, & Schrezenmeir, 2001; Urbancsek, Kazar, Mezes, & Neumann, 2001).
  - Supplementation with VSL#3 beginning on the first day of radiation, and continuing until the end of the radiation treatment period, led to a significant difference in the number of bowel movements and toxicity of diarrhea among 490 patients receiving pelvic radiation after surgery for sigmoid, rectal, or cervical cancer (Delia et al., 2007).
  - Supplementation with *Lactobacillus acidophilus* NDCO 1748 also significantly reduced diarrhea when administered to patients *during* radiation to the pelvis (Marteau et al., 2001).
  - Supplementation with *Lactobacillus rhamnosus* two weeks *after* radiation therapy reduced the need for diarrhea medication, and reduced the mean number of daily bowel movements among patients who had been experiencing diarrhea ≥ two weeks after receiving radiation to the abdomen or pelvis. However, the difference was not statistically significant when compared to the control group (Urbancsek et al., 2001).

Probiotic supplementation may prevent diarrhea resulting from radiation to the pelvis. Further research is needed to systematically determine the probiotic strain(s), dosage(s), and timing of administration (i.e., before, during, and/or after treatment) necessary to prevent and/or treat radiation-induced diarrhea (Delia et al., 2007; Marteau et al., 2001; Urbancsek et al., 2001).

- **Psyllium fiber supplementation for prevention of radiation-induced diarrhea:** Increased consumption of soluble fiber is routinely recommended for the treatment of diarrhea. (See the *Expert Opinion* section for further discussion related to soluble fiber.) One study found that 1–2 teaspoons of psyllium fiber (Metamucil®, Procter & Gamble) taken during pelvic radiation treatment for prostate or gynecologic cancer was effective in reducing the incidence and severity of radiation-induced diarrhea (Murphy, Stacey, Crook, Thompson, & Panetta, 2000).

Expert opinion, as evidenced by established clinical practice guidelines, supports the use of soluble fiber supplements for the treatment of diarrhea (Murphy et al., 2000; Singh, 2007). Further research is needed to define the type and dose of soluble fiber that is most effective in treating and/or preventing chemotherapy-induced and radiation-induced diarrhea.

TREATMENT INTERVENTIONS FOR RADIATION-INDUCED DIARRHEA

- **Octreotide:** 100 mcg SC three times daily is more effective than diphenoxylate 10 mg PO per day in patients with grade 2 or 3 diarrhea (Benson et al., 2004; Yavuz, Yavuz, Aydin, Can, & Kavgaci, 2002).

TREATMENT INTERVENTIONS FOR CHEMORADIOTHERAPY-INDUCED DIARRHEA

Octreotide 150 mcg SC three times daily results in near-complete resolution of diarrhea in patients with rectal carcinoma with grade 2 or 3 diarrhea receiving concomitant 5-fluorouracil (5-FU) and pelvic radiation therapy who are refractory to loperamide (Topkan & Karaoglu, 2007).

Benefits Balanced With Harms

Interventions for which clinicians and patients should weigh the beneficial and harmful effects according to individual circumstances and priorities

TREATMENT INTERVENTIONS FOR CHEMOTHERAPY-INDUCED DIARRHEA

- Amifostine 800 mg/m^2 infusion during 5-FU and calcium folinate infusion in patients with colorectal cancer when diarrhea recurred provided better protection than lower doses (500 g/m^2 or 150 mg/m^2). However, hypotension was significant with the 800 mg/m^2 dose (Tsavaris et al., 2003).

PREVENTION OF IRINOTECAN-INDUCED DIARRHEA

- **Neomycin:** Two studies addressed the use of neomycin for the prevention of irinotecan-induced diarrhea.
  - In a double-blind, randomized, placebo-controlled trial, a 45% lower incidence of grade 3 diarrhea was reported in the group receiving neomycin versus placebo. Neomycin 660 mg was administered orally three times per day for three consecutive days starting two days before chemotherapy. Treatment with neomycin did not result in a significantly shorter duration of diarrhea in days, *and* patients receiving neomycin had a 4.5-times higher risk for grade 2 nausea than those receiving placebo (De Jong et al., 2006).
  - In a nonrandomized study, seven evaluable patients received irinotecan alone in cycle 1 with resultant grade 2 diarrhea. In cycle 2, they were treated with irinotecan plus oral neomycin 1,000 mg three times per day for seven consecutive days starting two days before chemotherapy. Six out of seven patients had a decrease in diarrhea. By reducing the level of bacterial B-glucorinidase, neomycin plays a crucial role in reducing irinotecan-induced diarrhea without altering the efficacy of irinotecan. However, this is an extremely small study (Kehrer et al., 2001).

Effectiveness Not Established

Interventions for which insufficient or conflicting data or data of inadequate quality currently exist, with no clear indication of harm

PREVENTION OF IRINOTECAN-INDUCED DIARRHEA

At present, prophylactic antidiarrheal treatment is not a standard approach for irinotecan-based chemotherapy regimens. A few studies have investigated the potential benefit of prophylactic antidiarrheal therapy.

- **Oral alkalization (OA):** Three small studies addressed the use of oral alkalization for the prevention of irinotecan-induced diarrhea.
  - In one case-control study of 37 patients receiving irinotecan in combination with cisplatin, a complicated regimen of oral alkalization (OA) of the intestinal lumen in conjunction with control of defecation may have been beneficial when 0.5 g $NaHCO_3$ and 0.5 g magnesium oxide pc and hs, basic water (pH > 7.2) continuously for a total of 1,500–2,000 ml/day, and ursodeoxycholic acid 100 mg PO pc days 1–4 were given (Takeda et al., 2001).
  - Researchers in two other small studies utilizing OA along with irinotecan-based chemotherapy concluded that OA may be effective in ameliorating diarrhea. OA in one study consisted of 2 g of powdered $NaHCO_3$ diluted in 250 ml water; this solution was sipped during the days of irinotecan administration, starting in the morning (Moreno et al., 2006). In the other study, 2 g $NaHCO_3$, 2 g magnesium oxide, and 300 mg ursodexycholic acid were given PO before irinotecan and then every day for three days after (Maeda et al., 2004).
- **Budesonide:** In one small controlled trial, patients were randomly treated with budesonide (3 mg PO three times daily for a total of eight weeks during two cycles of irinotecan) versus placebo. Although a trend showed decreased incidence of diarrhea, budesonide failed to show a significant reduction in prevention of irinotecan-induced diarrhea and cannot be recommended without further investigation (Karthaus et al., 2005).
- **Charcoal:** Two small studies addressed the use of charcoal for the prevention of irinotecan-induced diarrhea.
  - 28 patients received 1,000 mg of activated charcoal plus 25 ml water the evening before irinotecan and then three times a day for 48 hours after irinotecan (only during the first treatment cycle with irinotecan). Results revealed decreased grade 3 and 4 diarrhea, decreased loperamide consumption, and increased irinotecan dose intensity (Michael et al., 2004).
  - Administration of 2 g of Kremezin® (Kureha Chemical), an oral adsorbent made of activated carbon (available in Japan), at the start of irinotecan, immediately after irinotecan, and three hours later significantly decreased the number of daily bowel movements during irinotecan treatments (Maeda et al., 2004).
- **Cholestyramine/levofloxacin:** In a small phase II trial, patients treated with levofloxacin 500 mg once daily and cholestyramine 4 g three times a day for three consecutive days, starting the day before each irinotecan administration, experienced decreased incidence of World Health Organization grade 3–4 diarrhea (Flieger et al., 2007, World Health Organization, n.d.).

Strategies for the prevention of irinotecan-induced diarrhea require further investigation (Benson et al., 2004).

PREVENTION OF CHEMOTHERAPY-INDUCED DIARRHEA

- **Probiotics:** Animal studies have suggested that the probiotic preparation VSL#3 effectively reduced CID when administered before and after chemotherapy treatment (Bowen et al., 2007). One randomized study of 150 adult patients with colorectal cancer receiving adjuvant chemotherapy in the postoperative period found that patients who received *Lactobacillus rhamnosus GG* supplementation ($1-2 \times 10^{10}$ per day) had less grade 3 or 4 diarrhea and less abdominal discomfort because of flatulence, borborygmia, or abdominal distention compared to patients who did not receive the probiotic supplements; both of these results were statistically significant (Osterlund et al., 2007). Although the authors of the study suggest that the probiotic may be a safe treatment to reduce the frequency of 5-FU chemotherapy–induced diarrhea, the study's limitations indicate the need for placebo-controlled, double-blinded, prospective, randomized studies including other chemotherapy agents in order to definitively conclude that the probiotic supplement reduces CID.

Further research is needed to determine whether probiotic preparations are effective in reducing CID.

- **Glutamine:** At present, glutamine supplementation is not a standard approach for the treatment of CID. Animal studies have suggested that low levels of glutamine can lead to atrophy of the small intestine with subsequent breakdown of the gut barrier (Daniele et al., 2001) and can increase gut permeability, resulting in bacterial translocation, malabsorption, and diarrhea (Savy, 2002). Therefore, several studies have investigated the potential benefit of glutamine supplementation. Examples of studies include the following.
  - Supplementation with 18 g of glutamine daily (divided doses of 6 g three times daily) reduced changes in intestinal absorption and intestinal permeability among patients with colorectal cancer receiving chemotherapy with 5-FU and folinic acid and led to a significant difference in the use of antidiarrheal medication (loperamide) among control versus experimental groups (Daniele et al., 2001).
  - A systematic review of five studies examining the effect of glutamine on CID reported conflicting results, leading the authors to conclude that further research is needed (Savarese, Savy, Vahdat, Wischmeyer, & Corey, 2003).

More research is needed to systematically examine the dosage of glutamine necessary to prevent and/or treat CID as well as to determine which patient populations are most likely to benefit from glutamine supplementation.

TREATMENT INTERVENTIONS FOR CHEMOTHERAPY-INDUCED DIARRHEA

- **Titration:** Upward titration of octreotide from 150 mcg to 500 mcg SC three times daily until symptoms are controlled may be more effective than standard doses in patients with CID who fail loperamide. The optimal dose of octreotide has not been determined (Benson et al., 2004).
- **Long-acting octreotide:** A 20–30 mg once-monthly IM injection may be given as secondary prophylaxis once patients have failed loperamide plus/minus Lomotil® (Pfizer Inc.) (Rosenoff, 2004).

PREVENTION OF RADIATION-INDUCED DIARRHEA

- **Glutamine:** At present, glutamine supplementation is not a standard approach for the treatment of radiation-induced diarrhea. However, studies are investigating the potential benefit of glutamine supplementation.
  - Animal studies suggest that glutamine inhibits bacterial translocation and decreases the risk of toxic radiation effects, such as diarrhea. However, human studies have not demonstrated a clear relationship, suggesting the need for further research (Savarese et al., 2003).
  - One randomized, double-blind, placebo-controlled study did not find statistically significant differences in incidence or severity of diarrhea episodes when patients undergoing pelvic radiation received 8 g of glutamine (divided doses of 4 g twice per day) during the one week of radiation and for two weeks after radiation was completed (Kozelsky et al., 2003).

More research is needed to investigate whether glutamine is protective against radiation-induced diarrhea, to systematically examine the dosage of glutamine necessary to prevent and/or treat radiation-induced diarrhea, and to determine which patient populations are most likely to benefit from glutamine supplementation.

TREATMENT INTERVENTIONS FOR RADIATION-INDUCED DIARRHEA

- **Antioxidant vitamins E and C:** 400 IU vitamin E and 500 mg vitamin C three times a day for eight weeks was administered in a nonrandomized, uncontrolled study of prostate and gynecologic patients experiencing postradiation proctitis, urgency, or fecal incontinence following pelvic radiation. Fourteen of 16 patients reported less diarrhea, and eight of those reported cessation of diarrhea (Kennedy et al., 2001).

Effectiveness Unlikely

Interventions for which lack of effectiveness has been demonstrated by negative evidence from a single rigorously conducted controlled trial, consistent negative evidence from well-designed controlled trials using small samples, or guidelines developed from evidence and supported by expert opinion

PREVENTION OF RADIATION-INDUCED DIARRHEA

- **Sulfasalazine:** This should not be used outside of a clinical trial in patients receiving pelvic radiation therapy (Benson et al., 2004).
- **Selenium supplementation:** Currently, no evidence supports that selenium supplementation can protect against diarrhea resulting from chemotherapy or radiation therapy (Dennert & Horneber, 2006).

TREATMENT INTERVENTIONS FOR RADIATION-INDUCED DIARRHEA

- **Pentosan polysulfate:** Marketed as Elmiron® (Ortho-McNeil Pharmaceutical, Inc.) for radiation-induced sequelae of the bladder, pentosan polysulfate was studied in doses of 300–600 mg/day versus placebo following radiation to the abdomen or pelvis. No significant difference occurred among the three arms of the study, and 20%–25% of the participants deteriorated in the first three months of the study (Pilepich et al., 2006).

Not Recommended for Practice

Interventions for which lack of effectiveness or harmfulness has been demonstrated by strong evidence from rigorously conducted studies, meta-analyses, or systematic reviews, or interventions where the costs, burden, or harms associated with the intervention exceed anticipated benefit

PREVENTION OF RADIATION-INDUCED DIARRHEA

- **Sucralfate:** This is not effective in preventing radiation-induced diarrhea and may aggravate some gastrointestinal (GI) symptoms (Benson et al., 2004; Martenson et al., 2000).

Expert Opinion

Low-risk interventions that are (1) consistent with sound clinical practice, (2) suggested by an expert in a peer-reviewed publication (journal or book chapter), and (3) for which limited evidence exists. An expert is an individual with peer-reviewed journal publications in the domain of interest.

ASSESSMENT OF PATIENTS WITH CHEMOTHERAPY-INDUCED DIARRHEA

- A high degree of vigilance is needed with regard to monitoring for GI toxicity in patients receiving irinotecan-based therapy and other intensive combination regimens (Benson et al., 2004).
- Assessment of symptoms must be rigorous and includes symptom duration and severity and constellation of signs and symptoms, including
  - Number of stools over baseline and stool composition, including presence of nocturnal diarrhea
  - Presence of added risk factors: fever, orthostatic symptoms (e.g., dizziness), abdominal pain/cramping, or weakness
  - Stool volume (although a valuable piece of information, may be impractical to determine)
  - Hydration status by physical examination (Benson et al., 2004).
- Patients with grade 3 or 4 CID or with grade 1 or 2 CID and the aforementioned added risk factors should have a stool workup (evaluation for blood, fecal leukocytes, *Clostridium difficile, Salmonella, Escherichia coli, Campylobacter,* and infectious colitis), complete blood count, and electrolyte profile (Benson et al., 2004).

EVALUATION OF DIETARY INTAKE

A review of the clinical guidelines indicates that the first step in the treatment of diarrhea should include evaluating dietary intake to identify foods or fluids that may be exacerbating diarrhea. Patients should be encouraged to adopt the following general diet strategies to promote resolution of diarrhea episodes and diet tolerance (American Institute for Cancer Research, 2007; Benson et al., 2004; Kornblau et al., 2000; Maroun et al., 2007; McCallum & Polisena, 2000).

- General diet strategies
  - Consume at least 8–10 servings (8 oz each) of liquid per day.
  - Drink liquids at room temperature.

- Eat small, frequent meals.
- Choose liquids such as Gatorade®, diluted fruit juice (50:50 juice and water), broth, or noncaffeinated soft drinks.
- Avoid substances that contain sorbitol, such as sugar-free candy and sugar-free chewing gum. (Note: Foods, beverages, and medications can contain sorbitol.)
- Patients should also avoid foods that exacerbate diarrhea, including
  - Foods high in insoluble fiber (e.g., raw fruits and vegetables, whole grain bread, nuts, popcorn, skins, seeds, legumes)
  - Greasy, fried, and high-fat foods
  - Foods and beverages that contain lactose
  - Large quantities of hyperosmotic liquids (e.g., fruit juice, sweetened fruit drinks)
  - Caffeinated beverages to (< 2–3 servings coffee, tea, or cola)
  - Alcohol.
- Patients should choose foods that bulk stools, including
  - High soluble fiber (pectin-containing) foods, such as applesauce, oatmeal, bananas, cooked carrots, and rice
  - Low insoluble fiber foods, such as rice, noodles, Cream of Wheat® (B&G Foods, Inc.), well-cooked eggs, bananas, white toast, canned or cooked fruit without skin, skinned turkey or chicken, fish, and mashed potatoes.
- Patients should choose foods that replete electrolytes, including
  - Foods high in sodium and potassium, such as bananas, peach nectar, apricot nectar, oranges, and potatoes.

TREATMENT OF CHEMOTHERAPY-INDUCED DIARRHEA

- Tincture of opium, a widely used antidiarrheal agent, may be a reasonable alternative as second-line therapy for CID. Two preparations are available, and because of the difference in morphine content, care must be taken not to confuse them.
  - **Deodorized tincture of opium**, the preferred preparation, contains the equivalent of 10 mg/ml morphine. The recommended dose is 10–15 drops in water every three to four hours.
  - **Camphorated tincture of opium (paregoric)**, a less concentrated preparation, contains the equivalent of 0.4 mg/ml morphine. The recommended dose is 1 tsp (5 ml) in water every three to four hours (Benson et al., 2004).

Definitions of the interventions are available at **www.ons.org/outcomes**.
Literature search completed through May 2008.

References

American Institute for Cancer Research. (2007). *Coping with the side effects of cancer treatment on your nutritional status.* Retrieved September 23, 2007, from http://www.aicr.org/site/PageServer?pagename=dc_cr_treatment#coping

Benson, A.B., III, Ajani, J.A., Catalano, R.B., Engelking, C., Kornblau, S.M., Martenson, J.A., Jr., et al. (2004). Recommended guidelines for the treatment of cancer treatment-induced diarrhea. *Journal of Clinical Oncology, 22*(14), 2918–2926.

Bowen, J.M., Stringer, A.M., Gibson, R.J., Yeoh, A.S., Hannam, S., & Keefe, D.M. (2007). VSL#3 probiotic treatment reduces chemotherapy-induced diarrhea and weight loss. *Cancer Biology and Therapy, 6*(9), 1449–1454.

Daniele, B., Perrone, F., Gallo, C., Pignata, S., De Martino, S., De Vivo, R., et al. (2001). Oral glutamine in the prevention of fluorouracil induced intestinal toxicity: A double blind, placebo controlled, randomised trial. *Gut, 48*(1), 28–33.

De Jong, F.A., Kehrer, D.F., Mathijssen, R.H., Creemers, G.J., de Bruijn, P., van Schaik, R.H., et al. (2006). Prophylaxis of irinotecan-induced diarrhea with neomycin and potential role for UGT1A1*28 genotype screening: A double-blind, randomized, placebo-controlled study. *Oncologist, 11*(8), 944–954.

Delia, P., Sansotta, G., Donato, V., Frosina, P., Messina, G., De Renzis, C., et al. (2007). Use of probiotics for prevention of radiation-induced diarrhea. *World Journal of Gastroenterology, 13*(6), 912–915.

Dennert, G., & Horneber, M. (2006). Selenium for alleviating the side effects of chemotherapy, radiotherapy and surgery in cancer patients. *Cochrane Database of Systematic Reviews* 2006, Issue 3. Art. No.: CD005037. DOI: 10.1002/14651858.CD005037.pub2.

Flieger, D., Klassert, C., Hainke, S., Keller, R., Kleinschmidt, R., & Fischback, W. (2007). Phase II clinical trial for prevention of delayed diarrhea with cholestyramine/levofloxacin in the second-line treatment with irinotecan biweekly in patients with metastatic colorectal carcinoma. *Oncology, 72*(1–2), 10–16.

Karthaus, M., Ballo, H., Abenhardt, W., Steinmetz, T., Geer, T., Schimke, J., et al. (2005). Prospective, double-blind, placebo-controlled, multicenter, randomized phase III study with orally administered budesonide for prevention of irinotecan (CPT-11)-induced diarrhea in patients with advanced colorectal cancer. *Oncology, 68*(4–6), 326–332.

Kehrer, D.F., Sparreboom, A., Verweij, J., de Bruijn, P., Nierop, C.A., van de Schraaf, J., et al. (2001). Modulation of irinotecan-induced diarrhea by cotreatment with neomycin in cancer patients. *Clinical Cancer Research, 7*(5), 1136–1141.

Kennedy, M., Bruninga, K., Mutlu, E.A., Losurdo, J., Choudhary, S., & Keshavarzian, A. (2001). Successful and sustained treatment of chronic radiation proctitis with antioxidant vitamins E and C. *American Journal of Gastroenterology, 96*(4), 1080–1084.

Kornblau, S., Benson, A.B., III, Catalano, R., Champlin, R.E., Engelking, C., Field, M., et al. (2000). Management of cancer treatment-related diarrhea: Issues and therapeutic strategies. *Journal of Pain and Symptom Management, 19*(2), 118–129.

Kozelsky, T.F., Meyers, G.E., Sloan, J.A., Shanahan, T.G., Dick, S.J., Moore, R.L., et al. (2003). Phase III double-blind study of glutamine versus placebo for the prevention of acute diarrhea in patients receiving pelvic radiation therapy. *Journal of Clinical Oncology, 21*(9), 1669–1674.

Maeda, Y., Ohune, T., Nakamura, M., Yamasaki, M., Kiribayashi, Y., & Murakami, T. (2004). Prevention of irinotecan-induced diarrhoea by oral carbonaceous adsorbent (Kremezin) in cancer patients. *Oncology Reports, 12*(3), 581–585.

Maroun, J.A., Anthony, L.B., Blais, N., Burkes, R., Dowden, S.D., Dranitsaris, G., et al. (2007). Prevention and management of chemotherapy-induced diarrhea in patients with colorectal cancer: A consensus statement by the Canadian Working Group on chemotherapy-induced diarrhea. *Current Oncology, 14*(1), 13–20.

Marteau, P.R., de Vrese, M., Cellier C.J., & Schrezenmeir, J. (2001). Protection from gastrointestinal diseases with the use of probiotics. *American Journal of Clinical Nutrition, 72*(Suppl. 2), 430S–436S.

Martenson, J.A., Bollinger, J.W., Sloan, J.A., Novotny, P.J., Urias, R.E., Michalak, J.C., et al. (2000). Sucralfate in the prevention of treatment-induced diarrhea in patients receiving pelvic radiation therapy: A North Central Cancer Treatment Group phase III double-blind placebo-controlled trial. *Journal of Clinical Oncology, 18*(6), 1239–1245.

McCallum, P., & Polisena, C. (Eds.). (2000). *The clinical guide to oncology nutrition.* Chicago: American Dietetic Association.

Michael, M., Brittain, M., Nagai, J., Feld, R., Hedley, D., Oza, A., et al. (2004). Phase II study of activated charcoal to prevent irinotecan-induced diarrhea. *Journal of Clinical Oncology, 22*(21), 4410–4417.

Moreno, V.V., Vidal, J.B., Alemany, H.M., Salvia, A.S., Serentill, M.L., Montero, I.C., et al. (2006). Prevention of irinotecan associated diarrhea by intestinal alkalization. A pilot study in gastrointestinal cancer patients. *Clinical and Translational Oncology, 8*(3), 208–212.

Murphy, J., Stacey, D., Crook, J., Thompson, B., & Panetta, D. (2000). Testing control of radiation-induced diarrhea with a psyllium bulking agent: A pilot study. *Canadian Oncology Nursing Journal, 10*(3), 96–100.

National Cancer Institute Cancer Therapy Evaluation Program. (2006). *Common terminology criteria for adverse events* (version 3.0). Bethesda, MD: National Cancer Institute. Retrieved November 13, 2007, from http://ctep.cancer.gov/protocolDevelopment/electronic_applications/docs/ctcaev3.pdf

Osterlund, P., Ruotsalainen, T., Korpela, R., Saxelin, M., Ollus, A., Valta, P., et al. (2007). Lactobacillus supplementation for diarrhoea related to chemotherapy of colorectal cancer: A randomised study. *British Journal of Cancer, 97*(8), 1028–1034.

Pilepich, M.V., Paulus, R., St. Clair, W., Barasacchio, R.A., Rostock, R., & Miller, R.C. (2006). Phase III study of pentosanpolysulfate (PPS) in treatment of gastrointestinal tract sequelae of radiotherapy. *American Journal of Clinical Oncology, 29*(2), 132–137.

Rosenoff, S. (2004). Resolution of refractory chemotherapy-induced diarrhea (CID) with octreotide long-acting formulation in cancer patients: 11 case studies. *Supportive Care in Cancer, 12*(8), 561–570.

Rosenoff, S.H., Gabrail, N.Y., Conklin, R., Hohneker, J.A., Berg, W.J., Ghulam, W., et al. (2006). A multicenter, randomized trial of long-acting octreotide for the optimum prevention of chemotherapy-induced diarrhea: Results of the STOP trial. *Journal of Supportive Oncology, 4*(6), 289–294.

Savarese, D.M., Savy, G., Vahdat, L., Wischmeyer, P.E., & Corey, B. (2003). Prevention of chemotherapy and radiation toxicity with glutamine. *Cancer Treatment Reviews, 29*(6), 501–513.

Savy, G.K. (2002). Glutamine supplementation: Heal the gut, help the patient. *Journal of Infusion Nursing, 25*(1), 65–69.

Singh, B. (2007). Psyllium as therapeutic and drug delivery agent. *International Journal of Pharmaceutics, 334*(1–2), 1–14.

Takeda, Y., Kobayashi, K., Akivama, Y., Soma, T., Handa, S., Kudoh, S., et al. (2001). Prevention of irinotecan (CPT-11)-induced diarrhea by oral alkalization combined with control of defecation in cancer patients. *International Journal of Cancer, 92*(2), 269–275.

Topkan, E., & Karaoglu, A. (2006). Octreotide in the management of chemoradiotherapy-induced diarrhea refractory to loperamide in patients with rectal carcinoma. *Oncology, 71*(5–6), 354–360.

Tsavaris, N., Kosmas, C., Vadiaka, M., Zonios, D., Papalambros, E., Papantoniou, N., et al. (2003). Amifostine, in a reduced dose, protects against severe diarrhea associated with weekly fluorouracil and folinic acid chemotherapy in advanced colorectal cancer: A pilot study. *Journal of Pain and Symptom Management, 26*(3), 849–854.

Urbancsek, H., Kazar, T., Mezes, I., & Neumann, K. (2001). Results of a double-blind, randomized study to evaluate the efficacy and safety of Antibiophilus in patients with radiation-induced diarrhoea. *European Journal of Gastroenterology and Hepatology, 13*(4), 391–396.

World Health Organization. (n.d.). *WHO toxicity criteria by grade.* Retrieved November 15, 2007, from http://www.fda.gov/cder/cancer/toxicityframe.htm

Yavuz, M.N., Yavuz, A.A., Aydin, F., Can, G., & Kavgaci, H. (2002). The efficacy of octreotide in the therapy of acute radiation-induced diarrhea: A randomized controlled study. *International Journal of Radiation Oncology, Biology, Physics, 54*(1), 195–202.

Zidan, J., Haim, N., Beny, A., Stein, M., Gez, E., & Kuten, A. (2001). Octreotide in the treatment of severe chemotherapy-induced diarrhea. *Annals of Oncology, 12*(2), 227–229.

CHAPTER **10**

Dyspnea

Problem

Dyspnea is "a subjective experience of breathing discomfort that consists of qualitatively distinct sensations that vary in intensity. The experience derives from interactions among multiple physiological, psychological, social and environmental factors, and may induce secondary physiological and behavioral responses" (American Thoracic Society, 1999, p. 322).

Incidence

At cancer diagnosis, dyspnea is estimated to occur in 15%–55% of people with cancer. During the last week of life, 18%–79% of people with cancer experience dyspnea (Ripamonti & Fusco, 2002). Dyspnea in people with cancer may be caused directly by the cancer, by manifestations of the cancer, or by its treatment, or it may be unrelated to the cancer.

Assessment

Dyspnea is a subjective experience; thus, self-report is the most reliable assessment method (Ripamonti & Bruera, 1997). A detailed assessment of dyspnea begins with questions focusing on the characteristics of the symptom in regard to onset, frequency, intensity, and nature of the respiratory changes (see Table 10-1), including use of a clinical measurement tool.

Clinical Measurement Tools

No single tool measures all of the dimensions of dyspnea. The choice of tool depends on the purpose of the assessment as well as the level of clinician and patient burden. The following clinical measurement tools for dyspnea are presented in Table 10-2.
1. Visual Analog Scale (see Figure 10-1)
2. Numeric Rating Scale (see Figure 10-2)
3. Cancer Dyspnea Scale

Table 10-1. Dyspnea Assessment Guide		
Assessment	Yes	No
Physical Status		
Tachycardia, tachypnea		
Use of accessory muscles		
Weight status		
Pallor indicating anemia		
Cyanosis with pulmonary origin		
Neurologic Status		
Memory or concentration problems		
Confusion		
Restlessness		
Psychosocial Status		
Anxiety, fear, depression		
Risk and Contributing Factors		
Anemia		
Congestive heart failure, cardiomyopathy		
Ascites and renal insufficiency caused or exacerbated by cancer treatment		
Chemotherapy, surgery, radiation therapy		
Other		
Laboratory data: Complete blood count, arterial blood gases, chest x-ray, echocardiogram, computed tomography scan of chest, ventilation and perfusion scan, pulmonary function tests, pulse oximetry		
Note. Based on information from Tyson, 2006.		

References

American Thoracic Society. (1999). Dyspnea. Mechanisms, assessment, and management: A consensus statement. *American Journal of Respiratory and Critical Care Medicine, 159*(1), 321–340.

Dorman, S., Byrne, A., & Edwards, A. (2007). Which measurement scales should we use to measure breathlessness in palliative care? A systematic review. *Palliative Medicine, 21*(3), 177–191.

Gift, A., & Narsavage, G. (1998). Validity of the numeric rating scale as a measure of dyspnea. *American Journal of Critical Care, 7*(3), 200–204.

Table 10-2. Clinical Measurement Tools for Dyspnea

Name of Tool	Number of Items	Domains	Reliability and Validity	Populations	Clinical Utility
Visual Analog Scale	1	Severity or intensity	Adequate reliability and validity established	Lung cancer	Unidimensional
Numeric Rating Scale	1	Severity or Intensity	Adequate reliability and validity established	Variety of cancer diagnoses	Unidimensional
Cancer Dyspnea Scale	12	Sense of effort, anxiety, discomfort related to dyspnea	Adequate reliability and validity established	Lung cancer	Easy to complete Multidimensional

Note. Based on information from Dorman et al., 2007; Gift & Narsavage, 1998; Joyce, 2005.

Figure 10-1. Visual Analog Dyspnea Scale

How much shortness of breath have you had in the last week?
Please indicate by marking the height on the column.

Shortness of breath as bad as can be

No shortness of breath

Note. From "Dyspnea" (p. 672), by A. Gift and A. Hoffman in M.E. Langhorne, J.S. Fulton, and S.E. Otto (Eds.), *Oncology Nursing* (5th ed.), 2007, St. Louis, MO: Elsevier Mosby. Copyright 2007 by Elsevier Mosby. Reprinted with permission.

Figure 10-2. Numeric Rating Scale for Dyspnea

On a scale from 0 to 10, indicate how much shortness of breath you have had in the past week where 0 = no shortness of breath and 10 = shortness of breath as the worst possible. Circle the number.

0   1   2   3   4   5   6   7   8   9   10

No shortness of breath   Worst possible

Note. From "Dyspnea" (p. 671), by A. Gift and A. Hoffman in M.E. Langhorne, J.S. Fulton, and S.E. Otto (Eds.), *Oncology Nursing* (5th ed.), 2007, St. Louis, MO: Elsevier Mosby. Copyright 2007 by Elsevier Mosby. Reprinted with permission.

Joyce, M. (2005). *Measuring oncology-nursing sensitive patient outcomes: Evidence-based summary.* Retrieved May 15, 2008, from http://www.ons.org/outcomes/measures/dyspnea.shtml

Ripamonti, C., & Bruera, E. (1997). Dyspnea: Pathophysiology and assessment. *Journal of Pain and Symptom Management, 13*(4), 220–330.

Ripamonti, C., & Fusco, F. (2002). Respiratory problems in advanced cancer. *Supportive Care in Cancer, 10*(3), 204–216.

Tyson, L.B. (2006). Dyspnea. In D. Camp-Sorrell & R.A. Hawkins (Eds.), *Clinical manual for the oncology advanced practice nurse* (2nd ed., pp. 153–157). Pittsburgh, PA: Oncology Nursing Society.

Case Study

J.B. is a 52-year-old woman with a history of resected, stage IIB, non-small cell lung cancer who was diagnosed one year ago with a large right lung mass (squamous cell carcinoma). A right pneumonectomy was performed, and after surgery she experienced breathlessness when walking up any incline or climbing stairs. She was followed for eight months without any evidence of disease recurrence.

In January 2007, J.B. developed a persistent cough productive of clear sputum. A computed tomography scan of the chest revealed lymph node enlargement, new left lower lobe opacity, three dense lesions in the liver, and an enlarged right adrenal gland. A positron-emission tomography scan showed intense metabolic activity in these areas.

J.B. had been married for 19 years. Her hobbies included long walks and gardening. She had worked in a bank since high school graduation and had recently been promoted to bank manager after completing her bachelor's degree at night. Her husband was a machinist, and they had two children who were out of the home and employed in the same community. She quit smoking one year ago. Her alcohol intake was occasional. She believed there was a higher power but did not attend church regularly.

Physical Assessment

Table 10-3 presents findings from a physical assessment of J.B. as well as a review of systems.

Table 10-3. Patient Physical Assessment and Review of Systems	
Physical Assessment	**Findings**
Temperature	36°C (oral)
Heart rate	97 regular (apical)
Respiratory rate	22
Systolic blood pressure (sitting)	110
Oxygen saturation	97%
Activity	At rest
Karnofsky performance score	80
Energy level—fatigue	Grade 1
Weight and appetite	Stable
Shortness of breath/dyspnea on exertion/chest pain	Breathlessness with activity
Cough	Productive of clear sputum
Neurologic symptoms	No
Pain	No
Coronary	Normal rate and rhythm
Lung	Vesicular breath sounds on the left

J.B. arrived for her first cycle of chemotherapy with carboplatin, paclitaxel, and bevacizumab. She told the infusion room nurse that her breathing was worse and stated that she felt okay while sitting but very breathless when she moved. Her vital signs were within normal limits, and her oxygen saturation on room air was 92% at rest and 90% on ambulation. Using a numeric rating scale to describe her dyspnea, J.B. rated it a 6. The infusion room nurse paged the advanced registered nurse practitioner (ARNP) to further evaluate the patient.

Based on the evidence cited in the *Recommended for Practice* section of the Oncology Nursing Society (ONS) Putting Evidence Into Practice (PEP) resource on dyspnea, J.B. would be monitored for deterioration of her oxygen saturations. The ARNP held J.B.'s chemotherapy because of the dyspnea.

The evidence supports the use of oral and parenteral opioids for the management of dyspnea in advanced cancer. J.B. was prescribed 15 mg of immediate-release morphine every four hours as needed. On a follow-up phone call, she stated that her breathing was better when she walked and she had used three to four pills in 24 hours. She rated her dyspnea as a 3. She was scheduled for her first chemotherapy in two days. The infusion room nurse continued to assess her dyspnea. If warranted, other interventions supported by evidence would be considered in conjunction with the patient's preferences and lifestyle, as well as the cost of the interventions.

Wendye M. DiSalvo, MSN, ARNP, AOCN®
Advanced Registered Nurse Practitioner
Dartmouth-Hitchcock Medical Center
Lebanon, NH

Dyspnea

2009 AUTHORS
Wendye M. DiSalvo, MSN, ARNP, AOCN®, and Margaret M. Joyce, PhD(c), RN, MSN, AOCN®
ONS STAFF: Heather Belansky, RN, MSN

2007 AUTHORS
Wendye M. DiSalvo, RN, ARNP, MS, AOCN®, Margaret M. Joyce, PhD(c), RN, AOCN®, Ann E. Culkin, RN, OCN®, Leslie B. Tyson, MS, APRN,BC, OCN®, and Kathleen Mackay, RN, BSN, OCN®
ONS STAFF: Barbara G. Lubejko, MS, RN

What can nurses do to assist people with cancer-related dyspnea?

The optimal treatment of dyspnea includes using specific therapies as appropriate to reverse the causes along with using palliative therapies to treat irreversible causes for symptomatic relief. The interventions discussed herein are palliative and are a result of a review of the literature focused solely on cancer-related dyspnea. Evidence from research that considers dyspnea attributed to other etiologies may be beneficial in cancer-related dyspnea but is beyond the scope of this resource.

Recommended for Practice

Interventions for which effectiveness has been demonstrated by strong evidence from rigorously designed studies, meta-analyses, or systematic reviews and for which expectation of harms is small compared with the benefits

IMMEDIATE-RELEASE ORAL OR PARENTERAL OPIOIDS

Evidence supports the use of oral and parenteral opioids for management of dyspnea in patients with terminal or advanced cancer because they reduce ventilatory demand by decreasing central respiratory drive. In three systematic reviews and several smaller studies, patients reported dyspnea relief with opioids (Allard, Lamontagne, Bernard, & Tremblay, 1999; Ben-Aharon, Gafter-Gvili, Paul, Leibovici, & Stemmer, 2008; Bruera, Macmillan, Pither, & MacDonald, 1990; Clemens & Klaschik, 2007; Jennings, Davies, Higgins, Gibbs, & Broadly, 2002; Mazzocato, Buclin, & Rapin, 1999; Viola et al., 2008).
- Morphine was the predominant opioid evaluated in the studies, but other opioids also were included.
- In general, patients who were opioid naïve were given smaller doses of opioid than those who were opioid tolerant. A wide range of doses was used in the studies.
- In patients already receiving opioids on a regular basis, supplemental oral and parenteral doses consisting of either 25% or 50% of the equivalent four-hour opioid dose (e.g., total 24-hour opioid dose divided into four-hour portions) have been assessed. One study found that supplemental opioid doses at 25% of the regular four-hour dose can reduce dyspnea for as long as four hours (Allard et al., 1999).

- Overall, the opioids were well tolerated, with the exception of reports of nausea and vomiting.
- More research is needed to define the most effective doses of oral and parenteral opioids and to determine those patients who are most likely to benefit from the use of opioids.

Likely to Be Effective

Interventions for which effectiveness has been demonstrated by supportive evidence from a single rigorously conducted controlled trial, consistent supportive evidence from well-designed controlled trials using small samples, or guidelines developed from evidence and supported by expert opinion

Expert consensus recommends the following palliative interventions to relieve cancer-related dyspnea (National Comprehensive Cancer Network [NCCN], 2008). The consensus guidelines for dyspnea are categorized by estimated life expectancy.

The life expectancy category labeled years to months to weeks includes the following measures to relieve symptoms.
- Temporary ventilator support if clinically indicated for severe reversible condition
- Oxygen therapy (See also palliative oxygen evidence [Bruera, de Stoutz, Velasco-Leiva, Schoeller, & Hanson, 1993; Bruera et al., 2003] listed in the *Effectiveness Not Established* section.)
- Benzodiazepines for anxiety
- Nonpharmacologic therapies such as
  - Increasing ambient airflow directed at the face or nose, such as generated by a fan
  - Providing cooler temperatures
  - Promoting relaxation and stress reduction
  - Providing educational, emotional, and psychosocial support for patients and family caregivers and referring to other disciplines as appropriate.

Interventions recommended for a dying patient experiencing dyspnea include the previous measures and the following.
- Reduce excessive secretions with scopolamine, hyoscyamine, or atropine.
- Implement oxygen therapy, if subjective report of relief (see palliative oxygen evidence [Bruera et al., 1993, 2003] listed in the *Effectiveness Not Established* section).
- Institute sedation as needed.
- Discontinue fluid support, and consider low-dose diuretics if fluid overload may be a contributing factor.

Benefits Balanced With Harms

Interventions for which clinicians and patients should weigh the beneficial and harmful effects according to individual circumstances and priorities

There are no interventions as of May 2008.

Effectiveness Not Established

Interventions for which insufficient or conflicting data or data of inadequate quality currently exist, with no clear indication of harm

PHARMACOLOGIC INTERVENTIONS

Extended-Release Morphine

One small study testing the regular administration of extended-release morphine failed to show a significant reduction in dyspnea for those who completed the study (Boyd & Kelly, 1997). In addition, of 15 patients entered in the study, 3 withdrew because of sedation and 3 died without showing a reduction in dyspnea. The high incidence of sedation and dizziness at 48 hours after initiation should raise concern, especially in opioid-naïve patients, and emphasizes the need to monitor patients carefully (Boyd & Kelly).

Midazolam Plus Morphine

Only one trial has been reported supporting the use of the combination of midazolam* plus morphine in patients with severe dyspnea in the last week of their lives (Navigante, Cerchietti, Castro, Lutteral, & Cabalar, 2006). Further research is needed before this regimen can be recommended.

Nebulized or Oral Transmucosal Fentanyl

Evidence is insufficient to recommend the use of nebulized or oral transmucosal fentanyl.* One small study reported a perceived benefit of nebulized fentanyl by the majority of patients (Coyne, Viswanathan, & Smith, 2002). However, the study has limitations. Case reports give anecdotal findings regarding the benefit of oral transmucosal fentanyl to relieve dyspnea (Benitez-Rosario, Martin, & Feria, 2005). Further research is needed before fentanyl in either form can be recommended.

Nebulized Furosemide

Evidence is insufficient to support the use of nebulized furosemide* in the treatment of dyspnea. As reported by one small controlled study (Wilcock et al., 2008), no beneficial effect of furosemide was reported compared to nebulized saline. However, in one uncontrolled study (Shimoyama & Shimoyama, 2002) and in three case reports (Kohara et al., 2003), the majority of patients reported that inhalation of furosemide decreased the sensation of dyspnea. Further rigorous research is required before this regimen can be recommended.

Nebulized Lignocaine (Lidocaine Hydrochloride)*

One small study evaluated nebulized lignocaine* in people with cancer experiencing breathlessness at rest (Wilcock, Corcoran, & Tattersfield, 1994). No benefit was seen with the inhaled lignocaine. In fact, the distress of breathing increased after inhalation of nebulized lignocaine.

Nebulized Opioids[†]

Currently, insufficient evidence exists to recommend the use of nebulized opioids in the treatment of dyspnea. Investigation into the use of inhaled nebulized opioids has yielded mixed results. Although some individual studies indicate the potential for efficacy (Bruera et al., 2005; Joyce, McSweeney, Carrieri-Kohlman, & Hawkins, 2004; Quigley, Joel, Patel, Baksh,

& Slevin, 2002; Tanaka et al., 1999), higher-level reviews have failed to show positive effects of nebulized opioids for the treatment of dyspnea and recommend further research with rigorous designs and larger samples (Charles, Reymond, & Israel, 2008; Jennings et al., 2002; Zeppetella, 1997).

Palliative Oxygen

Palliative oxygen is the use of oxygen to relieve the sensation of dyspnea, not necessarily to correct hypoxemia. At the present time, available data do not provide support for the use of palliative oxygen in people with advanced cancer. One meta-analysis (Uronis, Currow, McCrory, Samsa, & Abernethy, 2008) and three randomized controlled trials (two examined dyspnea at rest, and one examined dyspnea while walking) did not demonstrate a significant difference between air and oxygen even in the hypoxic subgroups. On average, patients improved symptomatically with both air and oxygen (Booth, Kelly, Cox, Adams, & Guz, 1996; Bruera et al., 2003; Philip et al., 2006), indicating that routine use of palliative oxygen would not demonstrate benefit to relieve the sensation of dyspnea. Notably, despite oxygen administration correcting hypoxemia, no significant correlation existed between dyspnea score and oxygen saturation levels, underscoring the subjective dimension of dyspnea (Booth et al.; Philip et al.; Uronis et al.).

One additional small, randomized trial demonstrated conflicting evidence that oxygen is beneficial in hypoxic patients experiencing dyspnea at rest. A study looking at the use of a different gas mixture (heliox 28%) in nonhypoxic dyspneic patients undergoing exercise indicated that the gas mixture may have some benefit (Ahmedzai, Laude, Robertson, Troy, & Vora, 2004).

NONPHARMACOLOGIC INTERVENTIONS

Acupuncture

One randomized controlled study involving 47 patients failed to show a beneficial effect of acupuncture on dyspnea in patients with advanced cancer (Vickers, Feinstein, Deng, & Cassileth, 2005). Another study evaluated 20 patients with cancer-related breathlessness who received acupuncture (Ahmedzai et al., 2004). The patients acknowledged an improvement in their breathlessness after the acupuncture, but the results may have been contaminated by the nurse remaining with the patient for 90 minutes post intervention. Further evaluation of acupuncture for cancer-related breathlessness is indicated.

COGNITIVE BEHAVIORAL APPROACH

One multicenter and three smaller studies examined the effect of specialized nursing interventions on the quality of life of patients with lung cancer experiencing breathlessness (Bredin et al., 1999; Connors, Graham, & Peel, 2007; Corner, Plant, A'Hern, & Bailey, 1996; Filshie, Penn, Ashley, & Davis, 1996). Interventions offered in the studies included the following.
- Assessment of breathlessness—what improves and what hinders
- Provision of information and support for patients and families in the management of breathlessness
- Exploration of the significance of breathlessness with patients, their disease, and their future
- Instruction in breathing control, relaxation, and distraction techniques
- Goal setting to enhance breathing and relaxation techniques as well as to enhance function, enable participation in social activities, and develop coping skills

- Identification of early signs of problems that need medical or pharmacotherapy intervention

Patients receiving these interventions reported a significant improvement in breathlessness, emotional and physical well-being, and performance status. A significant dropout rate in one trial because of disease progression demonstrated that patients who most benefit from this intervention have earlier-stage disease and higher performance status. Additional trials are needed to pinpoint which interventions are essential to improve the dyspnea outcome.

Effectiveness Unlikely

Interventions for which lack of effectiveness has been demonstrated by negative evidence from a single rigorously conducted controlled trial, consistent negative evidence from well-designed controlled trials using small samples, or guidelines developed from evidence and supported by expert opinion

There are no interventions as of May 2008.

Not Recommended for Practice

Interventions for which lack of effectiveness or harmfulness has been demonstrated by strong evidence from rigorously conducted studies, meta-analyses, or systematic reviews, or interventions where the costs, burden, or harms associated with the intervention exceed anticipated benefit

There are no interventions as of May 2008.

Expert Opinion

Low-risk interventions that are (1) consistent with sound clinical practice, (2) suggested by an expert in a peer-reviewed publication (journal or book chapter), and (3) for which limited evidence exists. An expert is an individual who has authored articles published in a peer-reviewed journal in the domain of interest.

Although limited evidence exists, experts recommend the following supportive interventions in patients experiencing cancer-related dyspnea (Campbell, 2004; Dudgeon, 2002; Gallo-Silver & Pollack, 2000; Hately, Laurence, Scott, Baker, & Thomas, 2003).
- Maximize treatments proven to be beneficial to individual patients, such as avoiding volume overload and using oxygen and nebulized bronchodilators.
- Use upright positioning that affords patients optimal lung capacity, especially with a coexisting diagnosis of chronic obstructive pulmonary disease.
- Educate patients about breathing exercises such as diaphragmatic breathing, altering breathing rhythm, and pursed lip breathing to optimize lung function (Dudgeon, 2002).
- Educate patients to recognize physical maneuvers that precipitate dyspnea. Employ interventions such as cognitive behavioral techniques (e.g., relaxation, imaging therapy) to decrease the anticipatory component associated with exertional dyspnea.

- Consider the use of assistive devices, such as a wheelchair and portable oxygen, to decrease physical activities that precipitate dyspnea.
- Expert opinion is conflicting regarding the use of benzodiazepines.* Some studies recommend it to treat anxiety associated with dyspnea (Hately et al., 2003; NCCN, 2008), whereas others claim that the use of an anxiolytic is not supported for relief of cancer-related dyspnea (Campbell, 2004; Gallo-Silver & Pollack, 2000).

* The use of this drug in the treatment of dyspnea has not been approved by the U.S. Food and Drug Administration and is considered off-label use.
† The use of the nebulized form of this drug in the treatment of dyspnea has not been approved by the U.S. Food and Drug Administration and is considered off-label use.

Definitions of the interventions are available at **www.ons.org/outcomes**.
Literature search completed through May 2008.

References

Ahmedzai, S.H., Laude, E., Robertson, A., Troy, G., & Vora, V. (2004). A double blind, randomized, controlled phase II trial of heliox28 gas mixture in lung cancer patients with dyspnoea on exertion. *British Journal of Cancer, 90*(2), 366–371.

Allard, P., Lamontagne, C., Bernard, P., & Tremblay, C. (1999). How effective are supplementary doses of opioids for dyspnea in terminally ill cancer patients? A randomized continuous sequential clinical trial. *Journal of Pain and Symptom Management, 17*(4), 256–265.

Ben-Aharon, I., Gafter-Gvili, A., Paul, M., Leibovici, L., & Stemmer, S.M. (2008). Interventions for alleviating cancer-related dyspnea: A systematic review. *Journal of Clinical Oncology, 26*(14), 2396–2404.

Benitez-Rosario, M.A., Martin, A.S., & Feria, M. (2005). Oral transmucosal fentanyl citrate in the management of dyspnea crises in cancer patients. *Journal of Pain and Symptom Management, 30*(5), 395–397.

Booth, S., Kelly, M.J., Cox, N.P., Adams, L., & Guz, A. (1996). Does oxygen help dyspnea in patients with cancer? *American Journal of Respiratory and Critical Care Medicine, 153*(5), 1515–1518.

Boyd, K.J., & Kelly, M. (1997). Oral morphine as symptomatic treatment of dyspnoea in patients with advanced cancer. *Palliative Medicine, 11*(4), 277–281.

Bredin, M., Corner, J., Krishnasamy, M., Plant, H., Bailey, C., & A'Hern, R. (1999). Multicentre randomised controlled trial of nursing intervention for breathlessness in patients with lung cancer. *BMJ, 318*(7188), 901–904.

Bruera, E., de Stoutz, N., Velasco-Leiva, A., Schoeller, T., & Hanson, J. (1993). Effects of oxygen on dyspnoea in hypoxaemic terminal-cancer patients. *Lancet, 342*(8862), 13–14.

Bruera, E., Macmillan, K., Pither, J., & MacDonald, R.N. (1990). Effects of morphine on the dyspnea of terminal cancer patients. *Journal of Pain and Symptom Management, 5*(6), 341–344.

Bruera, E., Sala, R., Spruyt, O., Palmer, J.L., Zhang, T., & Willey, J. (2005). Nebulized versus subcutaneous morphine for patients with cancer dyspnea: A preliminary study. *Journal of Pain and Symptom Management, 29*(6), 613–618.

Bruera, E., Sweeney, C., Willey, J., Palmer, J.L., Strasser, F., Morice, R.C., et al. (2003). Randomized controlled trial of supplemental oxygen versus air in cancer patients with dyspnea. *Palliative Medicine, 17*(8), 659–663.

Campbell, M.L. (2004). Terminal dyspnea and respiratory distress. *Critical Care Clinics, 20*(3), 403–417.

Charles, M.A., Reymond, L., & Israel, F. (2008). Relief of incident dyspnea in palliative cancer patients: A pilot, randomized, controlled trial comparing nebulized hydromorphone, systemic hydromorphone, and nebulized saline. *Journal of Pain and Symptom Management, 36*(1), 29–38.

Clemens, K.E., & Klaschik, E. (2007). Symptomatic therapy of dyspnea with strong opioids and its effect on ventilation in palliative care patients. *Journal of Pain and Symptom Management, 33*(4), 473–481.

Connors, S., Graham, S., & Peel, T. (2007). An evaluation of a physiotherapy led non-pharmacological breathlessness programme for patients with intrathoracic malignancy. *Palliative Medicine, 21*(4), 285–287.

Corner, J., Plant, H., A'Hern, R., & Bailey, C. (1996). Non-pharmacological intervention for breathlessness in lung cancer. *Palliative Medicine, 10*(4), 299–305.

Coyne, P.J., Viswanathan, R., & Smith, T.J. (2002). Nebulized fentanyl citrate improves patients' perception of breathing, respiratory rate, and oxygen saturation in dyspnea. *Journal of Pain and Symptom Management, 23*(2), 157–160.

Dudgeon, D.J. (2002). Managing dyspnea and cough. *Hematology/Oncology Clinics of North America, 16*(3), 557–577.

Filshie, J., Penn, K., Ashley, S., & Davis, C.L. (1996). Acupuncture for the relief of cancer-related breathlessness. *Palliative Medicine, 10*(2), 145–150.

Gallo-Silver, L., & Pollack, B. (2000). Behavioral interventions for lung cancer-related breathlessness. *Cancer Practice, 8*(6), 268–273.

Hately, J., Laurence, V., Scott, A., Baker, R., & Thomas, P. (2003). Breathlessness clinics within specialist palliative care settings can improve the quality of life and functional capacity of patients with lung cancer. *Palliative Medicine, 17*(5), 410–417.

Jennings, A.L., Davies, A.N., Higgins, J.P., Gibbs, J.S., & Broadley, K.E. (2002). A systematic review of the use of opioids in the management of dyspnoea. *Thorax, 57*(11), 939–944.

Joyce, M., McSweeney, M., Carrieri-Kohlman, V.L., & Hawkins, J. (2004). The use of nebulized opioids in the management of dyspnea: Evidence synthesis. *Oncology Nursing Forum, 31*(3), 551–561.

Kohara, H., Ueoka, H., Maeda, T., Takeyama, H., Saito, R., Shima, Y., et al. (2003). Effect of nebulized furosemide in terminally ill cancer patients with dyspnea. *Journal of Pain and Symptom Management, 26*(4), 962–967.

Mazzocato, C., Buclin, T., & Rapin, C.H. (1999). The effects of morphine on dyspnea and ventilatory function in elderly patients with advanced cancer: A randomized double-blind controlled trial. *Annals of Oncology, 10*(12), 1511–1514.

National Comprehensive Cancer Network. (2008). *NCCN Clinical Practice Guidelines in Oncology™: Palliative care* [v.1.2009]. Retrieved December 8, 2008, from http://www.nccn.org/professionals/physician_gls/PDF/palliative.pdf

Navigante, A.H., Cerchietti, L.C., Castro, M.A., Lutteral, M.A., & Cabalar, M.E. (2006). Midazolam as adjunct therapy to morphine in the alleviation of severe dyspnea perception in patients with advanced cancer. *Journal of Pain and Symptom Management, 31*(1), 38–47.

Philip, J., Gold, M., Milner, A., Di Iulio, J., Miller, B., & Spruyt, O. (2006). A randomized, double-blind, cross-over trial of the effect of oxygen on dyspnea in patients with advanced cancer. *Journal of Pain and Symptom Management, 32*(6), 541–550.

Quigley, C., Joel, S., Patel, N., Baksh, A., & Slevin, M. (2002). A phase I/II study of nebulized morphine-6-glucuronide in patients with cancer-related breathlessness. *Journal of Pain and Symptom Management, 23*(1), 7–9.

Shimoyama, N., & Shimoyama, M. (2002). Nebulized furosemide as a novel treatment for dyspnea in terminal cancer patients. *Journal of Pain and Symptom Management, 23*(1), 73–76.

Tanaka, K., Shima, Y., Kakinuma, R., Kubota, K., Ohe, Y., Hojo, F., et al. (1999). Effect of nebulized morphine in cancer patients with dyspnea: A pilot study. *Japanese Journal of Clinical Oncology, 29*(12), 600–603.

Uronis, H.E., Currow, D.C., McCrory, D.C., Samsa, G.P., & Abernethy, A.P. (2008). Oxygen for relief of dyspnoea in mildly- or non-hypoxaemic patients with cancer: A systematic review and meta-analysis. *British Journal of Cancer, 98*(2), 294–299.

Vickers, A.J., Feinstein, M.B., Deng, G.E., & Cassileth, B.R. (2005, August 18). Acupuncture for dyspnea in advanced cancer: A randomized, placebo-controlled pilot trial [ISRCTN89462491]. *BMC Palliative Care, 4*, 5.

Viola, R., Kiteley, C., Lloyd, N.S., Mackay, J.A., Wilson, J., & Wong, R.K. (2008). The management of dyspnea in cancer patients: A systematic review. *Supportive Care in Cancer, 16*(4), 329–337.

Wilcock, A., Corcoran, R., & Tattersfield, A.E. (1994). Safety and efficacy of nebulized lignocaine in patients with cancer and breathlessness. *Palliative Medicine, 8*(1), 35–38.

Wilcock, A., Walton, A., Manderson, C., Feathers, L., El Khoury, B., Lewis, M., et al. (2008). Randomised, placebo controlled trial of nebulised furosemide for breathlessness in patients with cancer. *Thorax, 63*(10), 872–875.

Zeppetella, G. (1997). Nebulized morphine in the palliation of dyspnoea. *Palliative Medicine, 11*(4), 267–275.

CHAPTER 11

Fatigue

Problem

Cancer-related fatigue is defined as "a distressing, persistent, subjective sense of physical, emotional, and/or cognitive tiredness or exhaustion related to cancer or cancer treatment that is not proportional to recent activity and interferes with usual functioning" (National Comprehensive Cancer Network [NCCN], 2008, p. FT-1).

Incidence

Fatigue is the most common symptom reported by patients with cancer during treatment. An estimated 80%–100% of people with cancer experience fatigue (Lawrence, Kupelnick, Miller, Devine, & Lau, 2004; Prue, Rankin, Allen, Gracey, & Cramp, 2006; Servaes, Verhagen, & Bleijenberg, 2002). Fatigue may be related directly to the cancer or its treatment and may continue for years after treatment is completed (Wang, 2008). Fatigue may occur as an isolated symptom or as one element in a cluster of symptoms such as pain, depression, sleep disturbance, and anemia (NCCN, 2008).

Assessment

Because fatigue is a subjective experience, it is best assessed by patient self-report. A detailed assessment of risk and contributing factors (see Table 11-1) and information obtained from a clinical measurement tool are essential for monitoring fatigue.

Clinical Measurement Tools

No matter what tool is used to measure fatigue, it should obtain comparable data at different points in time. This is essential in determining the effects of nursing interventions on the person's fatigue experience. The following clinical measurement tools for fatigue are presented in Table 11-2.

Table 11-1. Fatigue Assessment Guide		
Assessment	Yes	No
Physical Symptoms		
Shortness of breath		
Heart palpitations		
General lack of energy		
Risk and Contributing Factors		
Anemia		
Hypothyroidism		
Hypogonadism		
Adrenal insufficiency		
Cardiomyopathy		
Pulmonary dysfunction		
Fluid and electrolyte imbalances		
Nausea		
Pain		
Depressed mood		
Emotional distress		
Sleep disturbances		
Sedation secondary to specific classes of medications		

Note. Based on information from National Comprehensive Cancer Network, 2008; Newton, 2008.

1. Brief Fatigue Inventory (BFI) (see Figure 11-1)
2. Numeric Rating Scale (e.g., Oncology Nursing Society [ONS] Fatigue Scale [see Figure 11-2])
3. Revised Piper Fatigue Scale

References

Beck, S.L. (2004). *Measuring oncology-nursing sensitive patient outcomes: Evidence-based summary.* Retrieved April 17, 2008, from http://www.ons.org/outcomes/measures/fatigue .shtml

Butt, Z., Wagner, L.I., Beaumont, J.L., Paice, J.A., Peterman, A.H., Shevrin, D., et al. (2008). Use of a single-item screening tool to detect clinically significant fatigue, pain, distress, and anorexia in ambulatory cancer practice. *Journal of Pain and Symptom Management, 35*(1), 20–30.

Table 11-2. Clinical Measurement Tools for Fatigue

Name of Tool	Number of Items	Domains	Reliability and Validity	Populations	Clinical Utility
Brief Fatigue Inventory	9	Severity and impact of fatigue	Adequate reliability and validity established	Variety of cancer diagnoses, chronic cancer-related pain	Rapidly identifies patients with clinically significant fatigue
Numeric Rating Scale (e.g., Oncology Nursing Society Fatigue Scale)	1	Intensity	Less reliable than multiple-item fatigue measures. Established reliability and validity for fatigue screening.	Solid tumors	Easy to use
Revised Piper Fatigue Scale	22 plus 5 additional open-ended items	Behavioral/severity, affective, sensory, cognitive/mood	Adequate reliability and validity established	Variety of cancer diagnoses	Somewhat long for clinical use

Note. Based on information from Beck, 2004; Butt et al., 2008; Lee et al., 1991.

Lawrence, D.P., Kupelnick, B., Miller, K., Devine, D., & Lau, J. (2004). Evidence report on the occurrence, assessment, and treatment of fatigue in cancer patients. *Journal of the National Cancer Institute Monographs, 2004*(32), 40–50.

Lee, K.A., Hicks, G., & Nino-Murcia, G. (1991). Validity and reliability of a scale to assess fatigue. *Psychiatry Research, 36*(3), 291–298.

National Comprehensive Cancer Network. (2008). *NCCN Clinical Practice Guidelines in Oncology™: Cancer-related fatigue* [v.1.2008]. Retrieved April 17, 2008, from http://www.nccn.org/professionals/physician_gls/PDF/fatigue.pdf

Newton, S. (2008). Fatigue. In S. Newton, M. Hickey, & J. Marrs (Eds.), *Mosby's oncology nursing advisor* (pp. 361–364). St. Louis, MO: Elsevier Mosby.

Prue, G., Rankin, J., Allen, J., Gracey, J., & Cramp, F. (2006). Cancer-related fatigue: A critical appraisal. *European Journal of Cancer, 42*(7), 846–863.

Servaes, P., Verhagen, C., & Bleijenberg, G. (2002). Fatigue in cancer patients during and after treatment: Prevalence, correlates and interventions. *European Journal of Cancer, 38*(1), 27–43.

Wang, S.X. (2008). Pathophysiology of cancer-related fatigue. *Clinical Journal of Oncology Nursing, 12*(Suppl. 5), 11–20.

Figure 11-1. Brief Fatigue Inventory

Brief Fatigue Inventory

STUDY ID# _____   HOSPITAL # _____

Date: _____ / _____ / _____   Time: _____

Name _____ _____ _____
         Last   First   Middle Initial

Throughout our lives, most of us have times when we feel very tired or fatigued. Have you felt unusually tired or fatigued in the last week? Yes ▢ No ▢

1. Please rate your fatigue (weariness, tiredness) by circling the one number that best describes your fatigue right NOW.

0	1	2	3	4	5	6	7	8	9	10
No Fatigue										As bad as you can imagine

2. Please rate your fatigue (weariness, tiredness) by circling the one number that best describes your USUAL level of fatigue during past 24 hours.

0	1	2	3	4	5	6	7	8	9	10
No Fatigue										As bad as you can imagine

3. Please rate your fatigue (weariness, tiredness) by circling the one number that best describes your WORST level of fatigue during past 24 hours.

0	1	2	3	4	5	6	7	8	9	10
No Fatigue										As bad as you can imagine

4. Circle the one number that describes how, during the past 24 hours, fatigue has interfered with your:

A. General activity

0	1	2	3	4	5	6	7	8	9	10
Does not interfere										Completely Interferes

B. Mood

0	1	2	3	4	5	6	7	8	9	10
Does not interfere										Completely Interferes

C. Walking ability

0	1	2	3	4	5	6	7	8	9	10
Does not interfere										Completely Interferes

D. Normal work (includes both work outside the home and daily chores)

0	1	2	3	4	5	6	7	8	9	10
Does not interfere										Completely Interferes

E. Relations with other people

0	1	2	3	4	5	6	7	8	9	10
Does not interfere										Completely Interferes

F. Enjoyment of life

0	1	2	3	4	5	6	7	8	9	10
Does not interfere										Completely Interferes

Figure 11-2. Numeric Rating Scale

FATIGUE SCALE

Select the number that best describes how you feel today.

NO FATIGUE	MILD FATIGUE	MODERATE FATIGUE	EXTREME FATIGUE	THE WORST FATIGUE
0	1 2 3	4 5 6	7 8 9	10

Copyright © 2000 Oncology Nursing Society

Note. Copyright 2000 by Oncology Nursing Society. Used with permission.

Case Study

W.H. was a 53-year-old female diagnosed with stage T2 N0 MX invasive ductal breast cancer (grade III 2.5 × 2.5 × 2.3 cm tumor, estrogen receptor/progesterone receptor negative, HER2/neu negative). W.H.'s oncologist recommended AC-T (four cycles of doxorubicin/cyclophosphamide every three weeks followed by four cycles of paclitaxel every three weeks). W.H. was married and worked full-time managing a business. During chemotherapy teaching, W.H. mentioned how important it was for her to be able to continue working, stating that it would help her to "stay focused on something besides cancer." She also said that she did not have many hobbies and had always thrived on the intensity of her career, stating, "I'm kind of a control freak."

The topic of fatigue was covered during W.H.'s teaching about potential side effects from chemotherapy. Recognizing W.H.'s concern about having enough energy to continue working, W.H. and her nurse consulted the ONS Putting Evidence Into Practice (PEP) resource on fatigue to facilitate discussion about interventions that are effective in both preventing and treating fatigue during cancer treatment. After noting that multiple randomized controlled trials have shown exercise to be effective in limiting and managing fatigue, W.H. was quick to mention that she had never been one to exercise on a regular basis. Reading further, she learned that "exercise" can be something as simple as walking several times per week and said that she definitely was willing to give that a try.

Together, W.H. and her nurse also reviewed the interventions listed on the ONS PEP resource on fatigue that are likely to be effective. W.H. was not interested in learning relaxation techniques ("I can't see myself doing that") but said she would think about scheduling regular massages and trying to "slow down" at work. The nurse explained to W.H. the importance of screening for other factors that may be contributing to fatigue (interventions cited in the *Likely to Be Effective* section of the ONS PEP resource) and explained that this was a standard part of the nursing assessment at each visit in addition to measuring the intensity and impact of fatigue by completing the BFI.

W.H. found that working the day after receiving chemotherapy was difficult because of the delayed nausea, so she scheduled her chemotherapy for Thursdays, taking Fridays off. W.H. was proud of herself for taking this step (working less) in caring for herself. She also was walking at lunch with a friend several times per week and felt that the exercise helped her to reenergize.

Upon completion of the four cycles of doxorubicin and cyclophosphamide, W.H. admitted that she really struggles at work the week following her chemotherapy. She mentioned that she had a friend who "got a shot" during her chemotherapy to help with her fatigue. W.H.'s hemoglobin was 10.1 g/dl and her hematocrit was 29.4 g/dl. After reviewing the ONS PEP resource on fatigue, the nurse discussed with W.H. the risks and benefits of using erythropoiesis-stimulating agents (ESAs). The nurse facilitated further discussion with the patient and her oncologist during the visit.

Ultimately, W.H. was able to complete her treatment without further significant drop in hemoglobin and without adding an ESA. Her scores on the BFI remained at the mild fatigue level (1–3) throughout treatment except for the weeks after treatment, when her fatigue was at a moderate level (4–6). The patient and nurse continued to monitor the level of fatigue and its consequences for functioning as the patient completed her treatment and began the recovery process. The nurse provided anticipatory guidance that fatigue may persist for several months after the conclusion of treatment and continued to offer suggestions and reinforcement of the patient's efforts to adopt effective self-management behaviors.

Patricia Starr, RN, MSN, OCN®
Neuro-Oncology/CyberKnife® Care Coordinator
Waukesha Memorial Hospital
Waukesha, WI

Fatigue

2009 AUTHORS
Sandra A. Mitchell, PhD, CRNP, AOCN®, and Susan L. Beck, APRN, PhD, AOCN®, FAAN
ONS STAFF: Linda H. Eaton, MN, RN, AOCN®

2006 AUTHORS
Sandra A. Mitchell, MScN, CRNP, AOCN®, Susan L. Beck, PhD, APRN, AOCN®,
Linda Edwards Hood, MSN, RN, AOCN®, Katen Moore, MSN, APRN, AOCN®,
and Ellen R. Tanner, RN, BSN, OCN®
ONS STAFF: Linda H. Eaton, MN, RN, AOCN®

What interventions are effective in preventing and treating fatigue?

Recommended for Practice

Interventions for which effectiveness has been demonstrated by strong evidence from rigorously conducted studies, meta-analyses, or systematic reviews and for which expectation of harms is small compared with the benefits

EXERCISE

Fourteen meta-analyses or systematic reviews (Conn, Hafdahl, Porock, McDaniel, & Nielsen, 2006; Courneya & Friedenreich, 1999; Cramp & Daniel, 2008; Galvao & Newton, 2005; Jacobsen, Donovan, Vadaparampil, & Small, 2007; Knols, Aaronson, Uebelhart, Fransen, & Aufdemkampe, 2005; Labourey, 2007; Markes, Brockow, & Resch, 2006; McNeely et al., 2006; Oldervoll, Kaasa, Hjermstad, Lund, & Loge, 2004; Schmitz et al., 2005; Stevinson, Lawlor, & Fox, 2004; Stricker, Drake, Hoyer, & Mock, 2004; Thorsen, Courneya, Stevinson, & Fossa, 2008) support the benefits of exercise in the management of fatigue during and following cancer treatment in patients with breast cancer, prostate cancer, and mixed solid tumors and in recipients of hematopoietic stem cell transplantation. Although positive results for the outcome of fatigue have not been observed consistently across studies, and effect sizes were very small and in some cases were not statistically significant (Conn et al.; Jacobsen et al.; Markes et al.), the general pattern of results in 28 randomized controlled trials (RCTs) (N = 2,083 participants) indicates that exercising several times per week (including walking, cycling, swimming, resistance exercise, or a combination of aerobic and resistance exercise) can be effective in reducing fatigue during and following cancer treatment. Most of the studies reviewed suffer from methodologic shortcomings, and meta-analysis is limited by the fact that there is heterogeneity in the exercise characteristics and intervention dose, as well as diverse measures of outcomes and variation in the timing of outcome assessment. Moreover, few studies required that study participants have a clinically significant level of fatigue. As a result, the possibility exists that many participants were experiencing little or no fatigue at the time of study entry, thus limiting the ability to detect intervention effects. Much more research is needed to systematically assess the safety of exercise (both aerobic exercise and strength training) (Humpel & Iverson, 2005) and to tailor the type, intensity, frequency, and duration of physical exercise to different tumor types and stages of the disease and treatments. Further research is needed using larger samples, attention control groups (a feature of study design that tests the hypothesis that improvements in fatigue occurred not because of the intervention but rather are the result of the expectancy of improvement or as a result of the attention received during the course of the treatment), and blinding of the outcome assessor. The study design also should control for exercise motivation and preferences as well as participant adherence.

Likely to Be Effective

Interventions for which effectiveness has been demonstrated by supportive evidence from a single rigorously conducted controlled trial, consistent supportive evidence from well-designed controlled trials using small samples, or guidelines developed from evidence and supported by expert opinion

SCREENING FOR POTENTIAL ETIOLOGIC FACTORS AND MANAGING AS APPROPRIATE

There is expert consensus that patients with fatigue be screened for potentially treatable etiologic factors contributing to fatigue (National Comprehensive Cancer Network [NCCN], 2008) and managed as indicated. These treatable etiologic factors include concurrent distressing symptoms, including pain, nausea, and depression; hypothyroidism, hypogonadism, cardiomyopathy, adrenal insufficiency, pulmonary dysfunction, anemia, sleep disturbance, fluid and electrolyte imbalances, and emotional distress; and sedation secondary to specific classes of medications (e.g., opiates, antidepressants, antiemetics, antihistamines) or due to drug-drug interactions.

ENERGY CONSERVATION AND ACTIVITY MANAGEMENT

A nurse-delivered intervention focused on energy conservation and activity management (ECAM) was found to have a modest but significant effect in a large, multisite RCT in patients (predominantly with breast cancer) initiating chemotherapy or radiation (Barsevick et al., 2004). A pilot study by the same investigators showed a trend for ECAM to be superior using a historical control group (Barsevick, Whitmer, Sweeney, & Nail, 2002).

EDUCATION/INFORMATION PROVISION

A meta-analysis (Jacobsen et al., 2007), seven RCTs (Fawzy, 1995; Fillion et al., 2008; Gaston-Johansson et al., 2000; Given et al., 2002; Kim, Roscoe, & Morrow, 2002; Ream, Richardson, & Alexander-Dann, 2006; Yates et al., 2005), a matched-pairs controlled trial (Vilela et al., 2006), and two single-arm studies (Allison et al., 2004; Lindemalm, Strang, & Lekander, 2005) in patients with mixed solid and hematologic malignancies across all phases of the disease support a conclusion that educational interventions (including teaching, counseling, support, anticipatory guidance about fatigue patterns, coping skills training, and coaching) play a role in supporting positive coping in patients with fatigue and in reducing fatigue levels. In addition, the NCCN consensus panel guidelines recommend that patients and families be provided with anticipatory guidance about patterns of fatigue and recommendations for self-management, especially when beginning fatigue-inducing treatments (NCCN, 2008). These multifaceted psychoeducational interventions vary in content and delivery method. Thus, concluding which specific elements of such interventions are therapeutic is difficult. Moreover, six RCTs have demonstrated no statistically significant effect of psychoeducational interventions on fatigue outcomes. However, these trials in relatively small and heterogeneous samples may have been underpowered, and none of the studies used level of fatigue as a criterion of eligibility (Arving et al., 2007; Berglund et al., 2007; Brown et al., 2006; Godino, Jodar, Duran, Martinez, & Schiaffinio, 2006; Rummans et al., 2006; Williams & Schreier, 2005). Overall, study results support a conclusion that patients welcome psychoeducative interventions related to fatigue and that they can apply the skills to improve their self-management of fatigue. The potency of these interventions is modest, and they are not effective for all patients.

MEASURES TO OPTIMIZE SLEEP QUALITY

Seven studies (Berger et al., 2002, 2003; Davidson, Waisberg, Brundage, & MacLean, 2001; Dirksen & Epstein, 2008; Espie et al., 2008; Quesnel, Savard, Simard, Ivers, & Morin, 2003; Savard, Simard, Ivers, & Morin, 2005), including three RCTs, support the conclusion that a multicomponent cognitive-behavioral therapy (CBT) intervention designed to optimize sleep quality improves fatigue outcomes. The CBT intervention, delivered individually or in a group, generally included relaxation training, along with sleep consolidation strategies (avoiding long or late afternoon naps, limiting time in bed to actual sleep time), stimulus control therapy (go to bed only when sleepy, use bed/bedroom for sleep and sexual activities only, designate a consistent time to lie down and get up, avoid caffeine and stimulating activity in the evening), and strategies to reduce cognitive-emotional arousal (keep at least an hour to relax before going to bed and establish a pre-sleep routine to be used every night).

RELAXATION

Three RCTs (Cohen & Fried, 2007; Decker, Cline-Elsen, & Gallagher, 1992; Kim & Kim, 2005) found progressive muscle relaxation training, relaxation breathing and yoga-like positioning, and relaxation training with guided imagery delivered in a series of sessions to be effective in lowering fatigue scores. Although a meta-analysis of the effectiveness of relaxation training in reducing treatment-related symptoms in acute nonsurgical cancer treatment did not identify a statistically significant effect of relaxation on fatigue in pooled analyses, those results must be interpreted cautiously because only two of the three aforementioned studies described were included (Luebbert, Dahme, & Hasenbring, 2001).

MASSAGE, HEALING TOUCH, POLARITY THERAPY, AND HAPTOTHERAPY

Single studies provide evidence that massage and healing touch (combined in some studies with centering, breathing, and relaxing music) may be effective in reducing fatigue (Ahles et al., 1999; Cassileth & Vickers, 2004; Currin & Meister, 2008; Post-White et al., 2003). A controlled pilot study in a small sample of 15 women receiving radiation therapy for breast cancer (Roscoe, Matteson, Mustian, Padmanaban, & Morrow, 2005) demonstrated that polarity therapy (an intervention hypothesized to promote healing, relaxation, and well-being by unblocking and balancing energy flow and reestablishing homeostasis within the human energy field) also may be effective in reducing fatigue. On the other hand, in a small controlled trial, five sessions of haptotherapy (a form of complementary therapy that uses a massage-like touch together with an expressive-supportive conversation to help patients connect with feelings and improve coping) delivered over several weeks to patients undergoing outpatient chemotherapy did not result in improvement in fatigue (Van Den Berg, Visser, Schoolmeesters, Edelman, & Borne, 2006). A systematic review concluded that the mixed study results seen with therapeutic modalities that incorporate massage and healing touch may be due, in part, to methodologic limitations, including insufficient statistical power, nonrandomized designs, nonblinded outcomes assessment, and failure to account for participant attrition in statistical analysis (Myers, Walton, Bratsman, Wilson, & Small, 2008).

Benefits Balanced With Harms

Interventions for which clinicians and patients should weigh the beneficial and harmful effects according to individual circumstances and priorities

CORRECTION OF ANEMIA WITH ERYTHROPOIESIS-STIMULATING AGENTS

Data from eight meta-analyses or systematic reviews (Bohlius et al., 2006; Bokemeyer et al., 2007; Kimel, Leidy, Mannix, & Dixon, 2008; Mikhael, Melosky, Cripps, Rayson, & Kouroukis, 2007; Minton, Richardson, Sharpe, Hotopf, & Stone, 2008; Minton, Stone, Richardson, Sharpe, & Hotopf, 2008; Rizzo et al., 2008; Wilson et al., 2007) suggest that patients receiving erythropoiesis-stimulating agents (ESAs) to correct anemia less than 10 g/dl may experience increased vigor and diminished fatigue. Only limited evidence exists that ESAs improve fatigue when anemia is less severe. Although some data suggest that a target hemoglobin level of 11–12 g/dl will produce the greatest gains in fatigue and other quality-of-life outcomes (Stasi et al., 2005), better quality evidence is needed to unequivocally support the use of ESAs solely as an intervention to improve patient reported outcomes such as fatigue (Bottomley, Thomas, Van Steen, Flechtner, & Djulbegovic, 2002; Littlewood, Cella, & Nortier, 2002). Although both epoetin and darbepoetin are generally well tolerated, the use of these agents specifically for the management of fatigue must be considered in light of safety issues, including an increased risk of thrombotic events, hypertension, and concerns that ESAs may support or extend tumor growth in patients with head and neck cancer, breast cancer, non-small cell lung cancer, or cervical cancer. Particular caution should be exercised in the use of ESAs at higher doses, with dosing to target a hemoglobin $\geq$ 12 g/dl, and with protracted ESA treatment (Aapro, Scherhag, & Burger, 2008; Bennett et al., 2008; Melosky, 2008). ESAs may not be indicated to treat anemia associated with malignancy or the anemia of cancer in patients with solid or nonmyeloid hematologic malignancies (e.g., myeloma, chronic lymphocytic leukemia, non-Hodgkin lymphoma), or in patients at increased risk for thromboembolic complications (Rizzo et al., 2008). National clinical practice guidelines (NCCN, 2009; Rodgers, 2006) and the guidance of the U.S. Food and Drug Administration should be used to direct the management of patients receiving ESAs, including decisions about patient monitoring, treatment thresholds, dose reductions, treatment discontinuation, and the use of supplemental iron.

Effectiveness Not Established

Interventions for which insufficient or conflicting data or data of inadequate quality currently exist, with no clear indication of harm

STRUCTURED REHABILITATION

Three single-arm trials (Korstjens, Mesters, van der Peet, Gijsen, & van den Borne, 2006; Strauss-Blasche, Gnad, Ekmekcioglu, Hladschik, & Marktl, 2005; van Weert et al., 2006), a small RCT (Heim, v d Malsburg, & Niklas, 2007), and a systematic review (van Weert et al., 2008) suggest that structured rehabilitation programs result in statistically significant and sustained improvements in fatigue, particularly in patients who have completed treatment and are in the survivorship phase. The rehabilitation interventions studied were multicomponent interventions composed of a structured combination of intensive exercise, physical training, sports, psychoeducation, and physical modalities such as massage, mud packs, and manual lymph drainage. In some studies, these therapies were delivered over the course of a several-week inpatient rehabilitation hospital stay.

INDIVIDUAL AND GROUP PSYCHOTHERAPY

Improved fatigue outcomes resulting from individual or group psychotherapy have been demonstrated in two RCTs (Boesen et al., 2005; Fawzy et al., 1990). The addition of exercise to a group psychotherapy intervention (either stress management and relaxation training or expressive-supportive psychotherapy) was found to improve fatigue outcomes when compared to group psychotherapy alone (Courneya et al., 2003). Difficulty in disentangling the effect of the diverse components in these programs limits the conclusions that can be drawn, and in a multicenter RCT of supportive group psychotherapy in 158 women with metastatic breast cancer (Goodwin et al., 2001), a psychotherapy intervention did not result in a significant improvement in fatigue.

COGNITIVE-BEHAVIORAL THERAPY FOR FATIGUE

Two RCTs of CBT have been conducted in small heterogeneous samples, with mixed effects on the outcome of fatigue. In one RCT (N = 60 patients completing a course of chemotherapy), there was a trend toward greater improvement in fatigue over time in the group receiving CBT (p = 0.09) (Armes, Chalder, Addington-Hall, Richardson, & Hotopf, 2007). In another randomized trial of CBT in 112 fatigued cancer survivors, participants in the intervention group experienced clinically and statistically significant benefits in fatigue severity compared to the wait-list control group (Gielissen, Verhagen, Witjes, & Bleijenberg, 2006).

COGNITIVE-BEHAVIORAL THERAPY FOR CONCURRENT SYMPTOMS

Three RCTs and a small case series analysis have examined fatigue outcomes associated with CBT for concurrent symptoms such as pain or depression. Although outcomes of an RCT of CBT for cancer pain in 131 patients demonstrated improvement in the outcomes of pain, the differences in fatigue were not statistically significant (Dalton, Keefe, Carlson, & Youngblood, 2004). However, two RCTs (N = 200 patients with cancer with major depressive disorder [Strong et al., 2008] and N = 45 women with metastatic breast cancer [Savard et al., 2006]) and a small case series (N = 6 women with metastatic breast cancer [Levesque, Savard, Simard, Gauthier, & Ivers, 2004]) demonstrated that a CBT intervention for depression also resulted in statistically significant improvements in fatigue (p < 0.01).

EXPRESSIVE WRITING

A pilot study compared an expressive writing intervention (four weekly sessions in which participants wrote about their deepest thoughts and feelings) with a writing intervention where participants wrote about neutral issues related to health. No differences in fatigue were reported between the two groups, although post-intervention, the group that had received the expressive writing intervention reported greater vigor (de Moor et al., 2002).

HYPNOSIS

The effects of a 15-minute presurgery hypnosis session compared with nondirective empathic listening (attentional control) were examined in an RCT in 200 women undergoing excisional breast biopsy or lumpectomy. Patients in the hypnosis group reported significantly less fatigue ($p < 0.001$) (Montgomery et al., 2007) when discharged from the same-day surgery center. Despite the sample size and the inclusion of an attention control group, conclusions are limited by the fact that outcome assessors were not blinded to group assignment.

PAROXETINE

Four trials have examined the effectiveness of paroxetine in treating fatigue during and following cancer treatment, with mixed findings. In two large, multicenter, double-blinded, placebo-controlled RCTs (Morrow et al., 2003; Roscoe, Morrow, et al., 2005), paroxetine 20 mg PO daily did not have an effect on fatigue, although improvements in depression and overall mood were noted in the paroxetine treatment group. A recent meta-analysis pooling these results concluded that paroxetine has no benefit over placebo in the treatment of cancer-related fatigue (Minton, Richardson, et al., 2008; Minton, Stone, et al., 2008). However, two small trials have shown a trend toward a possible benefit for paroxetine in treating fatigue in women with hot flashes (N = 13) (Weitzner, Moncello, Jacobsen, & Minton, 2002) and patients receiving interferon alfa (N = 18) (Capuron et al., 2002).

METHYLPHENIDATE

Five prospective, open-label, single-arm trials with small samples and three placebo-controlled, double-blind RCTs have examined the use of methylphenidate (patient-controlled dosing or upward titration from 10 mg/day to 30 mg/day) in reducing fatigue. All five single-arm studies (Bruera, Driver, et al., 2003; Hanna et al., 2006; Sarhill et al., 2001; Schwartz, Thompson, & Masood, 2002; Sugawara et al., 2002) reported improvements in fatigue as a result of methylphenidate, although in one study (Sarhill et al.), more than half of the patients experienced side effects such as insomnia, agitation, anorexia, nausea and vomiting, or dry mouth, and in another study (Hanna et al.), 19% of patients withdrew because of adverse events. In the RCTs (Bruera et al., 2006; Butler et al., 2007; Mar Fan et al., 2007), methylphenidate had no effect on fatigue outcomes, although studies were generally underpowered. A meta-analysis combining the results of the Bruera et al. (2006) RCT with study results from another investigator that have been reported only in abstract form concluded that methylphenidate treatment compared with placebo was associated with a small but statistically significant ($Z = 1.96$; $p = 0.05$) reduction in cancer-related fatigue (Minton, Richardson, et al., 2008; Minton, Stone, et al., 2008).

DONEPEZIL

Donepezil 5 mg every morning has been evaluated in a double-blind, placebo-controlled RCT (N = 142) (Bruera et al., 2007) and in two uncontrolled, open-label trials (Bruera, Strasser, Shen, et al., 2003; Shaw et al., 2006). In both open-label trials, statistically significant improvements were reported in fatigue outcomes. However, in the RCT, fatigue outcomes were not significantly different between the donepezil-treated and placebo-control groups. Conclusions are limited by the paucity of RCTs, and this, together with small samples and short length of treatment, make it difficult to gauge conclusively the effects of donepezil on fatigue outcomes or its tolerability.

BUPROPION SUSTAINED-RELEASE

Bupropion-sustained release at a dose of 100–300 mg/day demonstrated preliminary efficacy in improving fatigue outcomes in two small, open-label, uncontrolled trials in 15 patients with various cancer diagnoses who were experiencing fatigue or depression with marked fatigue (Cullum, Wojciechowski, Pelletier, & Simpson, 2004) and 21 patients with mostly primary brain tumors, breast cancer, or a hematologic malignancy (Moss, Simpson, Pelletier, & Forsyth, 2005). Controlled studies are necessary to establish the efficacy of this intervention in a more homogeneous sample of patients with cancer and to determine whether this effect of bupropion is separate from its action as an antidepressant.

MODAFINIL

In a case report, the use of modafinil (at a dose of 100 mg QD or BID) was associated with improvements in daytime wakefulness and normalization of the sleep-wake cycle in two older adult patients with advanced cancer (Caraceni & Simonetti, 2004). No side effects were reported. In another case report, an older adult with postoperative lethargy and listlessness after resection of an intraventricular subependymoma experienced improved wakefulness and responsiveness after five days of treatment with modafinil 400 mg daily. The use of modafinil (at a dose of 100–400 mg in a daily or divided dose) also is supported by an expert opinion report (Cox & Pappagallo, 2001); however, controlled trials are needed.

VENLAFAXINE

A randomized, doubled-blinded, placebo-controlled crossover trial with 57 breast cancer survivors receiving venlafaxine 37.5 mg and 22 breast cancer survivors receiving 75 mg venlafaxine) found no improvement in fatigue overall at either dose of venlafaxine (Carpenter et al., 2007). However, a subgroup of 15 women with a ≥ 50% decrease in physiologic hot flashes experienced significant improvement in fatigue (p = 0.007). The side effects included dry mouth and constipation, and at 12-month follow-up, most study participants had discontinued venlafaxine treatment.

SERTRALINE

When the effects of sertraline on fatigue were studied in an RCT of 189 patients with advanced cancer, sertraline did not have a significant effect on fatigue in the absence of major depression (Stockler et al., 2007). Although the outcome of fatigue was not examined, a single-arm trial has suggested that sertraline improved anxiety, depression, and overall quality of life in depressed patients with cancer (Torta, Siri, & Caldera, 2008). RCTs examining whether sertraline improves fatigue outcomes in depressed patients with cancer are indicated.

TARGETED ANTI-CYTOKINE THERAPY

Two small pilot studies have examined the effects on fatigue of targeted anti-cytokine therapy with either infliximab or etanercept. In a small single-arm trial of infliximab 5 mg/kg, 9 of the 14 participants had improvements in their fatigue severity score (Tookman, Jones, Dewitte, & Lodge, 2008). However, treatment with infliximab was associated with five serious adverse events, including two serious infections attributed by the investigators as possibly related to treatment with infliximab. The effect on fatigue of etanercept 25 mg administered twice weekly in patients with advanced malignancy receiving docetaxel 43 mg/m^2 weekly was studied in a small cohort (N = 12). Patients receiving docetaxel plus etanercept reported significantly less fatigue than those patients receiving docetaxel alone (Monk et al., 2006). Small sample sizes, nonrandom group assignment, and the absence of a placebo control arm limit the conclusions that can be drawn.

REIKI

A small (N = 16), counterbalanced, crossover trial in patients who had recently completed treatment showed no benefit of Reiki on fatigue outcomes (Tsang, Carlson, & Olson, 2007). However, the small, heterogeneous sample and the fact that interaction and order effects were not examined limit the conclusions that can be drawn.

YOGA

Two RCTs and a single-arm pilot study have examined the effects of yoga on fatigue outcomes. In the small (N = 38) RCT comparing the effects of a seven-week yoga program to a wait-list control, no significant differences in fatigue were reported; however, the design did not control for the possible confounding effects of chemotherapy treatment (Cohen, Warneke, Fouladi, Rodriguez, & Chaoul-Reich, 2004). Additionally, in the single-arm trial (N = 13) of an eight-week yoga intervention, the intervention had no significant effect on fatigue, although a trend existed for increased yoga practice to be associated with decreased fatigue (p < 0.07) (Carson et al., 2007). Similarly, a 12-week yoga intervention also had no impact on fatigue in an RCT (N = 128) (Moadel et al., 2007). However, intervention group participants who were highly adherent with the yoga intervention experienced significant improvements in fatigue compared with those intervention group participants who were less adherent.

MINDFULNESS-BASED STRESS REDUCTION

The effects of mindfulness-based stress reduction on fatigue outcomes have been examined in four trials, with mixed results. An RCT comparing mindfulness-based stress reduction with a wait-list control (Speca, Carlson, Goodey, & Angen, 2000) and two single-arm studies (Carlson, Speca, Patel, & Goodey, 2003; Kieviet-Stijnen, Visser, Garssen, & Hudig, 2008), all with small samples, demonstrated no statistically significant effects on fatigue. However, another single-arm trial of a mindfulness-based stress reduction intervention in 63 participants with mixed tumors noted improvements in stress, mood disturbance, sleep quality, and fatigue (Carlson & Garland, 2005).

ACUPUNCTURE

In two RCTs (Gadsby, Franks, Jarvis, & Dewhurst, 1997; Molassiotis, Sylt, & Diggins, 2007) and a single-arm pilot study (Vickers, Straus, Fearon, & Cassileth, 2004), all with small samples, patients receiving traditional Chinese acupuncture or acupuncture-like transcutaneous electrical nerve stimulation tended to report less fatigue. Improvements may not be sustained once acupuncture is discontinued (Molassiotis et al.).

ART, MUSIC, OR ANIMAL-ASSISTED THERAPY

Art therapy (Bar-Sela, Atid, Danos, Gabay, & Epelbaum, 2007), music therapy (Bozcuk et al., 2006; Burns et al., 2008; Clark et al., 2006), and animal-assisted therapy (Johnson, Meadows, Haubner, & Sevedge, 2008) each have been studied in one or more small trials, and none has demonstrated positive effects on the outcome of fatigue. Studies were generally underpowered because of small sample sizes, and the interventions themselves may have been insufficiently potent. Nonrandom treatment assignment and the use of pre/post-test study designs rather than a comparison group further limit the conclusions that can be drawn.

DISTRACTION—VIRTUAL REALITY IMMERSION

A distractive intervention, virtual reality immersion (VRI), has been investigated in three randomized crossover trials (Schneider, Ellis, Coombs, Shonkwiler, & Folsom, 2003; Schneider & Hood, 2007; Schneider, Prince-Paul, Allen, Silverman, & Talaba, 2004), an RCT (Oyama, Kaneda, Katsumata, Akechi, & Ohsuga, 2000), and a single-arm pilot study (Oyama, Ohsuga, Tatsuno, & Katsumata, 1999). All but one (Schneider & Hood) of the trials studied fewer than 20 participants, and across studies, the results have been mixed. In one of the three randomized crossover trials, the patients who received the VRI intervention demonstrated a trend toward lower fatigue scores, although the differences did not reach statistical significance (Schneider et al.); however, in the largest crossover trial (N = 127) (Schneider & Hood), VRI had no effect on fatigue. Adequately powered RCTs are needed to further explore these preliminary results.

LEVOCARNITINE SUPPLEMENTATION

Four small, open-label, single-arm trials in patients with mixed advanced solid tumors receiving chemotherapy provide preliminary support for the safety and efficacy of levocarnitine supplementation in treating fatigue in nonanemic patients with cancer who have low serum carnitine levels (Cruciani et al., 2004, 2006; Gramignano et al., 2006; Graziano et al., 2002). Although the conclusions that can be drawn are limited by small sample sizes, nonrandomized study designs, and the absence of double-blinded controls, the results suggest that levocarnitine supplementation should be further studied as a possible intervention for fatigue in patients with cancer.

VITAMIN SUPPLEMENTATION

High-dose vitamin C supplementation has shown beneficial effects ($p < 0.01$) on fatigue in a single-arm, open-label trial in 39 terminally ill patients with advanced malignancies (Yeom, Jung, & Song, 2007). However, the sample was small (N = 39), and the study design did not provide for a comparison group or blinding. In a double-blind, crossover, placebo-controlled RCT in 40 women receiving a six-week course of breast irradiation, the use of a daily multivitamin was associated with worsened fatigue outcomes (de Souza Fêde et al., 2007). The investigators speculate that some of the ingredients in the multivitamin formula may have induced worsening fatigue. Moreover, confounds may have been introduced owing to the small sample size and the fact that the evaluation period in the study was extremely short, with a crossover at the midpoint of radiation therapy.

ADENOSINE 5' TRIPHOSPHATE INFUSION

A randomized, open-label study of 30-hour IV infusions of adenosine 5' triphosphate (ATP) administered every two to four weeks for 10 doses was conducted in 28 patients with advanced non-small cell lung cancer (Agteresch, Dagnelie, van der Gaast, Stijnen, & Wilson, 2000). Researchers reported a significant effect on fatigue, as measured by a single item on the Rotterdam Symptom Checklist. Mild infusional side effects such as chest discomfort and flushing resolved by slowing the rate of infusion. Conclusions are limited by the open-label design, the small sample size, and the fact that the investigators did not control for concomitant administration of corticosteroids to manage other disease-related symptoms such as cerebral edema, nausea, and dyspnea. The impact of continuous infusion therapy on quality of life was not assessed.

LECTIN-STANDARDIZED MISTLETOE EXTRACT

In two large retrospective cohort studies in women with breast cancer (Beuth, Schneider, & Schierholz, 2008; Schumacher et al., 2003), compared to those who were not using any complementary pharmacologic therapy or nutritional supplement, the administration of lectin-standardized mistletoe extract was associated with a significant reduction in fatigue, both while on postoperative treatment and during the post-treatment follow-up. Mistletoe extract was safe overall, with reported side effects of predominantly local and self-limited skin reactions such as erythema or itching. The fact that fatigue outcomes were collected via chart review rather than systematically by patient self-report limits the conclusions that can be drawn from these studies.

ESSIAC

A retrospective cohort study of 510 patients with breast cancer, with 32 (6.2%) reporting that they were using the herbal treatment Essiac to treat their breast cancer, found no significant differences in fatigue between those who were using Essiac and those who were not (Zick et al., 2006). The group using Essiac tended to be younger and with more advanced stages of breast cancer; however, this study did not control for these potential confounds.

CHINESE MEDICINAL HERBS

A Cochrane review of the effects of Chinese medicinal herbs on treatment side effects in women with breast cancer identified one study reporting a small but statistically significant improvement in fatigue in women receiving chemotherapy for breast cancer who also were receiving Chinese medicinal herbs compared to those women who did not receive this supplement (Zhang, Liu, Li, He, & Tripathy, 2007).

OMEGA-3 FATTY ACID SUPPLEMENTATION

Two single-arm, open-label trials (Cerchietti, Navigante, & Castro, 2007; Read et al., 2007) and one placebo-controlled RCT (Bruera, Strasser, Palmer, et al., 2003) examining the effects of supplementation with omega-3 fatty acids have shown preliminary evidence to suggest beneficial effects on fatigue outcomes, although overall, omega-3 fatty acid supplementation may not be well tolerated because of dysgeusia and oily diarrhea. In the studies where omega-3 fatty acids have been combined with other agents, disentangling the effects of specific agents on cancer-related fatigue and the side-effects profile is impossible. Additional research to establish the maximum tolerated dose of omega-3 fatty acid supplementation in patients with satisfactory performance status and limited gastrointestinal symptoms at baseline may be indicated as an initial step in further development of this therapy.

COMBINATION THERAPY: DIETARY SUPPLEMENTS AND LIPID REPLACEMENT/ ANTIOXIDANT SUPPLEMENTATION

Single studies in small, heterogeneous samples offer preliminary evidence that a dietary supplement such as soy protein (Jensen & Hessov, 1997), enteral food supplementation (Cerchietti et al., 2004), lipid replacement/antioxidant combination (Colodny et al., 2000), or a combination of polyphenols, antioxidants, vitamins, alpha-lipoic acid, and carbocysteine (alone or in combination with one or more pharmacologic agents such as celecoxib, medroxy progesterone acetate, l-carnitine, or thalidomide) (Mantovani et al., 2006, 2008) may be effective in reducing fatigue. Small sample sizes, nonrandomized, uncontrolled study designs, and the failure to control for baseline differences in fatigue between the study and comparison groups limit definitive conclusions. Moreover, with these combination therapies, disentangling the relative effects of a specific agent on the outcome of cancer-related fatigue and the overall tolerability of the regimen is impossible.

COMBINATION THERAPY: AROMATHERAPY, FOOT SOAK, AND REFLEXOLOGY

An open-label pilot study of a combination of an aromatherapy foot soak with lavender for 3 minutes and reflexology for 10 minutes with jojoba oil and lavender in 20 patients at the end of life found significant decreases in fatigue one and four hours after the treatment (Kohara et al., 2004).

Effectiveness Unlikely

Interventions for which lack of effectiveness has been demonstrated by negative evidence from a single rigorously conducted controlled trial, consistent negative evidence from well-designed controlled trials using small samples, or guidelines developed from evidence and supported by expert opinion

There are no interventions as of May 2008.

Not Recommended for Practice

Interventions for which lack of effectiveness or harmfulness has been demonstrated by strong evidence from rigorously conducted studies, meta-analyses, or systematic reviews, or interventions where the costs, burden, or harms associated with the intervention exceed anticipated benefit

There are no interventions as of May 2008.

Expert Opinion

Low-risk interventions that are (1) consistent with sound clinical practice, (2) suggested by an expert in a peer-reviewed publication (journal or book chapter), and (3) for which limited evidence exists. An expert is an individual with peer-reviewed journal publications in the domain of interest.

Although empirical evidence is limited, experts recommend that the following interventions be considered for patients experiencing fatigue during and following cancer treatment (Ahlberg, Ekman, Gaston-Johansson, & Mock, 2003; Bower et al., 2005; Cimprich, 1993; Cimprich & Ronis, 2003; Davis, Khoshknabi, & Yue, 2006; Iop, Manfredi, & Bonura, 2004; Lawrence, Kupelnick, Miller, Devine, & Lau, 2004; Levy, 2008; Mock, 2004; Mock et al., 2007; Mock & Olsen, 2003; Morrow, Shelke, Roscoe, Hickok, & Mustian, 2005; Mustian et al., 2007; Nail, 2002; NCCN, 2008; Radbruch et al., 2008; Shafqat et al., 2005; Sood & Moynihan, 2005; Stone & Minton, 2008).
- Work with patients and family caregivers to improve assessment of fatigue and identify management strategies.

- Promote open communication among patients, family members, and the caregiving team to facilitate discussions about the experience of fatigue and its effects on daily life.
- Consider attention-restoring activities, such as exposure to natural environments, and pleasant distractions such as music.
- Encourage a balanced diet with adequate intake of fluid, electrolytes, calories, protein, carbohydrates, fat, vitamins, and minerals.
- Consider treatment with low-dose corticosteroids.

Definitions of the interventions are available at **www.ons.org/outcomes**.
Literature search completed through May 2008.

References

Aapro, M., Scherhag, A., & Burger, H.U. (2008). Effect of treatment with epoetin-beta on survival, tumour progression and thromboembolic events in patients with cancer: An updated meta-analysis of 12 randomised controlled studies including 2,301 patients. *British Journal of Cancer, 99*(1), 14–22.

Agteresch, H.J., Dagnelie, P.C., van der Gaast, A., Stijnen, T., & Wilson, J.H. (2000). Randomized clinical trial of adenosine 5'-triphosphate in patients with advanced non-small-cell lung cancer. *Journal of the National Cancer Institute, 92*(4), 321–328.

Ahlberg, K., Ekman, T., Gaston-Johansson, F., & Mock, V. (2003). Assessment and management of cancer-related fatigue in adults. *Lancet, 362*(9384), 640–650.

Ahles, T.A., Tope, D.M., Pinkson, B., Walch, S., Hann, D., Whedon, M., et al. (1999). Massage therapy for patients undergoing autologous bone marrow transplantation. *Journal of Pain and Symptom Management, 18*(3), 157–163.

Allison, P.J., Edgar, L., Nicolau, B., Archer, J., Black, M., & Hier, M. (2004). Results of a feasibility study for a psycho-educational intervention in head and neck cancer. *Psycho-Oncology, 13*(7), 482–485.

Armes, J., Chalder, T., Addington-Hall, J., Richardson, A., & Hotopf, M. (2007). A randomized controlled trial to evaluate the effectiveness of a brief, behaviorally oriented intervention for cancer-related fatigue. *Cancer, 110*(6), 1385–1395.

Arving, C., Sjoden, P.O., Bergh, J., Hellbom, M., Johansson, B., & Glimelius, B. (2007). Individual psychosocial support for breast cancer patients: A randomized study of nurse versus psychologist interventions and standard care. *Cancer Nursing, 30*(3), E10–E19.

Bar-Sela, G., Atid, L., Danos, S., Gabay, N., & Epelbaum, R. (2007). Art therapy improved depression and influenced fatigue levels in cancer patients on chemotherapy. *Psycho-Oncology, 16*(11), 980–984.

Barsevick, A.M., Dudley, W., Beck, S., Sweeney, C., Whitmer, K., & Nail, L. (2004). A randomized clinical trial of energy conservation for patients with cancer-related fatigue. *Cancer, 100*(6), 1302–1310.

Barsevick, A.M., Whitmer, K., Sweeney, C., & Nail, L.M. (2002). A pilot study examining energy conservation for cancer treatment-related fatigue. *Cancer Nursing, 25*(5), 333–341.

Bennett, C.L., Silver, S.M., Djulbegovic, B., Samaras, A.T., Blau, C.A., Gleason, K.J., et al. (2008). Venous thromboembolism and mortality associated with recombinant erythropoietin and darbepoetin administration for the treatment of cancer-associated anemia. *JAMA, 299*(8), 914–924.

Berger, A.M., VonEssen, S., Kuhn, B.R., Piper, B.F., Agrawal, S., Lynch, J.C., et al. (2002). Feasibility of a sleep intervention during adjuvant breast cancer chemotherapy. *Oncology Nursing Forum, 29*(10), 1431–1441.

Berger, A.M., VonEssen, S., Kuhn, B.R., Piper, B.F., Agrawal, S., Lynch, J.C., et al. (2003). Adherence, sleep, and fatigue outcomes after adjuvant breast cancer chemotherapy: Results of a feasibility intervention study. *Oncology Nursing Forum, 30*(3), 513–522.

Berglund, G., Petersson, L.M., Eriksson, K.C., Wallenius, L., Roshanai, A., Nordin, K.M., et al. (2007). Between men: A psychosocial rehabilitation programme for men with prostate cancer. *Acta Oncologica, 46*(1), 83–89.

Beuth, J., Schneider, B., & Schierholz, J.M. (2008). Impact of complementary treatment of breast cancer patients with standardized mistletoe extract during aftercare: A controlled multicenter comparative epidemiological cohort study. *Anticancer Research, 28*(1B), 523–527.

Boesen, E.H., Ross, L., Frederiksen, K., Thomsen, B.L., Dahlstrom, K., Schmidt, G., et al. (2005). Psychoeducational intervention for patients with cutaneous malignant melanoma: A replication study. *Journal of Clinical Oncology, 23*(6), 1270–1277.

Bohlius, J., Wilson, J., Seidenfeld, J., Piper, M., Schwarzer, G., Sandercock, J., et al. (2006). Erythropoietin or darbepoetin for patients with cancer. *Cochrane Database of Systematic Reviews* 2006, Issue 3. Art. No.: CD003407. DOI: 10.1002/14651858.CD003407.pub4.

Bokemeyer, C., Aapro, M.S., Courdi, A., Foubert, J., Link, H., Osterborg, A., et al. (2007). EORTC guidelines for the use of erythropoietic proteins in anaemic patients with cancer: 2006 update. *European Journal of Cancer, 43*(2), 258–270.

Bottomley, A., Thomas, R., Van Steen, K., Flechtner, H., & Djulbegovic, B. (2002). Erythropoietin improves quality of life—A response. *Lancet Oncology, 3*(9), 527.

Bower, J.E., Ganz, P.A., Dickerson, S.S., Petersen, L., Aziz, N., & Fahey, J.L. (2005). Diurnal cortisol rhythm and fatigue in breast cancer survivors. *Psychoneuroendocrinology, 30*(1), 92–100.

Bozcuk, H., Artac, M., Kara, A., Ozdogan, M., Sualp, Y., Topcu, Z., et al. (2006). Does music exposure during chemotherapy improve quality of life in early breast cancer patients? A pilot study. *Medical Science Monitor, 12*(5), 200–205.

Brown, P., Clark, M.M., Atherton, P., Huschka, M., Sloan, J.A., Gamble, G., et al. (2006). Will improvement in quality of life (QOL) impact fatigue in patients receiving radiation therapy for advanced cancer? *American Journal of Clinical Oncology, 29*(1), 52–58.

Bruera, E., Driver, L., Barnes, E.A., Willey, J., Shen, L., Palmer, J.L., et al. (2003). Patient-controlled methylphenidate for the management of fatigue in patients with advanced cancer: A preliminary report. *Journal of Clinical Oncology, 21*(23), 4439–4443.

Bruera, E., El Osta, B., Valero, V., Driver, L.C., Pei, B.L., Shen, L., et al. (2007). Donepezil for cancer fatigue: A double-blind, randomized, placebo-controlled trial. *Journal of Clinical Oncology, 25*(23), 3475–3481.

Bruera, E., Strasser, F., Palmer, J.L., Willey, J., Calder, K., Amyotte, G., et al. (2003). Effect of fish oil on appetite and other symptoms in patients with advanced cancer and anorexia/cachexia: A double-blind, placebo-controlled study. *Journal of Clinical Oncology, 21*(1), 129–134.

Bruera, E., Strasser, F., Shen, L., Palmer, J.L., Willey, J., Driver, L.C., et al. (2003). The effect of donepezil on sedation and other symptoms in patients receiving opioids for cancer pain: A pilot study. *Journal of Pain and Symptom Management, 26*(5), 1049–1054.

Bruera, E., Valero, V., Driver, L., Shen, L., Willey, J., Zhang, T., et al. (2006). Patient-controlled methylphenidate for cancer fatigue: A double-blind, randomized, placebo-controlled trial. *Journal of Clinical Oncology, 24*(13), 2073–2078.

Burns, D.S., Azzouz, F., Sledge, R., Rutledge, C., Hincher, K., Monahan, P.O., et al. (2008). Music imagery for adults with acute leukemia in protective environments: A feasibility study. *Supportive Care in Cancer, 16*(5), 507–513.

Butler, J.M., Jr., Case, L.D., Atkins, J., Frizzell, G., Sanders, G., Griffin, P., et al. (2007). A phase III, double-blind, placebo-controlled prospective randomized clinical trial of d-threo-methylphenidate HCl in brain tumor patients receiving radiation therapy. *International Journal of Radiation Oncology, Biology, Physics, 69*(5), 1496–1501.

Capuron, L., Gumnick, J.F., Musselman, D.L., Lawson, D.H., Reemsnyder, A., Nemeroff, C.B., et al. (2002). Neurobehavioral effects of interferon-alpha in cancer patients: Phenomenology and paroxetine responsiveness of symptom dimensions. *Neuropsychopharmacology, 26*(5), 643–652.

Caraceni, A., & Simonetti, F. (2004). Psychostimulants: New concepts for palliative care from the modafinil experience? *Journal of Pain and Symptom Management, 28*(2), 97–99.

Carlson, L.E., & Garland, S.N. (2005). Impact of mindfulness-based stress reduction (MBSR) on sleep, mood, stress and fatigue symptoms in cancer outpatients. *International Journal of Behavioral Medicine, 12*(4), 278–285.

Carlson, L.E., Speca, M., Patel, K.D., & Goodey, E. (2003). Mindfulness-based stress reduction in relation to quality of life, mood, symptoms of stress, and immune parameters in breast and prostate cancer outpatients. *Psychosomatic Medicine, 65*(4), 571–581.

Carpenter, J.S., Storniolo, A.M., Johns, S., Monahan, P.O., Azzouz, G., Elam, J.L., et al. (2007). Randomized, double-blind, placebo-controlled crossover trials of venlafaxine for hot flashes after breast cancer. *Oncologist, 12*(1), 124–135.

Carson, J.W., Carson, K.M., Porter, L.S., Keefe, F.J., Shaw, H., & Miller, J.M. (2007). Yoga for women with metastatic breast cancer: Results from a pilot study. *Journal of Pain and Symptom Management, 33*(3), 331–341.

Cassileth, B.R., & Vickers, A.J. (2004). Massage therapy for symptom control: Outcome study at a major cancer center. *Journal of Pain and Symptom Management, 28*(3), 244–249.

Cerchietti, L.C., Navigante, A.H., & Castro, M.A. (2007). Effects of eicosapentaenoic and docosahexaenoic n-3 fatty acids from fish oil and preferential Cox-2 inhibition on systemic syndromes in patients with advanced lung cancer. *Nutrition and Cancer, 59*(1), 14–20.

Cerchietti, L.C., Navigante, A.H., Peluffo, G.D., Diament, M.J., Stillitani, I., Klein, S.A., et al. (2004). Effects of celecoxib, medroxyprogesterone, and dietary intervention on systemic syndromes in patients with advanced lung adenocarcinoma: A pilot study. *Journal of Pain and Symptom Management, 27*(1), 85–95.

Cimprich, B. (1993). Development of an intervention to restore attention in cancer patients. *Cancer Nursing, 16*(2), 83–92.

Cimprich, B., & Ronis, D.L. (2003). An environmental intervention to restore attention in women with newly diagnosed breast cancer. *Cancer Nursing, 26*(4), 284–292.

Clark, M., Isaacks-Downton, G., Wells, N., Redlin-Grazier, S., Eck, C., Hepworth, J.T., et al. (2006). Use of preferred music to reduce emotional distress and symptom activity during radiation therapy. *Journal of Music Therapy, 43*(3), 247–265.

Cohen, L., Warneke, C., Fouladi, R.T., Rodriguez, M.A., & Chaoul-Reich, A. (2004). Psychological adjustment and sleep quality in a randomized trial of the effects of a Tibetan yoga intervention in patients with lymphoma. *Cancer, 100*(10), 2253–2260.

Cohen, M., & Fried, G. (2007). Comparing relaxation training and cognitive-behavioral group therapy for women with breast cancer. *Research on Social Work Practice, 17*(3), 313–323.

Colodny, L., Lynch, K., Farber, C., Papsih, S., Phillips, K., Sanchez, M., et al. (2000). Results of a study to evaluate the use of Propax to reduce adverse effects of chemotherapy. *Journal of the American Nutraceutical Association, 3*(2), 17–25.

Conn, V.S., Hafdahl, A.R., Porock, D.C., McDaniel, R., & Nielsen, P.J. (2006). A meta-analysis of exercise interventions among people treated for cancer. *Supportive Care in Cancer, 14*(7), 699–712.

Courneya, K.S., & Friedenreich, C.M. (1999). Physical exercise and quality of life following cancer diagnosis: A literature review. *Annals of Behavioral Medicine, 21*(2), 171–179.

Courneya, K.S., Friedenreich, C.M., Sela, R.A., Quinney, H.A., Rhodes, R.E., & Handman, M.T. (2003). The group psychotherapy and home-based physical exercise (group-hope) trial in cancer survivors: Physical fitness and quality of life outcomes. *Psycho-Oncology, 12*(4), 357–374.

Cox, J.M., & Pappagallo, M. (2001). Modafinil: A gift to portmanteau. *American Journal of Hospice and Palliative Care, 18*(6), 408–410.

Cramp, F., & Daniel, J. (2008). Exercise for the management of cancer-related fatigue in adults. *Cochrane Database of Systematic Reviews* 2008, Issue 2. Art. No.: CD006145. DOI: 10.1002/14651858.CD006145 .pub2.

Cruciani, R.A., Dvorkin, E., Homel, P., Culliney, B., Malamud, S., Shaiova, L., et al. (2004, November). L-carnitine supplementation for the treatment of fatigue and depressed mood in cancer patients with carnitine deficiency: A preliminary analysis. *Annals of the New York Academy of Sciences, 1033,* 168–176.

Cruciani, R.A., Dvorkin, E., Homel, P., Malamud, S., Culliney, B., Lapin, J., et al. (2006). Safety, tolerability and symptom outcomes associated with L-carnitine supplementation in patients with cancer, fatigue, and carnitine deficiency: A phase I/II study. *Journal of Pain and Symptom Management, 32*(6), 551–559.

Cullum, J.L., Wojciechowski, A.E., Pelletier, G., & Simpson, J.S. (2004). Bupropion sustained release treatment reduces fatigue in cancer patients. *Canadian Journal of Psychiatry, 49*(2), 139–144.

Currin, J., & Meister, E.A. (2008). A hospital-based intervention using massage to reduce distress among oncology patients. *Cancer Nursing, 31*(3), 214–221.

Dalton, J.A., Keefe, F.J., Carlson, J., & Youngblood, R. (2004). Tailoring cognitive-behavioral treatment for cancer pain. *Pain Management Nursing, 5*(1), 3–18.

Davidson, J.R., Waisberg, J.L., Brundage, M.D., & MacLean, A.W. (2001). Nonpharmacologic group treatment of insomnia: A preliminary study with cancer survivors. *Psycho-Oncology, 10*(5), 389–397.

Davis, M.P., Khoshknabi, D., & Yue, G.H. (2006). Management of fatigue in cancer patients. *Current Pain and Headache Reports, 10*(4), 260–269.

de Moor, C., Sterner, J., Hall, M., Warneke, C., Gilani, Z., Amato, R., et al. (2002). A pilot study of the effects of expressive writing on psychological and behavioral adjustment in patients enrolled in a phase II trial of vaccine therapy for metastatic renal cell carcinoma. *Health Psychology, 21*(6), 615–619.

de Souza Fêde, A.B., Bensi, C.G., Trufelli, D.C., de Oliveira Campos, M.P., Pecoroni, P.G., Ranzatti, R.P., et al. (2007). Multivitamins do not improve radiation therapy-related fatigue: Results of a double-blind randomized crossover trial. *American Journal of Clinical Oncology, 30*(4), 432–436.

Decker, T.W., Cline-Elsen, J., & Gallagher, M. (1992). Relaxation therapy as an adjunct in radiation oncology. *Journal of Clinical Psychology, 48*(3), 388–393.

Dirksen, S.R., & Epstein, D.R. (2008). Efficacy of an insomnia intervention on fatigue, mood and quality of life in breast cancer survivors. *Journal of Advanced Nursing, 61*(6), 664–675.

Espie, C.A., Fleming, L., Cassidy, J., Samuel, L., Taylor, L.M., White, C.A., et al. (2008). Randomized controlled clinical effectiveness trial of cognitive behavior therapy compared with treatment as usual for persistent insomnia in patients with cancer. *Journal of Clinical Oncology, 26*(28), 4651–4658.

Fawzy, F.I. (1995). A short-term psychoeducational intervention for patients newly diagnosed with cancer. *Supportive Care in Cancer, 3*(4), 235–238.

Fawzy, F.I., Cousins, N., Fawzy, N.W., Kemeny, M.E., Elashoff, R., & Morton, D. (1990). A structured psychiatric intervention for cancer patients. I. Changes over time in methods of coping and affective disturbance. *Archives of General Psychiatry, 47*(8), 720–725.

Fillion, L., Gagnon, P., Leblond, F., Gelinas, C., Sayard, J., Dupuis, R., et al. (2008). A brief intervention for fatigue management in breast cancer survivors. *Cancer Nursing, 31*(2), 145–159.

Gadsby, J.G., Franks, A., Jarvis, P., & Dewhurst, F. (1997). Acupuncture-like transcutaneous electrical nerve stimulation within palliative care: A pilot study. *Complementary Therapies in Medicine, 5*(1), 13–18.

Galvao, D.A., & Newton, R.U. (2005). Review of exercise intervention studies in cancer patients. *Journal of Clinical Oncology, 23*(4), 899–909.

Gaston-Johansson, F., Fall-Dickson, J.M., Nanda, J., Ohly, K.V., Stillman, S., Krumm, S., et al. (2000). The effectiveness of the comprehensive coping strategy program on clinical outcomes in breast cancer autologous bone marrow transplantation. *Cancer Nursing, 23*(4), 277–285.

Gielissen, M.F., Verhagen, S., Witjes, F., & Bleijenberg, G. (2006). Effects of cognitive behavior therapy in severely fatigued disease-free cancer patients compared with patients waiting for cognitive behavior therapy: A randomized controlled trial. *Journal of Clinical Oncology, 24*(30), 4882–4887.

Given, B., Given, C.W., McCorkle, R., Kozachik, S., Cimprich, B., Rahbar, M.H., et al. (2002). Pain and fatigue management: Results of a nursing randomized clinical trial. *Oncology Nursing Forum, 29*(6), 949–956.

Godino, C., Jodar, L., Duran, A., Martinez, I., & Schiaffino, A. (2006). Nursing education as an intervention to decrease fatigue perception in oncology patients. *European Journal of Oncology Nursing, 10*(2), 150–155.

Goodwin, P.J., Leszcz, M., Ennis, M., Koopman, J., Vincent, L., Guther, H., et al. (2001). The effect of group psychosocial support on survival in metastatic breast cancer. *New England Journal of Medicine, 345*(24), 1719–1726.

Gramignano, G., Lusso, M.R., Madeddu, C., Massa, E., Serpe, R., Deiana, L., et al. (2006). Efficacy of l-carnitine administration on fatigue, nutritional status, oxidative stress, and related quality of life in 12 advanced cancer patients undergoing anticancer therapy. *Nutrition, 22*(2), 136–145.

Graziano, F., Bisonni, R., Catalano, V., Silva, R., Rovidati, S., Mencarini, E., et al. (2002). Potential role of le-vocarnitine supplementation for the treatment of chemotherapy-induced fatigue in non-anaemic cancer patients. *British Journal of Cancer, 86*(12), 1854–1857.

Hanna, A., Sledge, G., Mayer, M.L., Hanna, N., Einhorm, L., Monahan, P., et al. (2006). A phase II study of methylphenidate for the treatment of fatigue. *Supportive Care in Cancer, 14*(3), 210–215.

Heim, M.E., v d Malsburg, M.L., & Niklas, A. (2007). Randomized controlled trial of a structured training pro-gram in breast cancer patients with tumor-related chronic fatigue. *Onkologie, 30*(8–9), 429–434.

Humpel, N., & Iverson, D.C. (2005). Review and critique of the quality of exercise recommendations for can-cer patients and survivors. *Supportive Care in Cancer, 13*(7), 493–502.

Iop, A., Manfredi, A.M., & Bonura, S. (2004). Fatigue in cancer patients receiving chemotherapy: An analy-sis of published studies. *Annals of Oncology, 15*(5), 712–720.

Jacobsen, P.B., Donovan, K.A., Vadaparampil, S.T., & Small, B.J. (2007). Systematic review and meta-anal-ysis of psychological and activity-based interventions for cancer-related fatigue. *Health Psychology, 26*(6), 660–667.

Jensen, M.B., & Hessov, I. (1997). Randomization to nutritional intervention at home did not improve post-operative function, fatigue or well-being. *British Journal of Surgery, 84*(1), 113–118.

Johnson, R.A., Meadows, R.L., Haubner, J.S., & Sevedge, K. (2008). Animal-assisted activity among pa-tients with cancer: Effects on mood, fatigue, self-perceived health, and sense of coherence. *Oncology Nursing Forum, 35*(2), 225–232.

Kieviet-Stijnen, A., Visser, A., Garssen, B., & Hudig, W. (2008). Mindfulness-based stress reduction train-ing for oncology patients: Patients' appraisal and changes in well-being. *Patient Education and Coun-seling, 72*(3), 436–442.

Kim, S.D., & Kim, H.S. (2005). Effects of a relaxation breathing exercise on fatigue in hematopoietic stem cell transplantation patients. *Journal of Clinical Nursing, 14*(1), 51–55.

Kim, Y., Roscoe, J.A., & Morrow, G.R. (2002). The effects of information and negative affect on severity of side effects from radiation therapy for prostate cancer. *Supportive Care in Cancer, 10*(5), 416–421.

Kimel, M., Leidy, N.K., Mannix, S., & Dixon, J. (2008). Does epoetin alfa improve health-related quality of life in chronically ill patients with anemia? Summary of trials of cancer, HIV/AIDS, and chronic kidney disease. *Value Health, 11*(1), 57–75.

Knols, R., Aaronson, N.K., Uebelhart, D., Fransen, J., & Aufdemkampe, G. (2005). Physical exercise in can-cer patients during and after medical treatment: A systematic review of randomized and controlled clin-ical trials. *Journal of Clinical Oncology, 23*(16), 3830–3842.

Kohara, H., Miyauchi, T., Suehiro, Y., Ueoka, H., Takeyama, H., & Morita, T. (2004). Combined modality treat-ment of aromatherapy, footsoak, and reflexology relieves fatigue in patients with cancer. *Journal of Pal-liative Medicine, 7*(6), 791–796.

Korstjens, I., Mesters, I., van der Peet, E., Gijsen, B., & van den Borne, B. (2006). Quality of life of cancer survivors after physical and psychosocial rehabilitation. *European Journal of Cancer Prevention, 15*(6), 541–547.

Labourey, J.L. (2007). Physical activity in the management of cancer-related fatigue induced by oncological treatments. *Annales de Readaptation et de Medecine Physique, 50*(6), 445–459.

Lawrence, D.P., Kupelnick, B., Miller, K., Devine, D., & Lau, J. (2004). Evidence report on the occurrence, assessment, and treatment of fatigue in cancer patients. *Journal of the National Cancer Institute Mono-graphs, 2004*(32), 40–50.

Levesque, M., Savard, J., Simard, S., Gauthier, J.G., & Ivers, H. (2004). Efficacy of cognitive therapy for de-pression among women with metastatic cancer: A single-case experimental study. *Journal of Behavior Therapy and Experimental Psychiatry, 35*(4), 287–305.

Levy, M. (2008). Cancer fatigue: A review for psychiatrists. *General Hospital Psychiatry, 30*(3), 233–244.

Lindemalm, C., Strang, P., & Lekander, M. (2005). Support group for cancer patients. Does it improve their physical and psychological wellbeing? A pilot study. *Supportive Care in Cancer, 13*(8), 652–657.

Littlewood, T.J., Cella, D., & Nortier, J.W. (2002). Erythropoietin improves quality of life. *Lancet Oncology, 3*(8), 459–460.

Luebbert, K., Dahme, B., & Hasenbring, M. (2001). The effectiveness of relaxation training in reducing treatment-related symptoms and improving emotional adjustment in acute non-surgical cancer treatment: A meta-analytical review. *Psycho-Oncology, 10*(6), 490–502.

Mantovani, G., Maccio, A., Madeddu, C., Gramignano, G., Lusso, M.R., Serpe, R., et al. (2006). A phase II study with antioxidants, both in the diet and supplemented, pharmaconutritional support, progestagen, and anti-cyclooxygenase-2 showing efficacy and safety in patients with cancer-related anorexia/cachexia and oxidative stress. *Cancer Epidemiology, Biomarkers and Prevention, 15*(5), 1030–1034.

Mantovani, G., Maccio, A., Madeddu, C., Gramignano, G., Serpe, R., Massa, E., et al. (2008). Randomized phase III clinical trial of five different arms of treatment for patients with cancer cachexia: Interim results. *Nutrition, 24*(4), 305–313.

Mar Fan, H.G., Clemons, M., Xu, W., Chemerynsky, I., Breunis, H., Braganza, S., et al. (2007). A randomised, placebo-controlled, double-blind trial of the effects of d-methylphenidate on fatigue and cognitive dysfunction in women undergoing adjuvant chemotherapy for breast cancer. *Supportive Care in Cancer, 16*(6), 577–583.

Markes, M., Brockow, T., & Resch, K.L. (2006). Exercise for women receiving adjuvant therapy for breast cancer. *Cochrane Database of Systematic Reviews* 2006, Issue 4. Art. No.: CD005001. DOI: 10.1002/14651858.CD005001.pub2.

McNeely, M.L., Campbell, K.L., Rowe, B.H., Klassen, T.P., Mackey, J.R., & Courneya, K.S. (2006). Effects of exercise on breast cancer patients and survivors: A systematic review and meta-analysis. *Canadian Medical Association Journal, 175*(1), 34–41.

Melosky, B.L. (2008). Erythropoiesis-stimulating agents: Benefits and risks in supportive care of cancer. *Current Oncology, 15*(Suppl. 1), S10–S15.

Mikhael, J., Melosky, B., Cripps, C., Rayson, D., & Kouroukis, C.T. (2007). Canadian supportive care recommendations for the management of anemia in patients with cancer. *Current Oncology, 14*(5), 209–217.

Minton, O., Richardson, A., Sharpe, M., Hotopf, M., & Stone, P. (2008). A systematic review and meta-analysis of the pharmacological treatment of cancer-related fatigue. *Journal of the National Cancer Institute, 100*(16), 1155–1166.

Minton, O., Stone, P., Richardson, A., Sharpe, M., & Hotopf, M. (2008). Drug therapy for the management of cancer related fatigue. *Cochrane Database of Systematic Reviews* 2008, Issue 1. Art. No.: CD006704. DOI: 10.1002/14651858.CD006704.pub2.

Moadel, A.B., Shah, C., Wylie-Rosett, J., Harris, M.S., Patel, S.R., Hall, C.B., et al. (2007). Randomized controlled trial of yoga among a multiethnic sample of breast cancer patients: Effects on quality of life. *Journal of Clinical Oncology, 25*(28), 4387–4395.

Mock, V. (2004). Evidence-based treatment for cancer-related fatigue. *Journal of the National Cancer Institute Monographs, 2004*(32), 112–118.

Mock, V., Atkinson, A., Barsevick, A.M., Berger, A.M., Cimprich, B., Eisenberger, M.A., et al. (2007). Cancer-related fatigue. Clinical practice guidelines in oncology. *Journal of the National Comprehensive Cancer Network, 5*(10), 1054–1078.

Mock, V., & Olsen, M. (2003). Current management of fatigue and anemia in patients with cancer. *Seminars in Oncology Nursing, 19*(4, Suppl. 2), 36–41.

Molassiotis, A., Sylt, P., & Diggins, H. (2007). The management of cancer-related fatigue after chemotherapy with acupuncture and acupressure: A randomised controlled trial. *Complementary Therapies in Medicine, 15*(4), 228–237.

Monk, J.P., Phillips, G., Waite, R., Kuhn, J., Schaaf, L.J., Otterson, G.A., et al. (2006). Assessment of tumor necrosis factor alpha blockade as an intervention to improve tolerability of dose-intensive chemotherapy in cancer patients. *Journal of Clinical Oncology, 24*(12), 1852–1859.

Montgomery, G.H., Bovbjerg, D.H., Schnur, J.B., David, D., Goldfarb, A., Weltz, C.R., et al. (2007). A randomized clinical trial of a brief hypnosis intervention to control side effects in breast surgery patients. *Journal of the National Cancer Institute, 99*(17), 1304–1312.

Morrow, G.R., Hickok, J.T., Roscoe, J.A., Raubertas, R.F., Andrews, P.L., Flynn, P.J., et al. (2003). Differential effects of paroxetine on fatigue and depression: A randomized, double-blind trial from the University of Rochester Cancer Center Community Clinical Oncology Program. *Journal of Clinical Oncology, 21*(24), 4635–4641.

Morrow, G.R., Shelke, A.R., Roscoe, J.A., Hickok, J.T., & Mustian, K. (2005). Management of cancer-related fatigue. *Cancer Investigation, 23*(3), 229–239.

Moss, E.L., Simpson, J.S., Pelletier, G., & Forsyth, P. (2005). An open-label study of the effects of bupropion SR on fatigue, depression and quality of life of mixed-site cancer patients and their partners. *Psycho-Oncology, 15*(3), 259–267.

Mustian, K.M., Morrow, G.R., Carroll, J.K., Figueroa-Moseley, C.D., Jean-Pierre, P., & Williams, G.C. (2007). Integrative nonpharmacologic behavioral interventions for the management of cancer-related fatigue. *Oncologist, 12*(Suppl. 1), 52–67.

Myers, C.D., Walton, T., Bratsman, L., Wilson, J., & Small, B. (2008). Massage modalities and symptoms reported by cancer patients: Narrative review. *Journal of the Society for Integrative Oncology, 6*(1), 19–28.

Nail, L.M. (2002). Fatigue in patients with cancer. *Oncology Nursing Forum, 29*(3), 537.

National Comprehensive Cancer Network. (2008). *NCCN Clinical Practice Guidelines in Oncology™: Cancer-related fatigue* [v.1.2008]. Retrieved December 3, 2008, from http://www.nccn.org/professionals/physician_gls/PDF/fatigue.pdf

National Comprehensive Cancer Network. (2009). *NCCN Clinical Practice Guidelines in Oncology™: Cancer- and chemotherapy-induced anemia* [v.3.2009]. Retrieved December 3, 2008, from http://www.nccn.org/professionals/physician_gls/PDF/anemia.pdf

Oldervoll, L.M., Kaasa, S., Hjermstad, M.J., Lund, J.A., & Loge, J.H. (2004). Physical exercise results in the improved subjective well-being of a few or is effective rehabilitation for all cancer patients? *European Journal of Cancer, 40*(7), 951–962.

Oyama, H., Kaneda, M., Katsumata, N., Akechi, T., & Ohsuga, M. (2000). Using the bedside wellness system during chemotherapy decreases fatigue and emesis in cancer patients. *Journal of Medical Systems, 24*(3), 173–182.

Oyama, H., Ohsuga, M., Tatsuno, Y., & Katsumata, H. (1999). Evaluation of the psycho-oncological effectiveness of the bedside wellness system. *Cyberpsychology and Behavior, 2*(1), 81–84.

Post-White, J., Kinney, M.E., Savik, K., Gau, J.B., Wilcox, C., & Lerner, I. (2003). Therapeutic massage and healing touch improve symptoms in cancer. *Integrative Cancer Therapies, 2*(4), 332–344.

Quesnel, C., Savard, J., Simard, S., Ivers, H., & Morin, C.M. (2003). Efficacy of cognitive-behavioral therapy for insomnia in women treated for nonmetastatic breast cancer. *Journal of Consulting and Clinical Psychology, 71*(1), 189–200.

Radbruch, L., Strasser, F., Elsner, F., Goncalves, J.F., Loge, J., Kaasa, S., et al. (2008). Fatigue in palliative care patients—An EAPC approach. *Palliative Medicine, 22*(1), 13–32.

Read, J.A., Beale, P.J., Volker, D.H., Smith, N., Childs, A., & Clarke, S.J. (2007). Nutrition intervention using an eicosapentaenoic acid (EPA)-containing supplement in patients with advanced colorectal cancer. Effects on nutritional and inflammatory status: A phase II trial. *Supportive Care in Cancer, 15*(3), 301–307.

Ream, E., Richardson, A., & Alexander-Dann, C. (2006). Supportive intervention for fatigue in patients undergoing chemotherapy: A randomized controlled trial. *Journal of Pain and Symptom Management, 31*(2), 148–161.

Rizzo, J.D., Somerfield, M.R., Hagerty, K.L., Seidenfeld, J., Bohlius, J., Bennett, C.L., et al. (2008). Use of epoetin and darbepoetin in patients with cancer: 2007 American Society of Clinical Oncology/American Society of Hematology clinical practice guideline update. *Journal of Clinical Oncology, 26*(1), 132–149.

Rodgers, G.M. (2006). Guidelines for the use of erythropoietic growth factors in patients with chemotherapy-induced anemia. *Oncology, 20*(8, Suppl. 6), 12–15.

Roscoe, J.A., Matteson, S.E., Mustian, K.M., Padmanaban, D., & Morrow, G.R. (2005). Treatment of radiotherapy-induced fatigue through a nonpharmacological approach. *Integrative Cancer Therapies, 4*(1), 8–13.

Roscoe, J.A., Morrow, G.R., Hickok, J.T., Mustian, K.M., Griggs, J.J., Matteson, S.E., et al. (2005). Effect of paroxetine hydrochloride (Paxil) on fatigue and depression in breast cancer patients receiving chemotherapy. *Breast Cancer Research and Treatment, 89*(3), 243–249.

Rummans, T.A., Clark, M.M., Sloan, J.A., Frost, M.H., Bostwick, J.M., Atherton, P.J., et al. (2006). Impacting quality of life for patients with advanced cancer with a structured multidisciplinary intervention: A randomized controlled trial. *Journal of Clinical Oncology, 24*(4), 635–642.

Sarhill, N., Walsh, D., Nelson, K.A., Homsi, J., LeGrand, S., & Davis, M.P. (2001). Methylphenidate for fatigue in advanced cancer: A prospective open-label pilot study. *American Journal of Hospice and Palliative Care, 18*(3), 187–192.

Savard, J., Simard, S., Giguere, I., Ivers, H., Morin, C.M., Maunsell, E., et al. (2006). Randomized clinical trial on cognitive therapy for depression in women with metastatic breast cancer: Psychological and immunological effects. *Palliative and Supportive Care, 4*(3), 219–237.

Savard, J., Simard, S., Ivers, H., & Morin, C.M. (2005). Randomized study on the efficacy of cognitive-behavioral therapy for insomnia secondary to breast cancer, part I: Sleep and psychological effects. *Journal of Clinical Oncology, 23*(25), 6083–6096.

Schmitz, K.H., Holtzman, J., Courneya, K.S., Masse, L.C., Duval, S., & Kane, R. (2005). Controlled physical activity trials in cancer survivors: A systematic review and meta-analysis. *Cancer Epidemiology, Biomarkers and Prevention, 14*(7), 1588–1595.

Schneider, S.M., Ellis, M., Coombs, W.T., Shonkwiler, E.L., & Folsom, L.C. (2003). Virtual reality intervention for older women with breast cancer. *Cyberpsychology and Behavior, 6*(3), 301–307.

Schneider, S.M., & Hood, L.E. (2007). Virtual reality: A distraction intervention for chemotherapy. *Oncology Nursing Forum, 34*(1), 39–46.

Schneider, S.M., Prince-Paul, M., Allen, M.J., Silverman, P., & Talaba, D. (2004). Virtual reality as a distraction intervention for women receiving chemotherapy. *Oncology Nursing Forum, 31*(1), 81–88.

Schumacher, K., Schneider, B., Reich, G., Stiefel, T., Stoll, G., Bock, P.R., et al. (2003). Influence of postoperative complementary treatment with lectin-standardized mistletoe extract on breast cancer patients. A controlled epidemiological multicentric retrolective cohort study. *Anticancer Research, 23*(6D), 5081–5087.

Schwartz, A.L., Thompson, J.A., & Masood, N. (2002). Interferon-induced fatigue in patients with melanoma: A pilot study of exercise and methylphenidate. *Oncology Nursing Forum, 29*(7), E85–E90.

Shafqat, A., Einhorn, L.H., Hanna, N., Sledge, G.W., Hanna, A., Juliar, B.E., et al. (2005). Screening studies for fatigue and laboratory correlates in cancer patients undergoing treatment. *Annals of Oncology, 16*(9), 1545–1550.

Shaw, E.G., Rosdhal, R., D'Agostino, R.B., Jr., Lovato, J., Naughton, M.J., Robbins, M.E., et al. (2006). Phase II study of donepezil in irradiated brain tumor patients: Effect on cognitive function, mood, and quality of life. *Journal of Clinical Oncology, 24*(9), 1415–1420.

Sood, A., & Moynihan, T.J. (2005). Cancer-related fatigue: An update. *Current Oncology Reports, 7*(4), 277–282.

Speca, M., Carlson, L.E., Goodey, E., & Angen, M. (2000). A randomized, wait-list controlled clinical trial: The effect of a mindfulness meditation-based stress reduction program on mood and symptoms of stress in cancer outpatients. *Psychosomatic Medicine, 62*(5), 613–622.

Stasi, R., Amadori, S., Littlewood, T.J., Terzoli, E., Newland, A.C., & Provan, D. (2005). Management of cancer-related anemia with erythropoietic agents: Doubts, certainties, and concerns. *Oncologist, 10*(7), 539–554.

Stevinson, C., Lawlor, D.A., & Fox, K.R. (2004). Exercise interventions for cancer patients: Systematic review of controlled trials. *Cancer Causes and Control, 15*(10), 1035–1056.

Stockler, M.R., O'Connell, R., Nowak, A.K., Goldstein, D., Turner, J., Wilcken, N.R., et al. (2007). Effect of sertraline on symptoms and survival in patients with advanced cancer, but without major depression: A placebo-controlled double-blind randomised trial. *Lancet Oncology, 8*(7), 603–612.

Stone, P.C., & Minton, O. (2008). Cancer-related fatigue. *European Journal of Cancer, 44*(8), 1097–1104.

Strauss-Blasche, G., Gnad, E., Ekmekcioglu, C., Hladschik, B., & Marktl, W. (2005). Combined inpatient rehabilitation and spa therapy for breast cancer patients: Effects on quality of life and CA 15-3. *Cancer Nursing, 28*(5), 390–398.

Stricker, C.T., Drake, D., Hoyer, K.A., & Mock, V. (2004). Evidence-based practice for fatigue management in adults with cancer: Exercise as an intervention. *Oncology Nursing Forum, 31*(5), 963–976.

Strong, V., Waters, R., Hibberd, C., Murray, G., Wall, L., Walker, J., et al. (2008). Management of depression for people with cancer (SMaRT oncology 1), a randomised trial. *Lancet, 372*(9632), 40–48.

Sugawara, Y., Akechi, T., Shima, Y., Okuyana, T., Akizuki, N., Nakano, T., et al. (2002). Efficacy of methylpheni-date for fatigue in advanced cancer patients: A preliminary study. *Palliative Medicine, 16*(3), 261–263.

Thorsen, L., Courneya, K.S., Stevinson, C., & Fossa, S.D. (2008). A systematic review of physical activi-ty in prostate cancer survivors: Outcomes, prevalence, and determinants. *Supportive Care in Cancer, 16*(9), 987–997.

Tookman, A.J., Jones, C.L., Dewitte, M., & Lodge, P.J. (2008). Fatigue in patients with advanced cancer: A pilot study of an intervention with infliximab. *Supportive Care in Cancer, 16*(10), 1131–1140.

Torta, R., Siri, I., & Caldera, P. (2008). Sertraline effectiveness and safety in depressed oncological patients. *Supportive Care in Cancer, 16*(1), 83–91.

Tsang, K.L., Carlson, L.E., & Olson, K. (2007). Pilot crossover trial of Reiki versus rest for treating cancer-related fatigue. *Integrative Cancer Therapies, 6*(1), 25–35.

Van Den Berg, M., Visser, A., Schoolmeesters, A., Edelman, P., & Borne, B.V.D. (2006). Evaluation of hapto-therapy for patients with cancer treated with chemotherapy at a day clinic. *Patient Education and Coun-seling, 60*(3), 336–343.

van Weert, E., Hoekstra-Weebers, J., Otter, R., Postema, K., Sanderman, R., & van der Schans, C. (2006). Cancer-related fatigue: Predictors and effects of rehabilitation. *Oncologist, 11*(2), 184–196.

van Weert, E., Hoekstra-Weebers, J.E., May, A.M., Korstjens, I., Ros, W.J., & van der Schans, C.P. (2008). The development of an evidence-based physical self-management rehabilitation programme for cancer survivors. *Patient Education and Counseling, 71*(2), 169–190.

Vickers, A.J., Straus, D.J., Fearon, B., & Cassileth, B.R. (2004). Acupuncture for postchemotherapy fatigue: A phase II study. *Journal of Clinical Oncology, 22*(9), 1731–1735.

Vilela, L.D., Nicolau, B., Mahmud, S., Edgar, L., Hier, M., Black, M., et al. (2006). Comparison of psychoso-cial outcomes in head and neck cancer patients receiving a coping strategies intervention and control subjects receiving no intervention. *Journal of Otolaryngology, 35*(2), 88–96.

Weitzner, M.A., Moncello, J., Jacobsen, P.B., & Minton, S. (2002). A pilot trial of paroxetine for the treat-ment of hot flashes and associated symptoms in women with breast cancer. *Journal of Pain and Symp-tom Management, 23*(4), 337–345.

Williams, S.A., & Schreier, A.M. (2005). The role of education in managing fatigue, anxiety, and sleep disorders in women undergoing chemotherapy for breast cancer. *Applied Nursing Research, 18*(3), 138–147.

Wilson, J., Yao, G.L., Raftery, J., Bohlius, J., Brunskill, S., Sandercock, J., et al. (2007). A systematic review and economic evaluation of epoetin alfa, epoetin beta and darbepoetin alfa in anaemia associated with can-cer, especially that attributable to cancer treatment. *Health Technology Assessment, 11*(13), 1–220.

Yates, P., Aranda, S., Hargraves, M., Mirolo, B., Clavarino, A., McLachlan, S., et al. (2005). Randomized con-trolled trial of an educational intervention for managing fatigue in women receiving adjuvant chemother-apy for early-stage breast cancer. *Journal of Clinical Oncology, 23*(25), 6027–6036.

Yeom, C.H., Jung, G.C., & Song, K.J. (2007). Changes of terminal cancer patients' health-related quality of life after high dose vitamin C administration. *Journal of Korean Medical Science, 22*(1), 7–11.

Zhang, M., Liu, X., Li, J., He, L., & Tripathy, D. (2007). Chinese medicinal herbs to treat the side-effects of chemotherapy in breast cancer patients. *Cochrane Database of Systematic Reviews* 2007, Issue 2. Art. No.: CD004921. DOI: 10.1002/14651858.CD004921.pub2.

Zick, S.M., Sen, A., Feng, Y., Green, J., Olatunde, S., & Boon, H. (2006). Trial of essiac to ascertain its effect in women with breast cancer (TEA-BC). *Journal of Alternative and Complementary Medicine, 12*(10), 971–980.

CHAPTER **12**

Lymphedema

Problem

Lymphedema is the accumulation of lymph fluid in the body (American Cancer Society, 2006). The focus of this chapter is secondary lymphedema, a progressive, chronic swelling resulting from damage to the lymphatic vessels and/or lymph nodes. This leads to accumulation of fluid and other elements (i.e., subcutaneous fat, protein) in tissue spaces. Secondary lymphedema may lead to chronic inflammation and swelling, contributing to fibrosis, skin breakdown, and increased risk of infection (International Society of Lymphology [ISL], 2003).

Secondary lymphedema can occur in one or more limbs and can involve the corresponding quadrant of the trunk. Swelling also may affect the head and neck, breast, or genitalia. Although most commonly associated with cancer treatments, secondary lymphedema can occur after burns, trauma, venous disease, infection, inflammation, or immobility (Lymph Notes, 2006; Lymphoedema Framework, 2006).

Although not curable, lymphedema is most easily managed with early recognition and therapy. A delay in intervention may lead to more severe symptoms and decreased treatment efficacy (Lymphoedema Framework, 2006). Most research has focused on upper-extremity lymphedema, but many of the interventions may also be useful for lower-extremity lymphedema.

Incidence

Approximately 20% of women develop lymphedema after breast cancer treatment (Kalinowski, 2004). Factors related to the incidence and extent of lymphedema are the type of surgery, extent of lymph node dissection, and use of additional therapy to the area (i.e., nodal irradiation) (Coen, Taghaln, Kachnic, Assasad, & Powell, 2003; Meric et al., 2002; Sener et al., 2001; Swirsky & Nunnery, 1998; Tengrup, Tennvall-Nittby, Christiansson, & Laurin, 2000). Lymphedema can occur 1 to 20 years after surgery (Story, 2005).

Assessment

The most common method to assess for secondary lymphedema is patient self-report (Kalinowski, 2004). Detailed assessment (see Table 12-1) and use of a clinical measurement tool are important in determining the level of lymphedema. ISL (2003) provides staging criteria that are useful for describing the extent of lymphedema (see Table 12-2).

Clinical Measurement Tools

Circumferential measurement is the most commonly used objective assessment for lymphedema in the clinical setting (Gerber, 1998). Although water displacement

Table 12-1. Lymphedema Assessment Guide		
Assessment	Yes	No
Physical Symptoms		
Vital signs (fever may be indicative of infection)		
Weakness, decreased range of motion, stiffness, pain, numbness, paresthesia of the involved extremity		
Changes in fit of jewelry/clothing		
Feelings of heaviness in involved extremity		
Thickening, pitting, erythema, temperature of the involved extremity		
Swelling relieved with elevation or transient in nature		
Swelling not relieved by elevation		
Risk and Contributing Factors		
Age		
Menopausal status		
Diabetes		
Obesity		
Extent of lymph node biopsy and dissection		
Radiation therapy to the breast		
Radiation therapy to axilla		
Size of radiation field		
History of recurrent infection in the hand and arm		
Lack of exercise		
Overuse of an affected extremity		
Hematomas, seromas, cellulitis, wounds		
Tight or constrictive clothes		
Airplane travel		
Long-distance travel		

Note. Based on information from Brown, 2004; Cope, 2006; Marrs, 2007.

Table 12-2. International Society of Lymphology Staging Criteria	
Stage	**Criteria**
0	A latent or subclinical condition where swelling is not evident despite impaired lymph transport; it may exist months or years before overt edema occurs (stages I–III).
I	An early accumulation of fluid relatively high in protein content (e.g., in comparison with "venous" edema) and subsides with limb elevation; pitting may occur.
II	Elevation alone rarely reduces tissue swelling, and pitting is manifest. Late in stage II, the limb may or may not pit as tissue fibrosis supervenes.
III	Lymphostatic elephantiasis where pitting is absent and trophic skin changes such as acanthosis, fat deposits, and warty overgrowths develop

Note. Based on information from International Society of Lymphology, 2003.

is the gold standard for measuring lymphedema, it often is not appropriate for use in the clinical setting (Ridner, 2008). No matter what tool is used to measure lymphedema, it must be used to obtain comparable data at different points in time. The following clinical tools and techniques for measuring lymphedema are presented in Table 12-3.

1. Circumferential Measurement: A specially designed, nonstretch, flexible tape is placed at intervals of 4–10 cm from wrist to axilla to assess arm girth (Ridner, 2008). Lymphedema is diagnosed as a 2 cm difference or more in arm circumference between affected and unaffected limbs (Gerber, 1998). Measuring both arms of newly diagnosed women with breast cancer prior to, during, and following treatment is important in diagnosing early lymphedema (Coward, 1999). Extremity measurement comparison with the contralateral limb correlates with ISL's staging criteria as follows (Marrs, 2007).
    * Stage I: < 3 cm difference between extremities
    * Stage II: 3–5 cm difference between extremities
    * Stage III: > 5 cm difference between extremities
2. Bioelectrical Impedance Assessment: This technique uses electrical current to determine the amount of extracellular protein in the extremities (Cornish, Thomas, Ward, Hirst, & Bunce, 2002). Adhesive electrodes are placed on anatomical landmarks such as hands, wrists, and feet. Electrode placement varies depending on the impedance device being used (Ridner, 2008).
3. Perometer: The perometer is an infrared optoelectronic volumeter that estimates limb volume and records shape (Petlund, 1991; Stanton, Northfield, Holroyd, Mortimer, & Levick, 1997; Tierney, Aslam, Rennie, & Grace, 1996).
4. Lymphedema and Breast Cancer Questionnaire: The focus of this questionnaire is on the lymphedema symptom experience (Armer, Radina, Porock, & Culbertson, 2003).

Table 12-3. Lymphedema Clinical Measurement Tools

Name of Tool	Number of Items	Domains	Reliability and Validity	Populations	Clinical Utility
Bioelectrical Impedance Assessment	1	Resistance ratio because of protein in interstitial spaces	Unknown	Breast cancer	Takes less than five minutes to prepare and complete
Circumferential Measurement	1	Circumference	Problems with intra- and interrater reliability	Breast cancer	Quick and easy to use Requires minimal training or preparation
Lymphedema and Breast Cancer Questionnaire	19	Indicators of lymphedema, frequency, and management strategies	Adequate reliability and validity established	Breast cancer survivors	Nurse-administered structured interview
Perometer	1	Volume	Adequate reliability and validity established	Breast cancer	Quick and easy to use

Note. Based on information from Armer et al., 2003; Brown, 2004; Petlund, 1991; Ridner, 2008; Stanton et al., 1997; Tierney et al., 1996; Ward, 2006.

References

American Cancer Society. (2006). *Lymphedema: Understanding and managing lymphedema after cancer treatment.* Atlanta, GA: Author.

Armer, J.M., Radina, M.E., Porock, D., & Culbertson, S.D. (2003). Predicting breast cancer-related lymphedema using self-reported symptoms. *Nursing Research, 52*(6), 370–379.

Brown, J. (2004). A clinically useful method for evaluating lymphedema. *Clinical Journal of Oncology Nursing, 8*(1), 35–38.

Coen, J.J., Taghaln, A.G., Kachnic, L.A., Assasad, S.I., & Powell, S.N. (2003). Risk of lymphedema after regional nodal irradiation with breast conservation therapy. *International Journal of Radiation Oncology, Biology, Physics, 55*(5), 1209–1215.

Cope, D.G. (2006). Lymphedema. In D. Camp-Sorrell & R.A. Hawkins (Eds.), *Clinical manual for the oncology advanced practice nurse* (2nd ed., pp. 781–784). Pittsburgh, PA: Oncology Nursing Society.

Cornish, B.H., Thomas, B.J., Ward, L.C., Hirst, C., & Bunce, I.H. (2002). A new technique for the quantification of peripheral edema with application in both unilateral and bilateral cases. *Angiology, 53*(1), 41–47.

Coward, D.D. (1999). Lymphedema prevention and management knowledge in women treated for breast cancer. *Oncology Nursing Forum, 26*(6), 1047–1053.

Gerber, L.H. (1998). A review of measures of lymphedema. *Cancer, 83*(12, Suppl. American), 2803–2804.

International Society of Lymphology. (2003). The diagnosis and treatment of peripheral lymphedema. Consensus document of the International Society of Lymphology. *Lymphology, 36*(2), 84–91.

Kalinowski, B.H. (2004). Lymphedema. In C.H. Yarbro, M.H. Frogge, & M. Goodman (Eds.), *Cancer symptom management* (3rd ed., pp. 461–490). Sudbury, MA: Jones and Bartlett.

Lymph Notes. (2006). *Lymphedema glossary.* Retrieved January 9, 2008, from http://www.lymphnotes.com/gloss.php

Lymphoedema Framework. (2006). *Best practice for the management of lymphedema: An international perspective.* London: MEP Ltd.

Marrs, J. (2007). Lymphedema and implications for oncology nursing practice. *Clinical Journal of Oncology Nursing, 11*(1), 19–21.

Meric, F., Bucholz, T.A., Mirza, N.Q., Vlastos, G., Ames, F.C., Ross, M.I., et al. (2002). Long-term complications associated with breast-conservation surgery and radiotherapy. *Annals of Surgical Oncology, 9*(6), 543–549.

Petlund, C. (1991). Volumetry of limbs. In W.L. Olzewski (Ed.), *Lymph stasis: Pathophysiology, diagnosis and treatment* (pp. 443–451). Boca Raton, FL: CRC Press.

Ridner, S. (2008). *Measuring oncology-nursing sensitive patient outcomes: Evidence-based summary.* Retrieved January 5, 2008, from http://www.ons.org/outcomes/measures/lymphedema.shtml

Sener, S.F., Winchester, D.J., Martz, C.H., Feldman, J.L., Cavanaugh, J.A., Winchester, D.P., et al. (2001). Lymphedema after sentinel lymphadenectomy for breast carcinoma. *Cancer, 92*(4), 748–752.

Stanton, A.W., Northfield, J.W., Holroyd, B., Mortimer, P.S., & Levick, J.R. (1997). Validation of an optoelectronic limb volumeter (perometer). *Lymphology, 30*(2), 77–97.

Story, K.T. (2005). Alterations in circulation. In J.K. Itano & K.N. Taoka (Eds.), *Core curriculum for oncology nursing* (4th ed., pp. 364–379). St. Louis, MO: Elsevier.

Swirsky, J., & Nunnery, D.S. (1998). *Coping with lymphedema.* Garden City Park, NY: Avery Publishing.

Tengrup, I., Tennvall-Nittby, L., Christiansson, I., & Laurin, M. (2000). Arm morbidity after breast-conserving therapy for breast cancer. *Acta Oncologica, 39*(3), 393–397.

Tierney, S., Aslam, M., Rennie, K., & Grace, P. (1996). Infrared optoelectronic volumetry, the ideal way to measure limb volume. *European Journal of Vascular and Endovascular Surgery, 12*(4), 412–417.

Ward, L.C. (2006). Bioelectrical impedance analysis: Proven utility in lymphedema risk assessment and therapeutic monitoring. *Lymphatic Research and Biology, 4*(1), 51–56.

Case Study

M.S. was a 59-year-old woman diagnosed with stage IIA estrogen receptor/progesterone receptor positive/HER2 negative (T1 N1mic M0) left-sided breast cancer. She had a partial mastectomy with sentinel node biopsy, revealing micrometastases in one of two sentinel nodes. She had a full node dissection, revealing 16/16 negative nodes. Surgical margins were clear, and metastatic workup was negative.

During the immediate postsurgical period, she developed wound infection at the Jackson-Pratt drain site and was treated with oral antibiotics. She then received four cycles of docetaxel and cyclophosphamide, followed by breast irradiation (no nodal radiation therapy) and endocrine therapy with anastrozole.

Medical History

M.S. had a history of type 2 diabetes mellitus, hypertension, hyperlipidemia, polymyalgia rheumatic, fibromyalgia, and obesity (body mass index = 43.7). She reported allergies to penicillin, lisinopril, and metformin. Her risk factors for lymphedema were full axillary node dissection, breast irradiation, prior infection, and nail biting with chronic cuticle irritation.

Lymphedema Treatment Course

M.S. was initially diagnosed as having stage 0 lymphedema. She underwent baseline perometer measurement, with initial preoperative measure revealing 6% limb difference with left upper extremity greater than right. During her course of chemotherapy treatment on cycle 3, day 14 of docetaxel and cyclophosphamide, she developed herpes zoster in the T8 dermatome on the affected side. She was treated with antiviral therapy and did not develop a superimposed bacterial infection. However, on cycle 4, day 16 of treatment, M.S. developed cellulitis during her white blood cell nadir. She was treated with IV antibiotics, initially as an inpatient because of her fever and chills. She was discharged on oral antibiotics once blood cultures were negative and she was afebrile.

Despite two weeks of antibiotic therapy, perometer measurements revealed volume difference between affected and unaffected side to be 10% (increased from 6%). M.S. was seen by the certified lymphedema therapist, who recommended a plan to initiate phase I complete decongestive therapy (CDT) including both manual lymph drainage and compression bandaging once the infection cleared. Within two weeks of beginning therapy, her volume difference regressed to 7%, consistent with baseline. She was fitted for a compression garment (both sleeve and gauntlet) following completion of phase I CDT as part of the phase II maintenance program. M.S. had difficulty obtaining custom garments and developed recurrent cellulitis three and a half months after the initial infection. This led to an increase in her lymphedema, with a volume difference of 20%.

M.S.'s second episode of cellulitis/lymphangitis was characterized by a fever of 38.3°C (101°F), shaking chills, and rapid, diffuse erythema, which was thought to arise from an infected cuticle on the left hand. A blood culture obtained on the day of her clinic visit revealed one-quarter culture with gram-positive cocci. She was admitted to the hospital and treated with vancomycin until speciation was determined. Given her history of penicillin allergy, she was discharged on oral cephalexin after test dosing. She completed a 21-day course of cephalexin and has had no further infection at this time. She continued to use compression garments with variable compliance. Her last perometer measure showed a volume difference of 18%, and she is now four months post her most recent episode of cellulitis. Lymphedema education included lifestyle modification, diabetes control, and weight management. She continues to see a lymphedema specialist closer to home as part of her phase II CDT maintenance, but is overwhelmed at times by the rigors of multiple comorbid disease management.

Discussion

Multiple factors contribute to challenges in managing patients with lymphedema and those at risk for developing lymphedema. Should multiple episodes of cellulitis/lymphangitis develop, particularly given M.S.'s comorbid risks, prophylactic use of daily antibiotics may be indicated. The Oncology Nursing Society Putting Evidence Into Practice resource on lymphedema outlines recommendations for lymphedema intervention and management. Improved glucose control and modest weight reduction are imperative lifestyle modifications to decrease risk of lymphedema development and progression.

Marybeth Singer, MS, APN-BC, AOCN®, ACHPN
Nurse Practitioner, Gillette Center for Breast Oncology
Massachusetts General Hospital Cancer Center
Boston, MA

Lymphedema

2009 AUTHORS
Ellen G. Poage, MSN, ARNP, MPH, CLT-LANA, and Jane M. Armer, RN, PhD, FAAN
ONS STAFF: Heather Belansky, RN, MSN

2008 AUTHORS
Ellen G. Poage, MSN, FNP-C, MPH, CLT-LANA, Marybeth Singer, MS, APRN-BC, AOCN®, ACHPN,
M. Jeanne Shellabarger, RN, BSN, and Melanie D. Poundall, RN
RESEARCH CONSULTANT: Jane M. Armer, RN, PhD
ONS STAFF: Barbara G. Lubejko, RN, MS

What interventions are effective in reducing the risk for and treating secondary lymphedema?

Recommended for Practice

Interventions for which effectiveness has been demonstrated by strong evidence from rigorously conducted studies, meta-analyses, or systematic reviews and for which expectation of harms is small compared with the benefits

COMPLETE DECONGESTIVE THERAPY

Evidence at the highest level supports complete decongestive therapy (CDT) for the treatment of lymphedema (Browning, 1997; Lymphoedema Framework, 2006; Moseley, Carati, & Piller, 2007). In addition to reducing interstitial lymphatic fluid, CDT improves shoulder range of motion (Didem, Ufuk, Serdar, & Zumre, 2005) and decreases pain (Hamner & Fleming, 2007).

CDT, a two-phase therapy, involves multiple key components.
• Skin care
• Manual lymph drainage
• Compression: Low-stretch compression bandaging (phase I) and compression garments (phase II)
• Movement therapies including remedial exercise
• Patient education

CDT aims to decrease swelling and prepare patients for self-management and maintenance. Intensive therapy lasts 10–20 days (McNeely et al., 2004).
• Intensive CDT should begin when lymphedema is moderate to severe (Jeffs, 2006).
• Modified CDT (excluding one or two components) is indicated for mild to moderate lymphedema (Koul et al., 2007; Lymphoedema Framework, 2006).
• CDT is administered by a specialty-trained therapist.
• Early intervention with CDT is less costly and less burdensome and has better outcomes (Jeffs, 2006; McNeely et al., 2004).

COMPRESSION BANDAGING

The literature supports the use of compression bandaging (CB) to reduce swelling and gradient compression garments (sleeves, gloves, and gauntlets) to maintain reductions or prevent fluid accumulation. Specialized expertise is required for the initiation and monitoring of CB (McNeely et al., 2004).
- Short-stretch, multilayer bandages reduce the volume of lymphedema during the intensive treatment phase when used alone or in conjunction with other therapies (Jeffs, 2006; Lymphoedema Framework, 2006; McNeely et al., 2004).
- Maintenance therapy using nightly CB and compression garments decreases the risk of lymphedema recurrence (Lymphoedema Framework, 2006; Vignes, Porcher, Arrault, & Dupuy, 2007) and can stabilize lymphedema volume (Bani et al., 2007; Vignes et al.).

TREATMENT OF INFECTIONS

People with lymphedema are at increased risk for infection (Lymphoedema Framework, 2006). Criteria for hospitalization include (Lymphoedema Framework, 2006)
- Hypotension, tachycardia, fever, confusion, or vomiting
- Continuing symptoms despite oral antibiotics for 48 hours
- Unresolved local symptoms despite first- and second-line oral antibiotics.

Early detection and treatment of infection in lymphedematous limbs is critical to minimizing the risk for systemic infection. Oral penicillins, such as amoxicillin and dicloxacillin, should be started as soon as possible and continue for at least 14 days or until signs of inflammation have resolved. For patients with penicillin allergy, clindamycin may be used (Lymphoedema Framework, 2006).

Simple and manual lymph drainage should be avoided during acute infection with fever. If tolerated, reduced-level compression garments or CB may be applied. Long periods without compression should be avoided (Lymphoedema Framework, 2006), and aggressively initiating postinfection treatment to decrease edema is supported in the literature (Bernard, 2008).

Recurrent infections occur in up to 20% of patients (Bernard, 2008). The most frequent reason for failure is lack of compliance (nonadherence) with the prescribed drug regimen.

Likely to Be Effective

Interventions for which effectiveness has been demonstrated by supportive evidence from a single rigorously conducted controlled trial, consistent supportive evidence from well-designed controlled trials using small samples, or guidelines developed from evidence and supported by expert opinion

MAINTAINING OPTIMAL BODY WEIGHT

One important patient-related factor in women who develop lymphedema after breast cancer treatment is maintaining optimal body weight according to body mass index (BMI). Although isolating patient factors from treatment factors is not possible, evidence supports a BMI score > 30 as a risk factor for lymphedema (Mahamaneerat, Shyu, Stewart, & Armer, 2008; Ridner & Dietrich, 2008; Soran et al., 2006). One study age-matched its sample (N = 64) within three years and still found statistically significant group differences in BMI for lymphedema occurrence (Ridner & Dietrich). Although how body weight precisely affects lymphedema is not known, evidence indicates that it does influence lymphedema development and affects management. Likewise, efforts to reduce body weight may influence lymphedema volume and improve management. In one small study (N = 64), researchers compared weight loss by caloric reductions, with fat reduction alone, to a third control group with no dietary interventions (Shaw, Mortimer, & Judd, 2007). Although there seemed to be no difference in the groups (largely because of lack of dietary adherence), weight loss by whatever means appears to benefit arm volume (p = 0.002). In the end, results showed significant reductions in BMI (p = 0.008) with both intervention groups compared to control.

MANUAL LYMPH DRAINAGE

Systematic reviews and individual studies support the use of manual lymph drainage (MLD) for lymphedema treatment (Browning & Redman, 1997; Didem et al., 2005; Moseley et al., 2007). MLD practitioners require training at the specialist level. To find a qualified practitioner, visit www.clt-lana.org or www.lymphnet.org.

MLD has shown effectiveness in
- Early lymphedema (Jeffs, 2006)—One study found a significantly greater reduction in arm volume for those with mild lymphedema who received MLD with CB as compared to CB alone (McNeely et al., 2004).
- Breast/chest, head and neck, and genital lymphedema (Jeffs, 2006)—These areas are difficult to treat with CB.
- CDT programs modified because of a patient's premorbid condition and stage of disease (Jeffs, 2006; Koul et al., 2007).
- Situations where patients prefer modified treatment because of cost, time, and burden. One study indicated that although CDT is twice as effective in decreasing swelling, patients experience reduced but measurable reductions with MLD, compression garments, and self-care (Jeffs, 2006).
- Symptom relief—MLD can improve self-reported patient symptoms (Moseley et al., 2007).

SKIN CARE

Impeccable skin care is a cornerstone of lymphedema therapy (Lymphoedema Framework, 2006).
- Use neutral pH soaps to avoid drying.
- Apply emollients.
- Keep skin folds clean and dry.
- Inspect skin for cuts, scrapes, abrasions, and insect bites.
- Avoid using scented products.
- In hot climates, vegetable-based products are preferable to mineral oil- or petroleum-based products.

Benefits Balanced With Harms

Interventions for which clinicians and patients should weigh the beneficial and harmful effects according to individual circumstances and priorities

EXERCISE

Exercise and movement therapies play an important role in CDT by supporting cardiovascular health, muscle strength, and functional capacity. Integrating exercise requires an individualized approach (Lymphoedema Framework, 2006). Historically, heavy resistance training was discouraged, but current evidence is unclear (Ahmed, Thomas, Yee, & Schmitz, 2006; Bicego et al., 2006; Lymphoedema Framework). Risks and benefits should be discussed with individuals interested in exercise.

Potential benefits include
- Upper-extremity limb volume reduction (Moseley et al., 2007)
- Improvement in subjective symptoms, specifically limb heaviness, stiffness, and perceived volume (Moseley et al., 2007)
- Greater recovery of range of motion (de Rezende et al., 2006)
- Ability to regain premorbid level of functioning (Cinar et al., 2008; de Rezende et al., 2006).

Patient education may be an important component of exercise as indicated by one small study in which women who received an integrated exercise and education intervention experienced a lower rate of lymphedema (Box, Reul-Hirsh, Bullock-Saxton, & Furnival, 2002).

Studies have addressed fears that exercise will exacerbate or trigger lymphedema (Karadibak, Yavuzsen, & Saydam, 2008). One systematic review found no change in lymphedema for women who participated in aerobic and upper-extremity resistance training led by an exercise specialist (Bicego et al., 2006). Likewise, one review found that in studies where lymphedema was tracked as an adverse event, no incidence or exacerbation of lymphedema was attributed to the exercise (Cheema, Gaul, Lane, & Fiatarone Singh, 2008). Based on another review, the authors recommend that any exercise prescription should include components of frequency, intensity, time, and progression (Young-McCaughan & Arzola, 2007). Another study showed that women with mild to moderate lymphedema could forgo wearing a compression sleeve during low-intensity resistance activities (Johansson, Tibe, Weibull, & Newton, 2005).

PROPHYLACTIC ANTIBIOTICS FOR RECURRENT INFECTIONS

Recurrent infection occurs in nearly one-quarter of people with lymphedema who experience an initial cellulitis (Indelicato et al., 2006).
- For people who experience two to three infections per year, evaluate the benefits and risks of antibiotic prophylaxis. Recommended agents include penicillin or erythromycin (if penicillin allergy exists). Second-line prophylaxis includes clindamycin or clarithromycin (Lymphoedema Framework, 2006).
- During travel, an emergency supply of antibiotics, such as amoxicillin, that can be taken at the onset of symptoms may be indicated. For patients with penicillin allergy, clindamycin may be tried. For persistent symptoms or if fevers, chills, or constitutional symptoms develop, patients should be admitted to a hospital (Lymphoedema Framework, 2006).
- Cephalexin also may be used. For patients with penicillin allergy, ensure that they have had prior cephalexin without allergy (McNeely et al., 2004).

Effectiveness Not Established

Interventions for which insufficient or conflicting data or data of inadequate quality currently exist, with no clear indication of harm

COMPRESSION GARMENTS

Compression garments are used commonly in clinical practice to manage symptoms of lymphedema during the maintenance phase of CDT, after maximum limb volume reduction is achieved. They require careful patient fitting by a specialty-trained practitioner (Lymphoedema Framework, 2006).

Contraindications for compression garments include
- Arterial insufficiency
- Acute cardiac failure
- Extreme limb shape distortion
- Very deep skin folds
- Extensive skin ulceration
- Severe peripheral neuropathy
- Lymphorrhea (Lymphoedema Framework, 2006).

In a systematic review by Moseley et al. (2007), two studies with small samples evaluated the use of compression garments as a primary intervention. Johansson, Lie, Ekdahl, and Lindfeldt (1998) studied 12 patients who wore garments for two weeks with mean volume reduction of 5%. Swedborg (1984) studied 26 patients and found that 8% limb volume reduction occurred; however, only 12 patients remained in the study at six months, limiting generalization.

Another recent study evaluated early intervention utilizing compression garments in women with an increase in limb volume of 3% from baseline following breast cancer treatment (Stout Gergich et al., 2008). A mean volume decrease of 4.1% was achieved, lasting 4.8 months on average. Further research with a larger sample, randomized control design, and longer follow-up is warranted.

HYPERBARIC OXYGEN

One small study evaluating the effect of hyperbaric oxygen on lymphedema demonstrated improvement in lymphatic flow and subjective reporting of limb tissue softening (Gothard et al., 2004).

LOW-LEVEL LASER THERAPY

Low-level laser therapy (LLLT) has been evaluated for potential effectiveness in postmastectomy lymphedema. Early studies with small samples show a trend toward volume reduction, improvement of self-reported symptoms, and increased quality of life (Carati, Anderson, Gannon, & Piller, 2003; Kaviani, Fateh, Yousefi Nooraie, Alinagi-zadeh, & Ataie-Fashtami, 2006; Moseley et al., 2007). The exact mechanism of the effects of LLLT is unknown; however, hypotheses have included improved cellular repair and stimulation of the immune, lymphatic, and vascular systems. Further long-term follow-up in a true placebo-control design with a CDT arm is recommended.

The current studies are too small to offer generalizable information, and further studies with larger samples and more rigorous methodologic control are warranted.

NANOCRYSTALLINE SILVER DRESSING ON LYMPHATIC ULCERS

One small case report demonstrated meaningful improvement for a select population of patients (Forner-Cordero, Navarro-Monsoliu, Muñoz-Langa, Alcober-Fuster, & Rel-Monzó, 2007).

PNEUMATIC COMPRESSION PUMP

Limited evidence suggests that intermittent pneumatic compression (IPC) may be useful as part of comprehensive lymphedema treatment when it is ordered and performed by special- ty-trained clinicians. A systematic review found a 26% decrease in limb volume with pump therapy in addition to CDT (Moseley et al., 2007). However, improvement from IPC was not sustained in another study (Szuba, Achalu, & Rockson, 2002).

Pneumatic compression **should not be used** in patients with (Lymphoedema Framework, 2006)
- Chronic nonpitting lymphedema
- Known or suspected deep vein thrombosis or pulmonary embolus
- Uncontrolled or significant congestive heart failure
- Active erysipelas or cellulitis
- Ischemic vascular disease
- Severe peripheral neuropathy
- Edema at the proximal portion of the extremity
- Active metastatic disease affecting the limb.

SIMPLE LYMPH DRAINAGE

One small study found that simple lymph drainage (SLD) using an aromatherapy cream did not significantly reduce limb volume. However, patients reported improved symptom relief. Aromatherapy did not appear to add benefit (Barclay, Vestey, Lambert, & Balmer, 2006).

SURGICAL INTERVENTION

Limited evidence suggests that carefully selected patients may benefit from surgical reduc- tion, bypass of lymphatic obstructions, liposuction, lipectomy, microsurgical lymphatic ve- nous anastomoses, and lymphatic grafting. Safety and efficacy of these procedures and the populations that may benefit are unclear (Browning & Redman, 1997; Lymphoedema Frame- work, 2006).

Effectiveness Unlikely

Interventions for which lack of effectiveness has been demonstrated by negative evidence from a single rigorously conducted controlled trial, consistent negative evidence from well- designed controlled trials using small samples, or guidelines developed from evidence and supported by expert opinion

There are no interventions as of May 2008.

Not Recommended for Practice

Interventions for which lack of effectiveness or harmfulness has been demonstrated by strong evidence from rigorously conducted studies, meta-analyses, or systematic reviews, or interventions where the costs, burden, or harms associated with the intervention exceed anticipated benefit

DRUG THERAPY

Diuretics

No evidence supports the efficacy of diuretics in treating lymphedema. Although short courses may help to treat edema of mixed etiologies, lymphedema is a problem with protein displacement, not water (Lymphoedema Framework, 2006).

Benzopyrenes

Little evidence supports the use of benzopyrenes such as flavonoids, oxerutins, escins, coumarin, and ruscogen combined with hesperidin in the treatment of lymphedema (Lymphoedema Framework, 2006). Significant hepatotoxicity has been associated with the use of coumarin (Browning & Redman, 1997). A systematic review evaluated selected pharmaceuticals and reported a reduction in limb volume and improvement in limb heaviness (Moseley et al., 2007). While some agents showed variable reductions in limb volume, those with the greatest effect were in the combination trial with MLD. Numerous side effects, limited sample size, and conflicting results make recommendations difficult with current knowledge. The sustainability of improvement is not evaluable.

Expert Opinion

Low-risk interventions that are (1) consistent with sound clinical practice, (2) suggested by an expert in a peer-reviewed publication (journal or book chapter), and (3) for which limited evidence exists. An expert is an individual who has published articles in a peer-reviewed journal in the domain of interest.

BLOOD PRESSURE AND VENIPUNCTURE PRECAUTIONS

Expert opinion suggests that venipuncture and blood pressure (BP) measurements may increase the risk of lymphedema (National Lymphedema Network, 2008b).
- Avoid venipuncture, injections, and BP evaluations in at-risk and affected limbs.
- If venipuncture is unavoidable, strict asepsis may minimize risk.
- For BP measurements with bilateral lymphedema or at-risk arms, it is preferable to use a lower extremity to take the BP. If use of the lower extremity is not possible, use the less affected limb. If equally affected, use the nondominant arm. Avoid using an automated BP device. Manual cuffs should be inflated only to 20–40 mmHg above the patient's baseline BP.

AIR TRAVEL PRECAUTIONS

The following air travel precautions are recommended for people with or at risk for lymphedema (National Lymphedema Network, 2008a).
- Those with a history of lymphedema should utilize a correctly fitted compression garment, as changes in cabin pressure may trigger exacerbations.

- Individuals at risk for developing lymphedema should discuss with their healthcare providers the risks and benefits of wearing a compression garment or bandages during air travel.
- Use of a compression glove/gauntlet along with a compression sleeve may decrease the risk of swelling in hands and fingers.

Other air travel precautions include
- Exercising, deep breathing, standing, and moving around every 30 minutes
- Maintaining adequate fluid intake
- Avoiding carrying or moving heavy luggage.

PATIENT EDUCATION

Patients and caregivers should be taught to (Lymphoedema Framework, 2006)
- Take good care of skin and nails.
- Maintain optimal body weight.
- Eat a balanced diet.
- Avoid wearing tight clothing, watches, and jewelry.
- Avoid extremes in temperature.
- Use sunscreen and insect repellent.
- Wear compression garments if prescribed.
- Undertake exercise and diaphragmatic breathing exercises.
- Wear comfortable, supportive shoes.

For more information about lymphedema risk factors, refer to www.ons.org/outcomes and www.lymphnet.org/pdfDocs/nlnriskreduction.pdf.

Definitions of the interventions are available at **www.ons.org/outcomes**.
Literature search completed through May 2008.

The authors gratefully acknowledge Robin Shook, MS, for expert assistance in reference management and formatting.

References

Ahmed, R.L., Thomas, W., Yee, D., & Schmitz, K.H. (2006). Randomized controlled trial of weight training and lymphedema in breast cancer survivors. *Journal of Clinical Oncology, 24*(18), 2765–2772.

Bani, H.A., Fasching, P.A., Lux, M.M., Rauh, C., Willner, M., Eder, I., et al. (2007). Lymphedema in breast cancer survivors: Assessment and information provision in a specialized breast unit. *Patient Education and Counseling, 66*(3), 311–318.

Barclay, J., Vestey, J., Lambert, A., & Balmer, C. (2006). Reducing the symptoms of lymphoedema: Is there a role for aromatherapy? *European Journal of Oncology Nursing, 10*(2), 140–149.

Bernard, P. (2008). Management of common bacterial infections of the skin. *Current Opinion in Infectious Diseases, 21*(2), 122–128.

Bicego, D., Brown, K., Ruddick, M., Storey, D., Wong, C., & Harris, S.R. (2006). Exercise for women with or at risk for breast cancer-related lymphedema. *Physical Therapy, 86*(10), 1398–1405.

Box, R.C., Reul-Hirsch, H.M., Bullock-Saxton, J.E., & Furnival, C.M. (2002). Physiotherapy after breast cancer surgery: Results of a randomised controlled study to minimise lymphoedema. *Breast Cancer Research and Treatment, 75*(1), 51–64.

Browning, C. (1997). *Lymphoedema: Prevalence, risk factors and management: A review of research.* Kings Cross, Australia: NHMRC National Breast Cancer Center.

Carati, C.J., Anderson, S.N., Gannon, B.J., & Piller, N.B. (2003). Treatment of post-mastectomy lymphedema with low-level laser therapy. *Cancer, 98*(6), 1114–1122.

Cheema, B., Gaul, C.A., Lane, K., & Fiatarone Singh, M.A. (2008). Progressive resistance training in breast cancer: A systematic review of clinical trials. *Breast Cancer Research and Treatment, 109*(1), 9–26.

Cinar, N., Seckin, U., Kreskin, D., Bodur, H., Bozkurt, B., & Cengiz, O. (2008). The effectiveness of early rehabilitation in patients with modified radical mastectomy. *Cancer Nursing, 31*(2), 160–165.

de Rezende, L.F., Franco, R.L., de Rezende, M.F., Beletti, P.O., Morais, S.S., & Gurgel, M.S. (2006). Two exercise schemes in postoperative breast cancer: Comparison of effects on shoulder movement and lymphatic disturbance. *Tumori, 92*(1), 55–61.

Didem, K., Ufuk, Y.S., Serdar, S., & Zumre, A. (2005). The comparison of two different physiotherapy methods in treatment of lymphedema after breast surgery. *Breast Cancer Research and Treatment, 93*(1), 49–54.

Forner-Cordero, I., Navarro-Monsoliu, R., Munoz-Langa, J., Alcober-Fuster, P., & Rel-Monzo, P. (2007). Use of a nanocrystalline silver dressing on lymphatic ulcers in patients with chronic lymphoedema. *Journal of Wound Care, 16*(5), 235–239.

Gothard, L., Stanton, A., MacLaren, J., Lawrence, D., Hall, E., Mortimer, P., et al. (2004). Non-randomized phase II trial of hyperbaric oxygen therapy in patients with chronic arm lymphedema and tissue fibrosis after radiotherapy for early breast cancer. *Radiotherapy and Oncology, 70*(3), 217–224.

Hamner, J.B., & Fleming, M.D. (2007). Lymphedema therapy reduces the volume of edema and pain in patients with breast cancer. *Annals of Surgical Oncology, 14*(6), 1904–1908.

Indelicato, D.J., Grobmyer, S.R., Newlin, H., Morris, C.G., Haigh, L.S., Copeland, E.M., III, et al. (2006). Delayed breast cellulitis: An evolving complication of breast conservation. *International Journal of Radiation Oncology, Biology, Physics, 66*(5), 1339–1346.

Jeffs, E. (2006). Treating breast cancer-related lymphoedema at the London Haven: Clinical audit results. *European Journal of Oncology Nursing, 10*(1), 71–79.

Johansson, K., Lie, E., Edkahl, C., & Lindfeldt, J. (1998). A randomized study comparing manual lymph drainage with sequential pneumatic compression for treatment of postoperative arm lymphedema. *Lymphology, 31*(2), 56–64.

Johansson, K., Tibe, K., Weibull, A., & Newton, R.C. (2005). Low intensity resistance exercise for breast cancer patients with arm lymphedema with or without compression sleeve. *Lymphology, 38*(4), 167–180.

Karadibak, D., Yavuzsen, T., & Saydam, S. (2008). Prospective trial of intensive decongestive physiotherapy for upper extremity lymphedema. *Journal of Surgical Oncology, 97*(7), 572–577.

Kaviani, A., Fateh, M., Yousefi Nooraie, R., Alinagi-zadeh, M.R., & Ataie-Fashtami, L. (2006). Low-level laser therapy in management of postmastectomy lymphedema. *Lasers in Medical Science, 21*(2), 90–94.

Koul, R., Dufan, T., Russell, C., Guenther, W., Nugent, Z., Sun, X., et al. (2007). Efficacy of complete decongestive therapy and manual lymphatic drainage on treatment-related lymphedema in breast cancer. *International Journal of Radiation Oncology, Biology, Physics, 67*(3), 841–846.

Lymphoedema Framework. (2006). *Best practice for the management of lymphoedema.* London: MEP Ltd.

Mahamaneerat, W.K., Shyu, C.-R., Stewart, B.R., & Armour, J.M. (in press). Post-op swelling and lymphoedema following breast cancer treatment: A baseline-comparison BMI-adjusted approach. *Journal of Lymphoedema.*

McNeely, M.L., Magee, D.J., Lees, A.W., Bagnall, K.M., Haykowsky, M., & Hanson, J. (2004). The addition of manual lymph drainage to compression therapy for breast cancer related lymphedema: A randomized controlled trial. *Breast Cancer Research and Treatment, 86*(2), 95–106.

Moseley, A.L., Carati, C.J., & Piller, N.B. (2007). A systematic review of common conservative therapies for arm lymphoedema secondary to breast cancer treatment. *Annals of Oncology, 18*(4), 639–646.

National Lymphedema Network. (2008a). *NLN position paper: Air travel.* Retrieved May 15, 2008, from http://www.lymphnet.org/pdfDocs/nlnairtravel.pdf

National Lymphedema Network. (2008b). *NLN position paper: Lymphedema risk reduction practices.* Retrieved May 15, 2008, from http://www.lymphnet.org/pdfDocs/nlnriskreduction.pdf

Ridner, S.H., & Dietrich, M.S. (2008). Self-reported comorbid conditions and medication usage in breast cancer survivors with and without lymphedema. *Oncology Nursing Forum, 35*(1), 57–63.

Shaw, C., Mortimer, P., & Judd, P.A. (2007). Randomized controlled trial comparing a low-fat diet with a weight-reduction diet in breast cancer-related lymphedema. *Cancer, 109*(10), 1949–1956.

Soran, A., D'Angelo, G., Begovic, M., Ardic, F., Harlak, A., Samuel Wieand, H., et al. (2006). Breast cancer-related lymphedema—What are the significant predictors and how they affect the severity of lymphedema? *Breast Journal, 12*(6), 536–543.

Stout Gergich, N.L., Pfalzer, L.A., McGarvey, C., Springer, B., Gerber, L.H., & Soballe, P. (2008). Preoperative assessment enables the early diagnosis and successful treatment of lymphedema. *Cancer, 112*(12), 2809–2819.

Swedborg, I. (1984). Effects of treatment with an elastic sleeve and intermittent pneumatic compression in post-mastectomy patients with lymphoedema of the arm. *Scandinavian Journal of Rehabilitation Medicine, 16*(1), 35–41.

Szuba, A., Achalu, R., & Rockson, S.G. (2002). Decongestive lymphatic therapy for patients with breast carcinoma-associated lymphedema. *Cancer, 95*(11), 2260–2267.

Vignes, S., Porcher, R., Arrault, M., & Dupuy, A. (2007). Long-term management of breast cancer-related lymphedema after intensive decongestive physiotherapy. *Breast Cancer Research and Treatment, 101*(3), 285–290.

Young-McCaughan, S., & Arzola, S.M. (2007). Exercise intervention research for patients with cancer on treatment. *Seminars in Oncology Nursing, 23*(4), 264–274.

CHAPTER 13

Mucositis

Problem

Mucositis is an inflammatory and potentially ulcerative process that affects the mucous membranes of the body of individuals receiving chemotherapy and radiation therapy as treatments for cancer (i.e., mucotoxic chemotherapy, hyperfractionated radiotherapy to a field including the oral cavity, concurrent chemotherapy and radiation therapy) (Avritscher, Cooksley, & Elting, 2004; Brown & Wingard, 2004). Mucosal injury is the collective consequence of a number of concurrent and sequential biologic processes (Rubenstein et al., 2004). Although cancer treatments mainly attack cancer cells, healthy tissue such as the mucosa also may be damaged. It is classified based on the membranes involved (e.g., oral, gastrointestinal). The focus of this chapter is on content provided in the Oncology Nursing Society (ONS) Putting Evidence Into Practice (PEP) resource on mucositis.

Mucositis results in pain, dysphagia, diarrhea, and dysfunction, depending on the tissue affected. Oral mucositis results in severe discomfort and can impair patients' ability to eat, swallow, and talk. Mucositis is accompanied by a risk for life-threatening bacteremia and sepsis (Spielberger et al., 2004).

Incidence

Mucositis is a significant problem for patients with cancer, as approximately 40% will develop the condition due to the disease or during treatment (Beck, 2004). Patients with a high likelihood of being immunocompromised (e.g., lymphoma, leukemia) have a higher risk of developing mucositis. Other patients at high risk are those receiving radiation therapy to the head and neck and those undergoing stem cell transplantation. The likelihood of developing oral complications depends on the malignancy and the chemotherapy drug, dose, and delivery method. In addition to the risk for infections, this effect on the mucous membranes adds to patient distress in terms of pain, altered ability to eat, and bleeding. Depending on its severity, mucositis can cause difficulty eating and swallowing.

Assessment

Oncology nurses are challenged with the problem of mucositis and often work collaboratively with physicians to assess and effectively manage it through evidence-based interventions. A baseline assessment is helpful to stratify risk and to be better prepared to implement interventions earlier in the course of therapy. Table 13-1 presents common risk factors to assess for the development of mucositis.

Ongoing assessments prior to each cycle should include (a) diet and nutrition, (b) comfort, (c) bleeding, (d) tongue erosions or indentations, (e) saliva production, (f) mucosal dryness, (g) swallowing ability, (h) taste ability, (i) physical examination, and (j) other related symptoms.

Typically, the first symptom is a feeling of discomfort, with some redness and slight swelling of the lining of the mouth. Within a few days, small sores or ulcerations may appear. These can be painful. If this is the case, patients should be instructed to ask their physician to prescribe a numbing medication, which can help lessen the discomfort. Usually chemotherapy-induced mucositis improves within a two-week period.

Clinical Measurement Tools

The following clinical measurement tools for mucositis are presented in Table 13-2.
1. Common Terminology Criteria for Adverse Events (CTCAE) for mucositis and stomatitis (combined clinical examination and functional/symptomatic assessments) (National Cancer Institute Cancer Therapy Evaluation Program, 2006) (see Table 13-3)

Table 13-1. Baseline Assessment Areas for Mucositis		
Assessment	**Yes**	**No**
Age (very young and older patients are at increased risk)		
Gender (females > males)		
Poor oral health and hygiene		
Poor salivary function		
Low body mass index		
Renal toxicity (increased creatinine, increased toxicity)		
Smoking history		
Previous cancer treatment		
High risk: chemotherapy/biotherapy (drug, dose, schedule)		
High risk: radiation site/fractionization		
Combined modality (radiation plus chemotherapy/biotherapy)		
Blood/stem cell transplantation		
Note. Based on information from Beck, 2004; Eilers & Million, 2007; Jaroneski, 2006.		

2. Oral Assessment Guide (OAG) (Eilers, Berger, & Peterson, 1988) (see Table 13-4)
3. Oral Mucositis Assessment Scale

Table 13-2. Clinical Measurement Tools for Mucositis					
Name of Tool	**Number of Items**	**Domains**	**Reliability and Validity**	**Populations**	**Clinical Utility**
Common Terminology Criteria for Adverse Events	5-point grading scale for stomatitis and dysphagia, and 10-point pain scale	Stomatitis, dysphagia, and pain	Unknown	Unknown	Mean pain scores correlated with dysphagia, stomatitis, and the ability to eat. Studied in myeloablative chemotherapy Helpful to use separate patient-reported pain scale for monitoring progression of oral mucositis
Oral Assessment Guide	8	Signs (erythema), symptoms (pain, salivary changes), functional disturbances (ability to swallow, voice)	Face, content, and construct validity and interrater reliability established	Patients with high-dose chemotherapy for leukemia, patients receiving standard-dose chemotherapy	Easy to use in clinical setting with limited training Does not quantify amount of membrane breakdown or differentiate location of membrane changes Use of individual scores rather than total score provides more detailed data regarding changes in oral cavity.

(Continued on next page)

Table 13-2. Clinical Measurement Tools for Mucositis *(Continued)*

Name of Tool	Number of Items	Domains	Reliability and Validity	Populations	Clinical Utility
Oral Mucositis Assessment Scale	8 anatomic location assessments, and pain and difficulty swallowing using a 100-mm visual analog scale Categorical scale for ability to eat	Clinician component includes objective measures of mucositis erythema and ulceration or pseudomembrane in 8 anatomic locations of the oral cavity. Patient component includes subjective outcomes.	Face and content validity, interrater reliability established	Patients receiving chemotherapy and radiation therapy	Primarily a research tool; useful in multisite studies Multisite research data available Requires training and use of scale for scoring Scoring limited to mucous membrane changes and subjective report

Note. Based on information from Cella et al., 2003; Eilers, 2005; Hyland, 2004; Jaroneski, 2006; Sonis et al., 1999.

Table 13-3. Common Terminology Criteria for Adverse Events Grading Scale for Mucositis and Stomatitis

Grade	Criteria
1	Erythema of the mucosa
2	Minimal symptoms, normal diet, minimal respiratory symptoms but not interfering with function Patchy ulcerations or pseudomembranes Symptomatic but can eat and swallow a modified diet Respiratory symptoms interfering with function but not interfering with activities of daily living (ADLs)
3	Confluent ulcerations or pseudomembranes, bleeding with minor trauma Symptomatic and unable to adequately eat or hydrate orally Respiratory symptoms interfering with ADLs
4	Tissue necrosis; significant spontaneous bleeding, life-threatening consequences
5	Death

Note. Based on information from National Cancer Institute Cancer Therapy Evaluation Program, 2006.

			Numerical and Descriptive Ratings		
Category	**Tools for Assessment**	**Methods of Measurement**	**1**	**2**	**3**
Voice	Auditory	Converse with patient.	Normal	Deeper or raspy	Difficulty talking or painful
Swallow	Observation	Ask patient to swallow. To test gag reflex, gently place blade on back of tongue and depress.	Normal swallow	Some pain on swallow	Unable to swallow
Lips	Visual/palpatory	Observe and feel tissue.	Smooth and pink and moist	Dry or cracked	Ulcerated or bleeding
Tongue	Visual/palpatory	Feel and observe appearance of tissue.	Pink and moist and papillae present	Coated or loss of papillae with a shiny appearance with or without redness	Blistered or cracked
Saliva	Tongue blade	Insert blade into mouth, touching the center of the tongue and the floor of the mouth.	Watery	Thick or ropy	Absent
Mucous membranes	Visual	Observe appearance of tissue.	Pink and moist	Reddened or coated (increased whiteness) without ulcerations	Ulcerations with or without bleeding
Gingiva	Tongue blade and visual	Gently press tissue with tip of blade.	Pink and stippled and firm	Edematous with or without redness	Spontaneous bleeding or bleeding with pressure

Table 13-4. Oral Assessment Guide

(Continued on next page)

Table 13-4. Oral Assessment Guide (Continued)

Category	Tools for Assessment	Methods of Measurement	Numerical and Descriptive Ratings		
			1	2	3
Teeth or dentures (or denture-bearing area)	Visual	Observe appearance of teeth or denture-bearing area.	Clean and no debris	Plaque or debris in localized areas (between teeth if present)	Plaque or debris generalized along gum line or denture-bearing area

Note. Table courtesy of June Eilers, PhD, APRN-CNS, BC, The Nebraska Medical Center. Used with permission.

References

Avritscher, E.B.C., Cooksley, C.D., & Elting, L.S. (2004). Scope and epidemiology of cancer therapy-induced oral and gastrointestinal mucositis. *Seminars in Oncology Nursing, 20*(1), 3–10.

Beck, S.L. (2004). Mucositis. In C.H. Yarbro, M.H. Frogge, & M. Goodman (Eds.), *Cancer symptom management* (3rd ed., pp. 276–292). Sudbury, MA: Jones and Bartlett.

Brown, C.G., & Wingard, J. (2004). Clinical consequences of oral mucositis. *Seminars in Oncology Nursing, 20*(1), 16–21.

Cella, D., Pulliam, J., Fuchs, H., Miller, C., Hurd, D., Wingard, J.R., et al. (2003). Evaluation of pain associated with oral mucositis during the acute period after administration of high-dose chemotherapy. *Cancer, 98*(2), 406–412.

Eilers, J. (2005). *Measuring oncology nursing-sensitive patient outcomes: Evidence-based summary: Mucositis.* Retrieved August 31, 2008, from http://www.ons.org/outcomes/measures/mucositis.shtml

Eilers, J., Berger, A.M., & Petersen, M.C. (1988). Development, testing, and application of the Oral Assessment Guide. *Oncology Nursing Forum, 15*(3), 325–330.

Eilers, J., & Million, R. (2007). Prevention and management of oral mucositis in patients with cancer. *Seminars in Oncology Nursing, 23*(3), 201–212.

Hyland, S.A. (2004). Assessing the oral cavity. In M. Frank-Stromborg & J.S. Olsen (Eds.), *Instruments for clinical health-care research* (3rd ed., pp. 594–602). Sudbury, MA: Jones and Bartlett.

Jaroneski, L.A. (2006). The importance of assessment rating scales for chemotherapy-induced oral mucositis. *Oncology Nursing Forum, 33*(6), 1085–1092.

National Cancer Institute Cancer Therapy Evaluation Program. (2006). *Common terminology criteria for adverse events* (version 3.0). Bethesda, MD: National Cancer Institute. Retrieved August 31, 2008, from http://ctep.cancer.gov/protocolDevelopment/electronic_applications/docs/ctcaev3.pdf

Rubenstein, E.B., Peterson, D.E., Schubert, M., Keefe, D., McGuire, D., Epstein, J., et al. (2004). Clinical practice guidelines for the prevention and treatment of cancer therapy-induced oral and gastrointestinal mucositis. *Cancer, 100*(Suppl. 9), 2026–2046.

Sonis, S., Eilers, J., Epstein, J., LeVeque, F., Liggett, W., Mulaga, M., et al. (1999). Validation of a new scoring system for assessment of clinical trials research of oral mucositis induced by radiation or chemotherapy. *Cancer, 85*(10), 2103–2113.

Spielberger, R., Stiff, P., Bensinger, W., Gentile, T., Weisdorf, D., Kewalramani, T., et al. (2004). Palifermin for oral mucositis after intensive therapy for hematologic cancers. *New England Journal of Medicine, 351*(25), 2590–2598.

Case Study

Volunteering to work on an ONS PEP evidence-based practice resource provided support for changing clinical practice in a very large private practice in Miami, FL. Personal efforts to gather evidence to show physician partners why "magic mouthwash" should not be a routine recommendation were reinforced. Joining the ONS mucositis PEP resource team was the perfect opportunity to review the latest literature and provide the evidence-based information to fellow practitioners.

After the ONS PEP resource on mucositis was published, the multistep process for changing the standards in practice for managing mucositis was approached with vigor. Action steps included the following.

- Partnering with a physician in our group who was supportive of the project
- Identifying reasons why magic mouthwash prescriptions should not be used, including lack of evidence to support superior effectiveness over bland rinses and out-of-pocket cost to patients. (Magic mouthwash is a compound and not covered under many prescription plans. The solution can cost more than $50 per bottle. It also has a short expiration date once opened.)
- Recognizing that physicians sometimes prescribed magic mouthwash because they wanted to be able to give patients "something" prompted the development of a mucositis handout that could be given to patients instead of the mouthwash prescription. This handout was a collaborative effort with the local hospital and is available in English and Spanish. It contains recommendations for particular symptoms associated with mucositis and information on what mucositis is (see Figure 13-1).
- Presenting the idea of discontinuing all magic mouthwash prescriptions in the practice to the board of physicians, with the idea of substituting them with the mucositis handout and appropriate prescriptions for specific symptoms of mucositis. The board voted unanimously in favor of eliminating the prescriptions.
- Ensuring that the "old" prescription pads for magic mouthwash were removed from all three practice sites. This was accomplished by holding a contest within the practice. Every employee who turned in a magic mouthwash preprinted prescription pad received a raffle ticket (one ticket for each pad). The prize for the raffle was a $50 gift certificate to the restaurant of the employee's choice. Within one week, 101 preprinted magic mouthwash prescription pads (each full pad contained 50 prescriptions) had been turned in. The raffle was also an opportunity to communicate the practice change to all members of the clinical teams and to get them to actively participate in the change.

The project was a success in the practice setting because of the presentation of current evidence to the physicians with the aid of the ONS PEP resource on mucositis.

Cathy L. Maxwell, RN, OCN®
Director of Clinical Operations
Advanced Medical Specialties
Miami, FL

Figure 13-1. Mucositis Patient Handout

Mouth Care Tips
The following are mouth care tips for people at risk for mucositis or who have mucositis.
* Brush all tooth surfaces thoroughly for at least 90 seconds, at least twice daily, using a soft toothbrush. Rinse well. Store toothbrush in a clean, dry place.
* Do not use commercial mouthwashes because they contain alcohol, which is irritating to sensitive tissues. Unless otherwise instructed by your physician, use a mouthwash solution made with salt and baking soda (see following recipe). This solution reduces the acidity of oral fluids, dilutes mucus, and reduces the chances of a yeast infection (e.g., thrush) developing in the mouth.
* Floss at least once daily before bedtime or as advised by your doctor or nurse. Be careful when flossing to avoid cutting your gums. Do not floss if doing so causes pain.
* Use water-based moisturizers to protect lips.
* Drink plenty of water and other fluids with meals and between meals.
* Avoid tobacco, alcohol, and irritating foods (e.g., acidic, hot, rough, spicy). Cold foods such as flavored ice pops, ice cream, and applesauce may be easier to swallow and re- duce mouth discomfort.

Tell your doctor or nurse
* If you are unable to eat or swallow because of pain. Medication can be prescribed (e.g., pain medication, Gelclair® [EKR Therapeutics, Inc.], viscous xylocaine).
* If you notice white patches anywhere in your mouth, which might indicate an infection. Medication can be prescribed (e.g., fluconazole, nystatin, clotrimazole).
* If your gums bleed longer than usual for you. Your blood platelet count might be low.

Sore Mouth
If you have a sore mouth, do the following after meals and at bedtime.
* If your mouth is too sore to use a toothbrush, use a sponge swab (toothette) espe- cially made for this purpose. The swabs are available plain and with baking soda and can be purchased at your local pharmacy.
* Dip the sponge swab into about a half-cup of the mouthwash solution (see following recipe), and gently brush all surfaces of teeth, tongue, gums, and cheeks.
* Use as many swabs as necessary to clean thoroughly, dipping each swab only once into the solution.
* Rinse your mouth with the mouthwash solution.

Dry Mouth
If you have dry mouth, you may want to use a product such as Biotene® (Laclede Inc.) to help reduce dryness. Wait at least 30 minutes between using other mouth products and using the Biotene. This product contains enzymes that are inactivated if used immedi- ately before or after non-Biotene toothpastes or mouth washes. Oasis® Dry Mouth spray and Oasis Mouthwash (Gebauer Oral Care) are also recommended and available over the counter.

Homemade Mouthwash Recipe
Add ¼ teaspoon of table salt and ¼ teaspoon baking soda to one cup tap water and stir to mix.
Swish in mouth for at least 30 seconds, and then spit out, after meals and at bedtime. Discard the remainder of the solution. Make a fresh mixture for each use.

Note. Figure courtesy of Advanced Medical Specialties, Inc. Used with permission.

Mucositis

2009 AUTHORS
Debra J. Harris, RN, MSN, OCN®, and June G. Eilers, PhD, APRN-CNS, BC
ONS STAFF: Linda H. Eaton, MN, RN, AOCN®

2007 AUTHORS
Debra J. Harris, RN, MSN, OCN®, June G. Eilers, PhD, RN, BC, CS, Barbara J. Cashavelly, MSN, RN,
AOCN®, Cathy L. Maxwell, RN, OCN®, CCRC, and Amber Harriman, RN
RESEARCH CONSULTANT: Jane M. Armer, RN, PhD
ONS STAFF: Linda H. Eaton, MN, RN, AOCN®

What interventions are effective for managing oral mucositis in people receiving treatment for cancer?

Recommended for Practice

Interventions for which effectiveness has been demonstrated by strong evidence from rigorously designed studies, meta-analyses, or systematic reviews and for which expectation of harm is small compared with the benefits

ORAL CARE PROTOCOLS

Oral care protocols developed by multidisciplinary teams may reduce the severity of oral mucositis. These protocols should include educational components for patients and staff (McGuire, Correa, Johnson, & Wienandts, 2006; Multinational Association of Supportive Care in Cancer [MASCC], 2005; Rubenstein et al., 2004). Oral assessment with a validated tool should be conducted regularly to assess function, pain, and the oral cavity. The inclusion of dental professionals is recommended throughout treatment and follow-up (MASCC).

Basic oral care should include a soft toothbrush that is replaced regularly (MASCC, 2005; McGuire et al., 2006). See *Expert Opinion* section for other important aspects of oral care.

Likely to Be Effective

Interventions for which effectiveness has been demonstrated by supportive evidence from a single rigorously conducted controlled trial, consistent supportive evidence from well-designed controlled trials using small samples, or guidelines developed from evidence and supported by expert opinion

CRYOTHERAPY FOR PATIENTS RECEIVING BOLUS MUCOTOXIC CHEMOTHERAPY WITH SHORT HALF-LIFE (BOLUS 5-FLUOROURACIL, MELPHALAN)

Cryotherapy has a significant effect on the reduction of oral mucositis for patients receiving rapid infusions of either 5-fluorouracil (5-FU) or melphalan. The effectiveness is based on vasoconstriction of the circulation in the oral cavity and the short half-life of these agents. Consistent evidence is lacking to support the benefit of cryotherapy with other agents.

The optimum duration of cryotherapy requires further systematic investigation, as studies to date have been inconsistent. Recent studies indicate reduced oral mucositis with longer duration of cryotherapy after the completion of chemotherapy. Based on current knowledge, patients should hold ice or ice-cold water in their mouth for five minutes prior to the infusion, during the infusion, and for 30 minutes after completion of the infusion. Compliance with the cooling has been varied, and the use of cryotherapy presents concerns for individuals who do not tolerate cold in their oral cavity. Cryotherapy is not indicated in patients who are receiving oxaliplatin because of problems with exposure to cold (Aisa et al., 2005; Karagozoglu & Filiz Ulusoy, 2005; Kwong, 2004; Lilleby et al., 2006; Migliorati, Oberle-Edwards, & Schubert, 2006; Mori et al., 2006; Nikoletti, Hyde, Shaw, Myers, & Kristjanson, 2005; Papadeas, Naxakis, Riga, & Kalofonos, 2007; Scully, Sonis, & Diz, 2006; Sorensen, Skovsgaard, Bork, Damstrup, & Ingeberg, 2008; Svanberg, Birgegard, & Ohrn, 2007; Tartarone, Matera, Romano, Vigliotti, & Di Renzo, 2005).

PALIFERMIN FOR PATIENTS UNDERGOING HEMATOPOIETIC STEM CELL TRANSPLANTATION FOR HEMATOLOGIC MALIGNANCIES

Palifermin is a recombinant human keratinocyte growth factor that stimulates growth of epithelial cells. This drug has been shown to reduce severity and duration of oral mucositis in patients with hematologic malignancies receiving high-dose chemotherapy and total body irradiation with allogeneic or autologous stem cell transplantation. Palifermin is given at a dose of 60 mcg/kg/day IV for three days prior to the beginning of the conditioning regimen and for three days post-transplant for the prevention of oral mucositis. Because of the high cost of this agent, it should be used for patients most likely to develop severe mucositis. The most common side effects include mild rash and taste changes (MASCC, 2005; Scully et al., 2006; Speilberger et al., 2004; von Bultzingslowen et al., 2006). Further study of palifermin is needed to determine its use beyond the transplant setting.

One recent trial (Rosen et al., 2006) examined the use of palifermin at a dose of 40 mcg/kg/day given to patients with metastatic colorectal cancer receiving 5-FU and calcium leucovorin. Although the study did demonstrate a statistically significant reduction in grade 2 or higher mucositis, the results have been questioned because cryotherapy was not used despite its known benefits with 5-FU–induced mucositis (Haines, 2007; Langner et al., 2008; Loprinzi, Barton, & Sloan, 2006; Nasilowska-Adamska et al., 2007; Rosen et al.; Schmidt et al., 2008; Shea, Kewalramani, Mun, Jayne, & Dreiling, 2007).

Benefits Balanced With Harms

Interventions for which clinicians and patients should weigh the beneficial and harmful effects according to individual circumstances and priorities

There are no interventions as of May 2008.

Effectiveness Not Established

Interventions for which insufficient data or data of inadequate quality currently exist, with no clear indication of harm

ALLOPURINOL

Although initial small trials of allopurinol mouthwashes found some positive treatment findings for oral mucositis, these results were not confirmed in controlled trials (Clarkson, Worthington, & Eden, 2007; Kwong, 2004; Scully et al., 2006).

AMIFOSTINE

The role of amifostine in the management of oral mucositis has not been established. It is currently recommended to reduce esophagitis induced by concurrent chemotherapy and radiation in patients with non-small cell lung cancer and for the prevention of radiation proctitis in patients receiving standard dose radiation for rectal cancer (Antonadou, Pepelassi, Synodinou, Puglisi, & Throuvalas, 2002; Bensadoun, Schubert, Lalla, & Keefe, 2006; Rubenstein et al., 2004). Further studies are needed to establish the use of amifostine for management of oral mucositis.

ANTI-INFLAMMATORY RINSES

Anti-inflammatory rinses such as kamillosan liquidum, hydrocortisone, prostaglandin E1, and oral corticosteroids have been examined in small studies, none of which produced significant results. Poor study design and inadequate sample sizes prevent definitive conclusions regarding these agents (Shih, Miaskowski, Dodd, Stotts, & MacPhail, 2002).

ANTIMICROBIAL AGENTS

Many antimicrobial agents, including polymyxin, tobramycin, amphotericin B, fluconazole, and protegrin, have been studied in a variety of doses and combinations (Shih et al., 2002). No clear pattern of benefit has emerged, and little evidence exists to recommend the use of these agents (Donnelly, Bellm, Epstein, Sonis, & Symonds, 2003). One large placebo-controlled randomized trial has shown narrow-spectrum antibacterial lozenges to be effective in the radiation setting (Scully et al., 2006).

BENZYDAMINE HCL

Benzydamine is used in Europe and Canada but has not been approved by the U.S. Food and Drug Administration (FDA) for use in the United States. Benzydamine has been shown to produce a significant reduction in oral mucositis compared with placebo in patients receiving 0–5,000 cGy of radiation for head and neck cancer. This effect was not seen in patients receiving high single-day doses of radiation ≥ 22 cGy per day. Patients rinse with 15 ml benzydamine for two minutes four to eight times daily before and during radiation and for two weeks after completion of radiation (Epstein et al., 2001).

CAPHOSOL

Caphosol is a topical oral agent that lubricates the mucosa and theoretically helps to maintain the integrity of the oral cavity through its mineralizing potential. It contains high concentrations of calcium and phosphate ions. It has a U.S. patent as a prescription medical device. One randomized trial (N = 95) for prevention of mucositis in stem cell transplant recipients showed favorable effects when used in combination with fluoride as compared to the control group using only fluoride. Additional data are needed to support findings of this study (Papas et al., 2003).

CHLORHEXIDINE

Evidence related to the use of chlorhexidine for mucositis is mixed. Conflicting results may be related to lack of clarity regarding the presence of alcohol in the study agent. One recent study demonstrated a benefit of chlorhexidine rinse over normal saline and cryotherapy for severity and duration of mucositis (Sorensen et al., 2008). Trials that clearly state use of alcohol-free chlorhexidine have shown some benefit; therefore, evidence for alcohol-free formulations of chlorhexidine indicates that the effectiveness of the formulation is not established. **Chlorhexidine with alcohol has not been found to be effective in reducing mucositis. See *Not Recommended for Practice* section.**

FLUORIDE CHEWING GUM

Fluoride-containing sugar-free gum sweetened with xylitol may have antimicrobial effects and warrants further study. In one multicenter randomized trial (N = 145), participants were asked to chew five to six pieces of gum per day for 20 minutes per piece, a dose that has been shown to substantially increase salivary flow. Participants chewed gum on the first day of chemotherapy and continued for three days after the end of the course. This trial showed a decrease in severity of mucositis in patients who received less toxic chemotherapy regimens (Gandemer et al., 2007).

FLURBIPROFEN TOOTH PATCH

Flurbiprofen is an inhibitor of cyclooxygenase-2, which is thought to contribute to the development of oral mucositis. Flurbiprofen also has antiproliferative activity. One trial (N = 22) found a slight delay in the development of mucositis but no effect for prevention. Pain scores were higher in the flurbiprofen group. Study size and method of administration may have been inadequate to see effects for mucositis outcomes (Stokman, Spijkervet, Burlage, & Roodenburg, 2005).

GRANULOCYTE–COLONY-STIMULATING FACTOR (SUBCUTANEOUS)

Studies of granulocyte–colony-stimulating factor demonstrate conflicting results. Two randomized studies (Crawford, Tomita, Mazanet, Glaspy, & Ozer, 1999; Katano, Nakamura, Matso, Iyama, & Hisatsugu, 1995) showed reduction in oral mucositis incidence, whereas several other studies have not demonstrated any effects (Scully et al., 2006).

GELCLAIR

Gelclair® (EKR Therapeutics, Inc.) is a bioadherent substance that is diluted and applied to the mucosa as a viscous gel. It acts as a topical analgesic coating and may aid wound healing. It is approved as a medical device for treatment of oral mucositis. One small study (N = 20) found potential effects on pain during speaking; however, results were not statistically significant (Barber, Powell, Ellis, & Hewett, 2007).

GRANULOCYTE MACROPHAGE–COLONY-STIMULATING FACTOR (SUBCUTANEOUS)

Conflicting evidence exists for granulocyte macrophage–colony-stimulating factor (GM-CSF) for the treatment of oral mucositis. GM-CSF may or may not effectively treat mucositis. Study sample sizes were small, and patient dropout rate was high because of intolerable side effects (McAleese, Bishop, A'Hern, & Henk, 2006; Rossi, Rosati, Colarusso, & Manzione, 2003; Ryu et al., 2007; Scully et al., 2006; Shih et al., 2002; von Bultzingslowen et al., 2006).

HONEY

Two small studies (N = 40, N = 40) using pure natural honey in the radiation setting with head and neck cancer treatment found a statistically significant decrease in mucositis severity as well as weight loss, a frequent consequence of mucositis in this population. In each study, 20 ml of honey was applied to the mucosa before and after radiotherapy. The honey was swallowed slowly over time. This intervention was easy to use, cost effective, and pleasant for patients (Motallebnejad, Akram, Moghadamnia, Moulana, & Omidi, 2008; Rashad, Al-Gezawy, El-Gezawy, & Azzaz, 2008).

IMMUNOGLOBULIN

Studies using intramuscular injections of immunoglobulin have shown a reduction in oral mucositis; however, these studies are small (N = 22), and no studies of published data after 1997 were found during the literature search (Kwong, 2004; Shih et al., 2002).

L-ALANYL-L-GLUTAMINE

The effectiveness of glutamine in the treatment of oral mucositis has not been established. One small study (N = 29) using L-alanyl-L-glutamine 0.4 g/kg/day versus saline placebo demonstrated a moderate effect over mucositis intensity (p = 0.044). All patients in the study were given supplemental oral nutrition (Cerchietti et al., 2006). A pilot study (N = 32) failed to demonstrate that parenteral nutrition supplemented with glutamine 0.57 g/kg could reduce morphine use (Blijlevens, Donnelly, Naber, Schattenberg, & DePauw, 2005). A third study examined an oral form of glutamine (Saforis® [MGI Pharma] 2.5 g/5 ml three times per day versus placebo) in patients with breast cancer undergoing anthracycline-based chemotherapy. The study demonstrated improvement in incidence of World Health Organization grade > 2 mucositis (p = 0.026) and ability to eat solid food (p = 0.039) (Peterson, Jones, & Petit, 2006). Although some studies of glutamine have demonstrated promise, additional studies are required before effectiveness is clearly established. This agent currently is pending full FDA approval.

LOW-LEVEL LASER THERAPY

Seven small studies using low-level laser therapy (LLLT) have been conducted to date, demonstrating lack of toxicity and evidence of potential benefit for prevention, treatment, and pain control related to oral mucositis. Laser therapy requires specialized equipment and training, which is not widely available. Some researchers have suggested using LLLT where available to reduce the incidence of oral mucositis and associated pain in patients receiving chemotherapy or chemoradiation before hematopoietic stem cell transplantation (Antunes, Ferreira, de Matos, Pinheiro, & Ferreira, 2008; Arora, Pai, Maiya, Vidyasager, & Rajeev, 2008; Cruz et al., 2007; Genot & Klastersky, 2005; Genot-Klastersky et al., 2008; Jaguar et al., 2007; Maiya, Sagar, & Fernandes, 2006; Migliorati et al., 2006; Nes & Posso, 2005; Rubenstein et al., 2004; Schubert et al., 2007; Scully et al., 2006).

MULTIAGENT ("MAGIC" OR "MIRACLE") RINSES

Multiagent rinses typically include lidocaine, Benadryl®, and Maalox® or other similar agents. Some patients commented that the mouthwash made their mouth "numb," which is of concern for potential injury. Additionally, some formulations of these agents may contain alcohol, which should be avoided. Little evidence demonstrates the effectiveness of these rinses for mucositis (Dodd et al., 2000; Eilers, 2004).

ORAL ALOE VERA

Only one small study (N = 58) of aloe vera was identified. Although patients in the aloe vera arm had a lower maximal oral mucositis severity grade, this was not statistically significant. No other findings were statistically significant (Su et al., 2004).

PILOCARPINE

Early trials indicated that pilocarpine has some benefit in reducing the severity of oral mucositis; however, this was not demonstrated in a recent controlled trial. Side effects of this agent include tachycardia and palpitations (Awidi et al., 2001; Lockhart et al., 2005).

POVIDONE-IODINE (ORAL)

Although earlier trials demonstrated significant reductions in onset, incidence, total duration, and worst grade of oral mucositis with oral povidone-iodine (Eilers, 2004; Kwong, 2004; Shih et al., 2002), a more recent randomized controlled trial (RCT) (N = 132) did not. Additionally, povidone-iodine was found to be less tolerable than normal saline (Vokurka et al., 2005). Another trial examined an alcohol-free formulation of chlorhexidine, povidone-iodine, salt and sodium bicarbonate, and plain water rinses. This trial did show decreased incidence of severe mucositis with povidone-iodine over the other mouthwashes, which increased in significance over the six-week trial period (Madan, Sequeira, Shenoy, & Shetty, 2008). A small study (N = 40) also demonstrated a lower incidence of oral mucositis using povidone-iodine and a special toothbrush with suctioning (Yoneda et al., 2007). This agent is not to be used in patients with new granulation tissue, as it inhibits cell growth. Swallowing povidone-iodine is absolutely contraindicated.

TETRACAINE

One uncontrolled study (N = 50) demonstrated a reduction in oral cavity pain and fewer radiation treatment interruptions when treated with tetracaine gel applied approximately six times per day (Alterio et al., 2006).

ZINC SUPPLEMENTATION

One small RCT (N = 30) determined that no grade 4 oral mucositis developed in the zinc group, and mucositis development was delayed in that group (p < 0.01). Six weeks after the completion of radiation treatment, only one patient in the zinc group continued to have mucositis, whereas 10 of 12 patients in the placebo group did. In a second trial (N = 97), similar results were found. The optimal dose has yet to be determined (Ertekin, Koc, Karslioglu, & Sezen, 2003; Lin, Que, Lin, & Lin, 2006).

Effectiveness Unlikely

Interventions for which lack of effectiveness has been demonstrated by negative evidence from a single rigorously conducted controlled trial, consistent negative evidence from well-designed controlled trials using small samples, or guidelines developed from evidence and supported by expert opinion

ISEGANAN

Iseganan failed to show adequate effect for oral mucositis related to high doses of chemotherapy or radiation therapy for head and neck malignancy in two multisite RCTs of > 500 subjects each (Giles et al., 2004; Trotti et al., 2004).

MISOPROSTOL

Misoprostol failed to show any difference in extent, incidence, or duration of mucositis compared to placebo in a trial of patients with head and neck cancer treated with radiation. The study did not accrue adequate patients and had a 12% withdrawal rate because of increased level of oral/oropharyngeal soreness (Veness et al., 2006).

VITAMIN E (TOPICAL)

No statistically significant findings were demonstrated in a study of topical vitamin E in pediatric patients receiving doxorubicin-based chemotherapy. No differences were noted in pain scores, grade of mucositis, amount of opioid analgesia, topical oral analgesia, IV hydration, total parenteral nutrition, or episodes of febrile neutropenia compared with control (Sung et al., 2007).

WOBE-MUGOS E

Wobe-Mugos E contains proteolytic enzymes administered in oral tablets. In one trial (N = 69), treatment with this agent resulted in an earlier onset of mucositis and increased pain scores during treatment (Dorr & Herrmann, 2007).

Not Recommended for Practice

Interventions for which lack of effectiveness or harmfulness has been demonstrated by strong evidence from rigorously conducted studies, meta-analyses, or systematic reviews, or interventions for which the costs, burden, or harms associated with the intervention exceed anticipated benefit

CHLORHEXIDINE (ALCOHOL-BASED)

Chlorhexidine has had mixed reviews. Chlorhexidine with alcohol is not effective in reducing the severity of oral mucositis. In addition, it does not have significant effects on suppression of any type of oral flora (Shih et al., 2002). The MASCC (2005) guidelines indicate that chlorhexidine should not be used to treat established oral mucositis because its superiority to bland rinses has not been established (Rubenstein et al., 2004). Other reports indicate rinse-induced discomfort, taste alteration, and teeth staining (Cheng, Molassiotis, Chang, Wai, & Cheung, 2001; Dodd et al., 2000; Eilers, 2004; Pitten, Kiefer, Buth, Doelken, & Kramer, 2003). See *Effectiveness Not Established* section for chlorhexidine (alcohol-free) recommendation.

GM-CSF MOUTHWASH

GM-CSF mouthwash has not demonstrated any benefit in treating oral mucositis. The updated MASCC guidelines indicate that GM-CSF mouthwashes should not be used for the prevention of oral mucositis in the transplant setting (MASCC, 2005; Rubenstein et al., 2004). The recommendation also is supported in systematic reviews that discuss this agent (Kwong, 2004; Shih et al., 2002; von Bultzingslowen et al., 2006).

SUCRALFATE

Sucralfate has not demonstrated any benefit in treating oral mucositis and is not recommended for practice because of lack of tolerability related to nausea and other gastrointestinal effects, including rectal bleeding (Castagna et al., 2001; Dodd et al., 2003; Eilers, 2004; Etiz et al., 2000; Kwong, 2004; MASCC, 2005; Nottage et al., 2003; Rubenstein et al., 2004; Scully et al., 2006; Shih et al., 2002).

Expert Opinion

Low-risk interventions that are (1) consistent with sound clinical practice, (2) suggested by an expert in a peer-reviewed publication (journal or book chapter), and (3) for which limited evidence exists. An expert is an individual with peer-reviewed journal publications in the domain of interest.

Although RCTs are lacking, experts agree that routine basic oral care is an important element of care for prevention and management of oral mucositis. In fact, it would be regarded as unethical to withhold basic oral care as one arm of a research study in order to validate the benefit of such care.

An oral care protocol consisting of at least the following elements should be included for all patients receiving treatment that places them at risk for developing oral mucositis (Cheng, Chang, & Yuen, 2004; Cheng et al., 2001; Dodd et al., 2000, 2003; Eilers, 2004; Kwong, 2004; MASCC, 2005; Rubenstein et al., 2004; Scully et al., 2006; Shih et al., 2002).

Clinicians:
- Collaborate with a multidisciplinary team in all phases of treatment.
- Conduct a systematic oral assessment at least daily or at each patient visit. In the outpatient setting, teach patients to perform oral assessment daily as well as when to report assessment findings to the clinician.
- Provide written instruction and education regarding oral care to patients. Verify understanding with return explanation and demonstration.

Patient Instructions:
- Brush all tooth surfaces for at least 90 seconds at least twice daily using a soft toothbrush. Allow toothbrush to air dry before storing.
- Floss at least once daily or as advised by the clinician.
- Rinse mouth four times a day with a bland rinse (see below).
- Avoid tobacco, alcohol, and irritating foods (acidic, hot, rough, spicy).
- Use water-based moisturizers to protect lips.
- Maintain adequate hydration.

BLAND RINSES

Rinses are used to remove loose debris and aid with oral hydration. Bland rinses include 0.9% saline (normal saline), sodium bicarbonate, and a saline and sodium bicarbonate mixture. Any of these rinses can be administered at room temperature or refrigerated, and all are inexpensive. Patients should be instructed to swish a tablespoon of the rinse in the oral cavity for at least 30 seconds and then expectorate. Sodium bicarbonate reduces the acidity of oral fluids, dilutes accumulating mucus, and discourages yeast colonization (Dodd et al., 2000; Eilers, 2004; Rubenstein et al., 2004; Scully et al., 2006; Shih et al., 2002).

Definitions of the interventions are available at **www.ons.org/outcomes**. Literature search completed through May 2008.

References

Aisa, Y., Mori, T., Kudo, M., Yashima, T., Kondo, S., Yokoyama, A., et al. (2005). Oral cryotherapy for the prevention of high-dose melphalan-induced stomatitis in allogeneic hematopoietic stem cell transplant recipients. *Supportive Care in Cancer, 13*(4), 266–269.

Alterio, D., Jereczek-Fossa, B.A., Zuccotti, G.F., Leon, M.E., Omodeo Sale, E.O., Pasetti, M., et al. (2006). Tetracaine oral gel in patients treated with radiotherapy for head-and-neck cancer: Final results of a phase II study. *International Journal of Radiation Oncology, Biology, Physics, 64*(2), 392–395.

Antonadou, D., Pepelassi, M., Synodinou, M., Puglisi, M., & Throuvalas, N. (2002). Prophylactic use of amifostine to prevent radiochemotherapy-induced mucositis and xerostomia in head-and-neck cancer. *International Journal of Radiation Oncology, Biology, Physics, 52*(3), 739–747.

Antunes, H.S., Ferreira, E.M., de Matos, V.D., Pinheiro, C.T., & Ferreira, C.G. (2008). The impact of low power laser in the treatment of conditioning-induced oral mucositis: A report of 11 clinical cases and their review. *Medicina Oral, Patología Oral y Cirugía Bucal, 13*(3), 189–192.

Arora, H., Pai, K.M., Maiya, A., Vidyasager, M.S., & Rajeev, A. (2008). Efficacy of He-Ne laser in the prevention and treatment of radiotherapy-induced oral mucositis in oral cancer patients. *Oral Surgery, Oral Medicine, Oral Pathology, Oral Radiology, and Endodontics, 105*(2), 180–186.

Awidi, A., Homsi, U., Kakail, R.I., Mubarak, A., Hassan, A., Kelta, M., et al. (2001). Double-blind, placebo-controlled cross-over study of oral pilocarpine for the prevention of chemotherapy-induced oral mucositis in adult patients with cancer. *European Journal of Cancer, 37*(16), 2010–2014.

Barber, C., Powell, R., Ellis, A., & Hewett, J. (2007). Comparing pain control and ability to eat and drink with standard therapy vs. Gelclair: A preliminary, double centre, randomised controlled trial on patients with radiotherapy-induced oral mucositis. *Supportive Care in Cancer, 15*(4), 427–440.

Bensadoun, R.J., Schubert, M.M., Lalla, R.V., & Keefe, D. (2006). Amifostine in the management of radiation-induced and chemo-induced mucositis. *Supportive Care in Cancer, 14*(6), 566–572.

Blijlevens, N.M., Donnelly, J.P., Naber, A.H., Schattenberg, A.V., & DePauw, B.E. (2005). A randomised, double-blinded, placebo-controlled, pilot study of parenteral glutamine for allogeneic stem cell transplant patients. *Supportive Care in Cancer, 13*(10), 790–796.

Castagna, L., Benhamou, E., Pedraza, E., Luboinski, M., Forni, M., Brandes, I., et al. (2001). Prevention of mucositis in bone marrow transplantation: A double blind randomised controlled trial of sucralfate. *Annals of Oncology, 12*(7), 953–955.

Cerchietti, L.C., Navigante, A.H., Lutteral, M.A., Castro, M.A., Kirchuck, R., Bonomi, M., et al. (2006). Double-blinded, placebo-controlled trial on intravenous L-alanyl-L-glutamine in the incidence of oral mucositis following chemoradiotherapy in patients with head-and-neck cancer. *International Journal of Radiation Oncology, Biology, Physics, 65*(5), 1330–1337.

Cheng, K.K., Chang, A.M., & Yuen, M.P. (2004). Prevention of oral mucositis in pediatric patients treated with chemotherapy: A randomized crossover trial comparing two protocols of oral care. *European Journal of Cancer, 40*(8), 1208–1216.

Cheng, K.K., Molassiotis, A., Chang, A.M., Wai, W.C., & Cheung, S.S. (2001). Evaluation of an oral care protocol intervention in the prevention of chemotherapy-induced oral mucositis in pediatric cancer patients. *European Journal of Cancer, 37*(16), 2056–2063.

Clarkson, J.E.,Worthington, H.V., & Eden, O.B. (2007). Interventions for treating oral mucositis for patients with cancer receiving treatment. *Cochrane Database of Systematic Reviews* 2007, Issue 2. Art. No.: CD001973. DOI: 10.1002/14651858.CD001973.pub3.

Crawford, J., Tomita, D.K., Mazanet, R., Glaspy, J., & Ozer, H. (1999). Reduction of oral mucositis by fil-grastim (r-metHuG-CSF) in patients receiving chemotherapy. *Cytokines, Cellular and Molecular Therapy, 5*(4), 187–193.

Cruz, L.B., Ribeiro, A.S., Rech, A., Rosa, L.G., Castro, C.G., & Brunetto, A.L. (2007). Influence of low-energy laser in the prevention of oral mucositis in children with cancer receiving chemotherapy. *Pediatric Blood and Cancer, 48*(4), 435–440.

Dodd, M.J., Dibble, S.L., Miaskowski, C., MacPhail, L., Greenspan, D., Paul, S.M., et al. (2000). Randomized clinical trial of the effectiveness of 3 commonly used mouthwashes to treat chemotherapy-induced mucositis. *Oral Surgery, Oral Medicine, Oral Pathology, Oral Radiology, and Endodontics, 90*(1), 39–47.

Dodd, M.J., Miaskowski, C., Greenspan, D., MacPhail, L., Shih, A., Shiba, G., et al. (2003). Radiation-induced mucositis: A randomized clinical trial of micronized sucralfate versus salt and soda mouthwashes. *Cancer Investigation, 21*(1), 21–33.

Donnelly, J.P., Bellm, L.A., Epstien, J.B., Sonis, S.T., & Symonds, R.P. (2003). Antimicrobial therapy to prevent or treat oral mucositis. *Lancet Infectious Diseases, 3*(7), 405–412.

Dorr, W., & Herrmann, T. (2007). Efficacy of Wobe-Mugos E for reduction of oral mucositis after radiotherapy: Results of a prospective, randomized, placebo-controlled, triple-blind phase III multicenter study. *Strahlentherapie und Onkologie, 183*(3), 121–127.

Eilers, J. (2004). Nursing interventions and supportive care for the prevention and treatment of oral mucositis associated with cancer treatment. *Oncology Nursing Forum, 31*(Suppl. 4), 13–23.

Epstein, J.B., Silverman, S., Paggiarino, D.A., Crockett, S., Schubert, M.M., Senzer, N.N., et al. (2001). Benzydamine HCl for prophylaxis of radiation-induced oral mucositis: Results from a multicenter, randomized, double-blind, placebo-controlled clinical trial. *Cancer, 92*(4), 875–885.

Ertekin, M.V., Koc, M., Karslioglu, I., & Sezen, O. (2003). Zinc sulfate in the prevention of radiation-induced oropharyngeal mucositis: A prospective, placebo-controlled, randomized study. *International Journal of Radiation Oncology, Biology, Physics, 58*(1), 167–174.

Etiz, D., Erkal, H.S., Serin, M., Kucuk, B., Hepari, A., Elhan, A.H., et al. (2000). Clinical and histopathological evaluation of sucralfate in prevention of oral mucositis induced by radiation therapy in patients with head and neck malignancies. *Oral Oncology, 36*(1), 116–120.

Gandemer, V., Le Deley, M., Dollfus, C., Auvrignon, A., Bonnaure-Mallet, M., Duval, M., et al. (2007). Multicenter randomized trial of chewing gum for preventing oral mucositis in children receiving chemotherapy. *Journal of Pediatric Hematology/Oncology, 29*(2), 86–94.

Genot, M., & Klastersky, J. (2005). Low-level laser for prevention and therapy of oral mucositis induced by chemotherapy or radiotherapy. *Current Opinion in Oncology, 17*(3), 236–240.

Genot-Klastersky, M.T., Klastersky, J., Awada, F., Awada, A., Crombez, P., Martinez, M.D., et al. (2008). The use of low-energy laser (LEL) for the prevention of chemotherapy- and/or radiotherapy-induced oral mucositis in cancer patients: Results from two prospective studies. *Supportive Care and Cancer, 16*(12), 1381–1387.

Giles, F.J., Rodriguez, R., Weisdorf, D., Wingard, J.R., Martin, P.J., Fleming, T.R., et al. (2004). A phase III, randomized, double-blind, placebo-controlled study of iseganan for the reduction of stomatitis in patients receiving stomatotoxic chemotherapy. *Leukemia Research, 28*(6), 559–565.

Haines, I. (2007). Questions about the role of palifermin in fluorouracil-based therapy for metastatic colorectal cancer. *Journal of Clinical Oncology, 25*(19), E24–E25. Retrieved December 12, 2008, from http://jco.ascopubs.org/cgi/repring/25/19/e24

Jaguar, G.C., Prado, J.D., Nishimoto, I.N., Pinheiro, M.C., deCastro, D.O., Jr., da Cruz Perez, D.E., et al. (2007). Low-energy laser therapy for prevention of oral mucositis in hematopoetic stem cell transplantation. *Oral Diseases, 13*(6), 538–543.

Karagozoglu, S., & Filiz Ulusoy, M.F. (2005). Chemotherapy: The effect of oral cryotherapy on the development of mucositis. *Journal of Clinical Nursing, 14*(6), 754–765.

Katano, M., Nakamura, M., Matsuo, T., Iyama, A., & Hisatsugu, T. (1995). Effect of granulocyte colony-stimulating factor (G-CSF) on chemotherapy-induced oral mucositis. *Surgery Today, 25*(3), 202–206.

Kwong, K.K. (2004). Prevention and treatment of oropharyngeal mucositis following cancer therapy: Are there new approaches? *Cancer Nursing, 27*(3), 183–205.

Langner, S., Staber, P.B., Schub, N., Gramatzki, M., Grothe, W., Behre, G., et al. (2008). Palifermin reduces incidence and severity of oral mucositis in allogeneic stem-cell transplant recipients. *Bone Marrow Transplantation, 42*(4), 275–279.

Lilleby, K., Garcia, P., Gooley, T., McDonnnell, P., Taber, R., Holmberg, L., et al. (2006). A prospective, randomized study of cryotherapy during administration of high-dose melphalan to decrease the severity and duration of oral mucositis in patients with multiple myeloma undergoing autologous peripheral blood stem cell transplantation. *Bone Marrow Transplantation, 37*(11), 1031–1035.

Lin, L.C., Que, J., Lin, L.K., & Lin, F.C. (2006). Zinc supplementation to improve mucositis and dermatitis in patients after radiotherapy for head-and-neck cancers: A double-blind, randomized study. *International Journal of Radiation Oncology, Biology, Physics, 65*(3), 745–750.

Lockhart, P.B., Brennan, M.T., Kent, M.L., Packman, C.H., Norton, H.J., Fox, P.C., et al. (2005). Randomized controlled trial of pilocarpine hydrochloride for the moderation of oral mucositis during autologous blood stem cell transplantation. *Bone Marrow Transplantation, 35*(7), 713–720.

Loprinzi, C., Barton, D., & Sloan, J. (2006). Whose opinion counts? *Journal of Clinical Oncology, 24*(33), 5183–5185.

Madan, P.D., Sequeira, P.S., Shenoy, K., & Shetty, J. (2008). The effect of three mouthwashes on radiation-induced oral mucositis in patients with head and neck malignancies: A randomized control trial. *Journal of Cancer Research Therapies, 4*(1), 3–8.

Maiya, G., Sagar, M., & Fernandes, D. (2006). Effect of low level helium-neon (He-Ne) laser therapy in the prevention and treatment of radiation induced mucositis in head and neck cancer patients. *Indian Journal of Medical Research, 124*(4), 399–402.

McAleese, J.J., Bishop, K.M., A'Hern, R., & Henk, J.M. (2006). Randomized phase II study of GM-CSF to reduce mucositis caused by accelerated radiotherapy of laryngeal cancer. *British Journal of Radiology, 79*(943), 608–613.

McGuire, D., Correa, M., Johnson, J., & Wienandts, P. (2006). The role of basic oral care and good clinical practice principles in the management of oral mucositis. *Supportive Care in Cancer, 14*(6), 541–547.

Migliorati, C.A., Oberle-Edwards, L., & Schubert, M. (2006). The role of alternative and natural agents, cryotherapy and/or laser for management of alimentary mucositis. *Supportive Care in Cancer, 14*(6), 533–540.

Mori, T., Aisa, Y., Yamazaki, R., Mihara, A., Ikeda, Y., & Okamoto, S. (2006). Cryotherapy for the prevention of high-dose melphalan-induced oral mucositis [Letter to the editor]. *Bone Marrow Transplantation, 38*(9), 637–638.

Motallebnejad, M., Akram, S., Moghadamnia, A., Moulana, Z., & Omidi, S. (2008). The effect of topical application of pure honey on radiation-induced mucositis: A randomized clinical trial. *Journal of Contemporary Dental Practice, 9*(3), 40–47.

Multinational Association of Supportive Care in Cancer. (2005). *Summary of evidence-based clinical practice guidelines for care of patients with oral and gastrointestinal mucositis (2005 update).* Retrieved July 10, 2006, from http://www.mascc.org/media/Resource_centers/Guidelines_mucositis.doc

Nasilowska-Adamska, B., Rzepeci, P., Manko, J., Czyz, A., Markieweicz, M., Federowicz, I., et al. (2007). The influence of palifermin (Kepivance) on oral mucositis and acute graft versus host disease in patients with hematological diseases undergoing hematopoietic stem cell transplant. *Bone Marrow Transplantation, 40*(10), 983–988.

Nes, A.G., & Posso, M.B. (2005). Patients with moderate chemotherapy-induced mucositis: Pain therapy using low intensity lasers. *International Nursing Review, 52*(1), 68–72.

Nikoletti, S., Hyde, S., Shaw, T., Myers, H., & Kristjanson, L.J. (2005). Comparison of plain ice and flavoured ice for preventing oral mucositis associated with the use of 5-fluorouracil. *Journal of Clinical Nursing, 14*(6), 750–753.

Nottage, M., McLachlan, S.A., Brittain, M.A., Oza, A., Hedley, D., Feld, R., et al. (2003). Sucralfate mouthwash for prevention and treatment of 5-fluorouracil-induced mucositis: A randomized, placebo-controlled trial. *Supportive Care in Cancer, 11*(1), 41–47.

Papadeas, E., Naxakis, S., Riga, M., & Kalofonos. C. (2007). Prevention of 5-fluorouracil–related stomatitis by oral cryotherapy: A randomized controlled study. *European Journal of Oncology Nursing, 11*(1), 60–65.

Papas, A.S., Clark, R.E., Martuscelli, G., O'Loughlin, K.T., Johansen, E., & Miller, K.B. (2003). A prospective, randomized trial for the prevention of mucositis in patients undergoing hematopoietic stem cell transplantation. *Bone Marrow Transplantation, 31*(8), 705–712.

Peterson, D.E., Jones, J.B., & Petit, R.G., II. (2006). Randomized, placebo-controlled trial of Saforis for prevention and treatment of oral mucositis in breast cancer patients receiving anthracycline-based chemotherapy. *Cancer, 109*(2), 322–331.

Pitten, F.A., Kiefer, T., Buth, C., Doelken, G., & Kramer, A. (2003). Do cancer patients with chemotherapy-induced leukopenia benefit from an antiseptic chlorhexidine-based oral rinse? A double-blind, block-randomized, controlled study. *Journal of Hospital Infection, 53*(4), 283–291.

Rashad, U.M., Al-Gezawy, S.M., El-Gezawy, E., & Azzaz, A.N. (2008, May 19). Honey as topical prophylaxis against radiochemotherapy-induced mucositis in head and neck cancer. *Journal of Laryngology and Otology*, pp. 1–6 (Epub ahead of print, http://journals.cambridge.org/action/displayAbstract?aid=1879532).

Rosen, L.S., Abdi, E., Davis, I.D., Gutheil, J., Schnell, F.M., Zalcberg, J., et al. (2006). Palifermin reduces the incidence of oral mucositis in patients with metastatic colorectal cancer treated with fluorouracil-based chemotherapy. *Journal of Clinical Oncology, 24*(433), 5194–5200.

Rossi, A., Rosati, G., Colarusso, D., & Manzione, L. (2003). Subcutaneous granulocyte–macrophage colony-stimulating factor in mucositis induced by an adjuvant 5-fluorouracil plus leucovorin regimen. *Oncology, 64*(4), 353–360.

Rubenstein, E.B., Peterson, D.E., Schubert, M., Keefe, D., McGuire, D., Epstein, J., et al. (2004). Clinical practice guidelines for the prevention and treatment of cancer therapy–induced oral and gastrointestinal mucositis. *Cancer, 100*(Suppl. 9), 2026–2046.

Ryu, J.K., Swann, S., LeVeque, F., Scarantino, C.W., Johnson, D., Chen, A., et al. (2007). The impact of concurrent granulocyte macrophage-colony stimulating factor on radiation-induced mucositis in head and neck cancer patients: A double-blind placebo-controlled prospective phase III study by Radiation Therapy Oncology Group 9901. *International Journal of Radiation Oncology, Biology, Physics, 67*(3), 643–650.

Schmidt, E., Thoennissen, N.H., Rudat, A., Bieker, R., Schliemann, C., Mesters, R.M., et al. (2008). Use of palifermin for the prevention of high-dose methotrexate-induced oral mucositis. *Annals of Oncology, 19*(9), 1644–1649.

Schubert, M.M., Eduardo, F.P., Guthrie, K.A., Franquin, J., Bensadoun, R.J., Migliorati, C.A., et al. (2007). A phase III randomized double-blind placebo-controlled clinical trial to determine the efficacy of low level laser therapy for the prevention of oral mucositis in patients undergoing hematopoietic cell transplantation. *Supportive Care in Cancer, 15*(10), 1145–1154.

Scully, C., Sonis, S., & Diz, P.D. (2006). Oral mucositis. *Oral Diseases, 12*(3), 229–241.

Shea, T.C., Kewalramani, T., Mun, Y., Jayne, G., & Dreiling, L.K. (2007). Evaluation of single-dose palifermin to reduce oral mucositis in fractionated total-body irradiation and high-dose chemotherapy with autologous peripheral blood progenitor cell transplantation. *Journal of Supportive Oncology, 5*(4, Suppl. 2), 60–61.

Shih, A., Miaskowski, C., Dodd, M.J., Stotts, N.A., & MacPhail, L. (2002). A research review of the current treatments for radiation-induced oral mucositis in patients with head and neck cancer. *Oncology Nursing Forum, 29*(7), 1063–1078.

Sorensen, J.B., Skovsgaard, T., Bork, E., Damstrup, L., & Ingeberg, S. (2008). Double-blind, placebo-controlled, randomized study of chlorhexidine prophylaxis for 5-fluorouracil–based chemotherapy-induced oral mucositis with nonblinded randomized comparison to oral cooling (cryotherapy) in gastrointestinal malignancies. *Cancer, 112*(7), 1600–1606.

Spielberger, R., Stiff, P., Bensinger, W., Gentile, T., Weisdorf, D., Kewalramani, T., et al. (2004). Palifermin for oral mucositis after intensive therapy for hematologic cancers. *New England Journal of Medicine, 351*(25), 2590–2598.

Stokman, M.A., Spijkervet, F.K., Burlage, F.R., & Roodenburg, J.L. (2005). Clinical effects of flurbiprofen tooth patch on radiation-induced oral mucositis. A pilot study. *Supportive Care in Cancer, 13*(1), 42–48.

Su, C.K., Mehta, V., Ravikumar, L., Shah, R., Pinto, H., Halpern, J., et al. (2004). Phase II double-blind randomized study comparing oral aloe vera versus placebo to prevent radiation-related mucositis in patients with head-and-neck neoplasms. *International Journal of Radiation Oncology, Biology, Physics, 60*(1), 171–177.

Sung, L., Tomlinson, G.A., Greenberg, M.L., Koren, G., Judd, P., Ota, S., et al. (2007). Serial controlled N-of-1 trials of topical vitamin E as prophylaxis for chemotherapy-induced oral mucositis in paediatric patients. *European Journal of Cancer, 43*(8), 1269–1275.

Svanberg, A., Birgegard, G., & Ohrn, K. (2007). Oral cryotherapy reduces mucositis and opioid use after myeloablative therapy—A randomized controlled trial. *Supportive Care in Cancer, 15*(10), 1155–1161.

Tartarone, A., Matera, R., Romano, G., Vigliotti, M.L., & Di Renzo, N. (2005). Prevention of high-dose melphalan-induced mucositis by cryotherapy. *Leukemia and Lymphoma, 46*(4), 633–634.

Trotti, A., Garden, A., Warde, P., Symonds, P., Langer, C., Redman, R., et al. (2004). A multinational, randomized phase III trial of iseganan HCl oral solution for reducing the severity of oral mucositis in patients receiving radiotherapy for head-and-neck malignancy. *International Journal of Radiation Oncology, Biology, Physics, 58*(3), 674–681.

Veness, M.J., Foroudi, F., Gebski, V., Timms, I., Sathiyaseelan, Y., Cakir, B., et al. (2006). Use of topical misoprostol to reduce radiation-induced mucositis: Results of a randomized, double-blind, placebo-controlled trial. *Australasian Radiology, 50*(5), 468–474.

Vokurka, S., Bystricka, E., Koza, V., Scudlova, J., Pavlicova, V., Valentova, D., et al. (2005). The comparative effects of povidone-iodine and normal saline mouthwashes on oral mucositis in patients after high-dose chemotherapy and APBSCT: Results of a randomized multicentre study. *Supportive Care in Cancer, 13*(7), 554–558.

von Bultzingslowen, I., Brennan, M.T., Spijkervet, F.K., Logan, R., Stringer, A., Raber-Durlacher, J.E., et al. (2006). Growth factors and cytokines in the prevention and treatment of oral and gastrointestinal mucositis. *Supportive Care in Cancer, 14*(6), 519–527.

Yoneda, S., Imai, S., Hanada, N., Yamazaki, T., Senpuku, H., Ota, Y., et al. (2007). Effects of oral care on development of oral mucositis and microorganisms in patients with esophageal cancer. *Japanese Journal of Infectious Diseases, 60*(1), 23–28.

CHAPTER 14

Pain

Problem

Nociceptive pain is caused by an injury to body tissues. The injury may be a cut, bruise, bone fracture, crush injury, burn, or anything that damages tissues. This type of pain is usually aching, sharp, or throbbing. Most pain is nociceptive pain. Pain receptors for tissue injury (nociceptors) are located mostly in the skin or in the internal organs (Pfizer Inc., 2007).

Neuropathic pain results from damage to the peripheral or central nervous system (Challapalli et al., 2005). The pain is characterized by dysesthesia, hyperesthesia, or a shooting or lancinating sensation, resulting from nerve injury or compression (Ross et al., 2005).

Incidence

An estimated 50% of people receiving treatment for cancer and 80%–90% of people with advanced disease experience moderate pain (Miaskowski, 2005). The majority of pain experienced by patients with cancer originates directly from the tumor. It may also occur as a result of cancer treatment. However, pain may be unrelated to both treatment and the tumor (Paice, 2004).

Assessment

Pain assessment begins with screening individuals for risk and contributing factors in addition to physical, psychosocial, and neurologic symptoms (see Table 14-1). An extensive history and physical examination should be obtained, including diagnostic evaluation if needed (Paice, 2004). A clinical measurement tool is used to quantify specific pain characteristics and is essential in measuring the effect of nursing interventions on these pain characteristics.

Clinical Measurement Tools

Many tools are available to measure the various dimensions of pain. When selecting a tool, the level of clinician and patient burden should be considered in addition to the purpose of the measurement. The following clinical measurement tools for pain are presented in Table 14-2.

1. Brief Pain Inventory (short form) (see Figure 14-1)
2. Numeric Rating Scale (see Figure 14-2)
3. Visual Analog Scale (see Figure 14-3)

Table 14-1. Pain Assessment Guide		
Assessment	**Yes**	**No**
Physical Symptoms		
Onset, location(s), quality, intensity, duration of pain		
Aggravating and relieving factors		
Previous pain treatment		
Nonverbal: writhing, moaning, guarding, grimacing, restlessness		
Psychosocial Symptoms		
Effect of pain on other aspects of the person's life		
Significant past experience of pain and effect on patient		
Meaning of pain to patient and family		
Typical coping responses to stress or pain		
Knowledge about pain management		
Changes in mood related to pain (i.e., depression, anxiety)		
Neurologic Symptoms		
Perform pertinent neurologic examination if head and neck pain or neck and back pain		
Risk and Contributing Factors		
Tumor location (i.e., bone cancer, central nervous system lesions)		
Neuropathies secondary to primary or metastatic tumor, abdominal tumors related to visceral tumors, obstruction, and/or ascites		
Cancer treatment		
Note. Based on information from Aiello-Laws, 2008; D'Arcy, 2007; Paice, 2004.		

References

Aiello-Laws, L.B. (2008). Pharmacologic treatment of adult cancer pain: Evidence-based nursing interventions. *Oncology Nursing News, 2*(2), 9–11.

Challapalli, V., Tremont-Lukats, I.W., McNicol, E.D., Lau, J., & Carr, D.B. (2005). Systemic administration of local anesthetic agents to relieve neuropathic pain. *Cochrane Database of Systematic Reviews* 2005, Issue 4. Art. No.: CD003345. DOI: 10.1002/14651858.CD003345.pub2.

Table 14-2. Clinical Measurement Tools for Pain

Name of Tool	Number of Items	Domains	Reliability and Validity	Populations	Clinical Utility
Brief Pain Inventory (short form)	9	Experience of pain, location, intensity, pain medications, pain relief, and interference with daily activity	Adequate reliability and validity established	Various cancer diagnoses	Multidimensional Easy for most patients to complete
Numeric Rating Scale	1	Intensity Also can be used to assess pain relief, frequency, duration, unpleasantness, or distress	Adequate reliability and validity established	Various cancer diagnoses	Two-point or 33% decrease in score is clinically meaningful.
Visual Analog Scale	1	Intensity	Adequate reliability and validity established	Various cancer diagnoses	May be more difficult to understand and complete than other single-item pain ratings

Note. Based on information from Jensen, 2003; Kwekkeboom, 2005; Paice, 2004.

D'Arcy, Y. (2007). *Pain management: Evidence-based tools and techniques for nursing professionals.* Marblehead, MA: HCPro, Inc.

Jensen, M.P. (2003). The validity and reliability of pain measures in adults with cancer. *Journal of Pain, 4*(1), 2–21.

Kwekkeboom, K. (2005). *Measuring oncology-nursing sensitive patient outcomes: Evidence-based summary.* Retrieved April 28, 2008, from http://www.ons.org/outcomes/measures/pain.shtml

Miaskowski, C. (2005). The next step to improving cancer pain management. *Pain Management Nursing, 6*(1), 1–2.

Paice, J.A. (2004). Pain. In C.H. Yarbro, M.H. Frogge, & M. Goodman (Eds.), *Cancer symptom management* (3rd ed., pp. 77–96). Sudbury, MA: Jones and Bartlett.

Pfizer, Inc. (2007). Celebrex [Package insert]. Retrieved June 26, 2007, from http://pfizer.com/pfizer/download/uspi_celebrex.pdf

Ross, J.R., Goller, K., Hardy, J., Riley, J., Broadley, K., A'hern, R., et al. (2005). Gabapentin is effective in the treatment of cancer-related neuropathic pain: A prospective, open-label study. *Journal of Palliative Medicine, 8*(6), 1118–1126.

Figure 14-1. Brief Pain Inventory (Short Form)

STUDY ID #:_ _ _ _ _ _ _ _ _ _   DO NOT WRITE ABOVE THIS LINE   HOSPITAL #:_ _ _ _ _ _ _ _ _ _

Brief Pain Inventory (Short Form)

Date:_ _ _ _/_ _ _ _/_ _ _ _   Time:_ _ _ _ _ _ _

Name:_ _ _ _ _ _ _ _ _ _ _ _ _ _ _ _ _ _ _ _ _ _ _ _ _ _ _ _ _ _ _ _ _ _ _ _ _ _ _ _ _ _ _ _ _ _

                Last   First   Middle Initial

1. Throughout our lives, most of us have had pain from time to time (such as minor headaches, sprains, and toothaches). Have you had pain other than these every-day kinds of pain today?

        1. Yes   2. No

2. On the diagram, shade in the areas where you feel pain. Put an X on the area that hurts the most.

3. Please rate your pain by circling the one number that best describes your pain at its worst in the last 24 hours.

    0   1   2   3   4   5   6   7   8   9   10
    No   Pain as bad as
    Pain   you can imagine

4. Please rate your pain by circling the one number that best describes your pain at its least in the last 24 hours.

    0   1   2   3   4   5   6   7   8   9   10
    No   Pain as bad as
    Pain   you can imagine

5. Please rate your pain by circling the one number that best describes your pain on the average.

    0   1   2   3   4   5   6   7   8   9   10
    No   Pain as bad as
    Pain   you can imagine

6. Please rate your pain by circling the one number that tells how much pain you have right now.

    0   1   2   3   4   5   6   7   8   9   10
    No   Pain as bad as
    Pain   you can imagine

(Continued on next page)

Figure 14-1. Brief Pain Inventory (Short Form) *(Continued)*

STUDY ID #:_____ DO NOT WRITE ABOVE THIS LINE HOSPITAL #:_____

Date:____/____/____   Time:_____
Name:_____ _____ _____
             Last   First   Middle Initial

7.   What treatments or medications are you receiving for your pain?

8.   In the last 24 hours, how much relief have pain treatments or medications provided? Please circle the one percentage that most shows how much relief you have received.

    0%   10%   20%   30%   40%   50%   60%   70%   80%   90%   100%
    No   Complete
    Relief   Relief

9.   Circle the one number that describes how, during the past 24 hours, pain has interfered with your:

A.   General Activity
0   1   2   3   4   5   6   7   8   9   10
Does not   Completely
Interfere   Interferes

B.   Mood
0   1   2   3   4   5   6   7   8   9   10
Does not   Completely
Interfere   Interferes

C.   Walking Ability
0   1   2   3   4   5   6   7   8   9   10
Does not   Completely
Interfere   Interferes

D.   Normal Work (includes both work outside the home and housework)
0   1   2   3   4   5   6   7   8   9   10
Does not   Completely
Interfere   Interferes

E.   Relations with other people
0   1   2   3   4   5   6   7   8   9   10
Does not   Completely
Interfere   Interferes

F.   Sleep
0   1   2   3   4   5   6   7   8   9   10
Does not   Completely
Interfere   Interferes

G.   Enjoyment of life
0   1   2   3   4   5   6   7   8   9   10
Does not   Completely
Interfere   Interferes

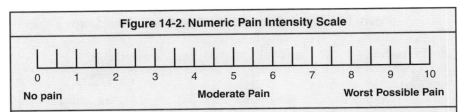

Figure 14-2. Numeric Pain Intensity Scale

0   1   2   3   4   5   6   7   8   9   10

No pain   **Moderate Pain**   **Worst Possible Pain**

Note. Reprinted from *Pain Management: Evidence-Based Tools and Techniques for Nursing Professionals* (p. 37), by Y. D'Arcy, © 2007 HCPro, Inc., 200 Hoods Lane, Marblehead, MA 01945 781/639-1872. www.hcpro.com. Used with permission.

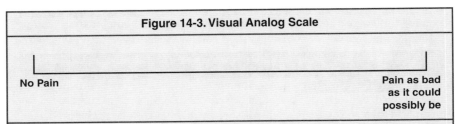

Figure 14-3. Visual Analog Scale

No Pain   **Pain as bad as it could possibly be**

Note. Reprinted from *Pain Management: Evidence-Based Tools and Techniques for Nursing Professionals* (p. 36), by Y. D'Arcy, © 2007 HCPro, Inc., 200 Hoods Lane, Marblehead, MA 01945 781/639-1872. www.hcpro.com. Used with permission.

Case Study

K.L. was a 48-year-old woman with metastatic adenocarcinoma of the breast admitted for uncontrolled pain, nausea, and vomiting. She had known metastases to the lung, liver, right humerus, and left femur. Her past treatments have included bilateral mastectomy with lymph node dissection and chemotherapy consisting of doxorubicin, cyclophosphamide, and paclitaxel. In addition, she had received radiation to her humerus and femur. Last week, she decided that she wanted no more chemotherapy and wanted palliative care only. K.L. was divorced and had two children, ages 10 and 12. She had no prescription coverage and limited financial resources.

K.L. reported lower-back pain radiating down her left thigh to her outer left calf and to her greater, second, and third toes. She described the pain in her lower back as a "deep ache" and "constant." The pain radiating down her leg was described as "intermittent, burning, shooting, and like electricity." She rated her pain as a 20 on a 0–10 scale where 0 = no pain and 10 = greatest amount of pain possible. At home, she was taking hydromorphone 4 mg PO every four hours as needed. She had taken 24 mg in the last 24 hours. She stated that the pain medication helped decrease her pain to an 8 but did not alleviate the pain shooting down her leg. She complained of nausea and vomiting and stated, "It is hard to eat or drink when I am so nauseated." Her last bowel movement was yesterday, and she stated it was hard. She denied changes in bladder function. Her gait was stable, and she denied lower extremity weakness. She had a prescription for prochlorperazine 20 mg PO every six hours PRN. She had taken 40 mg in the past 24 hours and was taking no other medications. On admission, her blood was drawn and was within normal limits except for elevated liver function tests. A magnetic resonance imaging (MRI) scan of her spine revealed a compression fracture in L5.

The pain assessment guidelines on the Oncology Nursing Society (ONS) Putting Evidence Into Practice (PEP) resource on pain aided in the diagnosis of the L5 compression fracture by helping to localize and characterize the pain as nociceptive (bone metastases) and neuropathic (spinal cord compression). The assessment pointed to the need for an MRI, which confirmed the L5 compression fracture. Radiation and steroids were initiated. As recommended by the ONS PEP resource, K.L.'s opioids were changed to an around-the-clock schedule with a PRN breakthrough dose. To manage the neuropathic pain, gabapentin was started at 1,800 mg per day in three divided doses. To manage her nausea, prochlorperazine was discontinued, and she was started on around-the-clock metoclopramide. She was instructed to eat small, frequent meals, increase her fluids, and eat a high-fiber diet. A bowel regimen including a stool softener was initiated, and she was instructed to avoid bulk-forming laxatives. A social worker was consulted to assist with financial issues and to provide her with resources to assist her children in coping with their mother's illness.

Lisa Hartkopf Smith, RN, MS, AOCN®, CNS
Oncology Clinical Nurse Specialist
Riverside Methodist Hospitals
Columbus, OH

Pain

2009 AUTHORS
Lisa B. Aiello-Laws, RN, MSN, APNG, AOCNS®, and Suzanne W. Ameringer, PhD, RN
ONS STAFF: Linda H. Eaton, MN, RN, AOCN®

2007 AUTHORS
Lisa B. Aiello-Laws, RN, MSN, APNG, Nancy A. Delzer, MSN, RN, AOCN®, BC-PCM,
Mary E. Peterson, RN, OCN®, and Janice K. Reynolds, RN, BSN, OCN®
RESEARCH CONSULTANTS: Marie A. Bakitas, DNSc, ARNP, AOCN®, FAAN,
and Christine A. Miaskowski, RN, PhD, FAAN
ONS STAFF: Kristine B. LeFebvre, MSN, RN, AOCN®

What are the pharmacologic interventions for nociceptive and neuropathic cancer pain in adults?

Overview: Although chemotherapy, hormonal therapy, and biologic response modifiers are "pharmacological agents that result in pain reduction through tumor shrinkage" (National Comprehensive Cancer Network [NCCN], 2008), this resource focuses only on primary nonopioids, opioids, and coanalgesics.

General principles: Combinations of nonopioids, opioids, and coanalgesics should be considered for effective management of acute and persistent nociceptive and neuropathic pain that occurs as a result of cancer or cancer treatment (American Pain Society [APS], 2005; *Merck Manuals*, n.d.; NCCN, 2008).

Recommended for Practice

Interventions for which effectiveness has been demonstrated by strong evidence from rigorously conducted studies, meta-analyses, or systematic reviews and for which expectation of harms is small compared with the benefits

NOCICEPTIVE PAIN

Nonopioids

Acetaminophen: This drug is an analgesic and antipyretic but lacks clinically useful peripheral anti-inflammatory activity, demonstrates no antiplatelet effect, and does not damage gastric mucosa (APS, 2005). As an effective analgesic in mild pain, it also can be used in conjunction with opioids to reduce or maintain opioid dose (dose-sparing effect) (APS; NCCN, 2008).
- Acetaminophen is well-tolerated up to recommended doses of 4 g/day (3 g/day in frail older adults) (NCCN, 2008).
- Chronic daily usage of 4 g/day in adults increases hepatic toxicity.
- Dose should not exceed 2.5 g/day in people who drink 2 oz of alcohol daily.
- Patients should be cautioned about taking over-the-counter drugs containing acetaminophen or other drugs that cause hepatotoxicity.
- Acute overdose can cause renal and hepatic damage.

Nonsteroidal anti-inflammatory drugs (NSAIDs): NSAIDs are effective for many types of cancer-related pain, especially pain caused by inflammation (e.g., bone metastasis, postoperative pain). Unless contraindicated, NSAIDs should be used routinely to manage acute and persistent pain (APS, 2005). NSAIDs have the potential to cause decreased platelet aggregation, gastrointestinal (GI) discomfort, and renal and cardiac toxicity (APS; NCCN, 2008). All prescription NSAIDs may increase the chance of a heart attack or stroke. **Bleeding and ulcers can occur without warning and may cause death** (McNichol, Strassels, Goudas, Lau, & Carr, 2005).

- NSAIDs do not produce physical or psychological dependence.
- Ketorolac is the only parenteral NSAID.
- NSAIDs have a ceiling dose effect. If a patient does not respond to one NSAID at a maximum therapeutic dose, consider a trial of a different one (APS, 2005).
- NSAIDs can be safely given to older adults but should be monitored for potential toxicity through measurement of blood pressure, blood urea nitrogen, creatinine, complete blood count, and fecal occult blood (NCCN, 2008).
- Efficacy of cyclooxygenase-2 selective NSAIDs has been demonstrated primarily in non-cancer populations (APS, 2005; Pfizer Inc., 2007).

Opioids

Opioids are recommended for moderate to severe acute and persistent nociceptive pain (American Geriatrics Society Panel on Persistent Pain in Older Persons, 2002; APS, 2005; NCCN, 2008; Nicholson, 2007; Reid, Martin, Sterne, Davies, & Hanks, 2006; Wiffen & McQuay, 2007). They bind directly to opioid receptors and do not have a ceiling dose effect (APS).

- **For persistent pain,** administer a long-acting opioid around the clock (ATC) (Currow, Plummer, Cooney, Gorman, & Glare, 2007).
- **For breakthrough pain,** add an immediate-release opioid on a PRN basis (Mercadante et al., 2008; Wiffen & McQuay, 2007).
- Titrate opioid doses to achieve pain relief with minimal side effects. Increase dose of long-acting opioids if frequent doses of immediate-release opioids are needed or when a long-acting opioid fails to relieve pain at the pharmacologic peak or end of dose (Mercadante, Villari, Ferrera, & Casuccio, 2006; NCCN, 2008; Wallace et al., 2008; Wootton, 2004; Zeppetella & Ribeiro, 2006).
- Calculate the increase in long-acting opioid dose based on total ATC and PRN doses taken in the previous 24 hours. Increase both ATC and breakthrough doses using an equianalgesic table (APS, 2005; Wallace et al., 2008).
- Most clinical circumstances require use of only one opioid at an appropriate dosage to manage pain rather than inadequate doses of multiple opioids (Maltoni et al., 2005).
- Use the least invasive, easiest, and safest route first (NCCN, 2008; Swarm et al., 2007). The oral route is preferred. Equal effectiveness exists between IV and subcutaneous opioids (APS, 2005; Grosset et al., 2005). **Caution:** Avoid intramuscular administration because it is painful and absorption is unreliable (APS).
- Oral transmucosal formulations are effective immediate-release opioids (Freye, Levy, & Braun, 2007; Mercadante et al., 2007; Slatkin, Xie, Messina, & Segal, 2007).
- Adverse effects differ among opioids; consider switching if adverse effects are significant (NCCN, 2008; Rodriguez et al., 2007; Swarm et al., 2007).
- Regardless of administration route, patients should be monitored closely, primarily during a change in the drug, route, or dose.

Fentanyl: Transdermal fentanyl is an effective alternative to morphine for patients in whom the oral route cannot be used (Herr, Bjoro, Steffensmeier, & Rakel, 2006; Reid et al., 2006; Tassinari et al., 2008). Transdermal opioids are not recommended for acute pain but are appropriate for patients whose opioid needs are stable and who cannot take oral opioids (Reid et al.). Recent evidence suggests wide intra- and interindividual variability in the absorption of transdermal fentanyl (Smith & Coyne, 2005). Factors found to be associated with effective titration are patient age (older patients may require a lower dose) and pain type (patients with neuropathic pain may require a higher dose) (Hagen, Fisher, Victorino, & Farrar, 2007). Oral transmucosal fentanyl (e.g., oral transmucosal fentanyl citrate [OTFC], fentanyl buccal tablet [FBT]) is effective for breakthrough (episodic) pain (Mercadante, Arcuri, Fusco, et al., 2005). Buccal fentanyl absorption does not appear to differ in patients with mucositis (Darwish, Kirby, Robertson, Tracewell, & Jiang, 2007). Plasma concentrations peak in about 5–10 minutes. OTFC and FBT are not bioequivalent, so extreme caution must be used when converting from transmucosal to buccal form. Do not use in patients who are opioid naïve or who have only been on a low-dose opioid (Weinbroum, 2005).

Methadone: Methadone appears to be a useful alternative to other opioid analgesics and may be useful as part of an opioid rotation strategy (Colella et al., 2006; Elsner, Radbruch, Loick, Gartner, & Sabatowski, 2005; Wiffen & McQuay, 2007). Methadone has both an immediate and a long-acting analgesic effect. Although methadone is similar to morphine, its pharmacokinetics and pharmacodynamics make dose titration difficult, with a risk of toxic drug accumulation (Koshy, Kuriakose, Sebastian, & Koshy, 2005). Methadone appears to be a useful and more affordable alternative to some other choices. The following unique aspects of methadone should be noted (APS, 2005).

- Methadone may cause QT prolongation and torsades de pointes. Electrocardiogram monitoring is recommended with methadone doses > 150 mg/day and in patients with either risk factors for QT prolongation or symptoms that may be attributable to arrhythmia (APS, 2005).
- Overdosing can result when converting from other opioids to methadone because equianalgesic potency can range from 4:1 to 12:1, depending on the dose of the original opioid. Clinicians should be skilled in performing equianalgesic calculations (see *Expert Opinion* section).
- Methadone has a large number of drug-drug interactions. Some increase and some decrease the bioavailability of methadone.

Opioid side effect management: The most common side effects of opioids are constipation, sedation, and nausea and vomiting (APS, 2005; Komurcu et al., 2007; Pan et al., 2007). Other side effects include respiratory depression, dry mouth, pruritus, and myoclonus (APS; Centeno & Vara, 2005). Always initiate a bowel regimen (softener + laxative) when the patient is started on an opioid to prevent constipation (American Geriatrics Society Panel on Persistent Pain in Older Persons, 2002; APS; Mercadante, Arcuri, Fusco, et al., 2005; NCCN, 2008; Nicholson, 2007; Zeppetella & Ribeiro, 2006) (see the ONS PEP resource on constipation). Consider prophylactic antiemetics when initiating opioids (NCCN).

Coanalgesics

Corticosteroids: To manage acute and persistent cancer pain, corticosteroids may be effective (Mercadante et al., 2007). Side effects of chronic, long-term use include weight gain, osteoporosis, Cushing syndrome, proximal myopathy, euphoria, increased appetite, and psychosis. Corticosteroids may increase the risk of GI bleed, especially when used with NSAIDs or anticoagulants, and should not be routinely used in conjunction with these medications. However, benefits often outweigh risks in patients with life-limiting, progressive disease. Doses should be tapered; rapid withdrawal can exacerbate pain and adrenal insufficiency (APS, 2005).

Local anesthetics: Topical or injectable local anesthetics are effective in reducing pain associated with procedures such as lumbar puncture, bone marrow aspirate, and port access (APS, 2005).

NEUROPATHIC PAIN

General principles: Pharmacologic management of neuropathic pain should be guided by the following general principles.
- The effectiveness of analgesics is variable; drugs and doses must be individualized.
- Coanalgesics should be administered as a single agent initially—although some patients may require combinations of coanalgesics.
- With most coanalgesics, the onset of pain relief is delayed, and it may take weeks for the coanalgesic to produce analgesia. Consider using short-acting opioid analgesics to provide pain relief.
- Although a drug class is considered as part of first- or second-line treatment (see following information), not all members of the class are recommended for neuropathic pain.
  - First-line treatments include certain antidepressants (i.e., tricyclic antidepressants and dual reuptake inhibitors of both serotonin and norepinephrine), calcium channel $\alpha2$-δ ligands (i.e., gabapentin, pregabalin), topical lidocaine, and opioid analgesics and tramadol (the latter in patients with moderate to severe pain [Arbaiza & Vidal, 2007] or in patients refractory to the other first-line medications).
  - Second-line treatments include certain other anticonvulsant and antidepressant medications, cannabinoids, mexiletine, N-methyl-D-aspartate receptor antagonists, and topical capsaicin (*Merck Manuals,* n.d.).
- Consider referral to a pain specialist if neuropathic pain persists.

Coanalgesics

Anticonvulsants: Anticonvulsants are effective for the treatment of trigeminal neuralgia, postherpetic neuralgia, glossopharyngeal neuralgia, and post-traumatic neuralgia. Gabapentin is the best studied and best tolerated (APS, 2005; NCCN, 2008; Pergolizzi et al., 2006). **Caution:** Not all anticonvulsants are recommended. For example, phenytoin has been found to be effective against neuropathic pain yet has many side effects (e.g., confusion, ataxia) and requires close monitoring of serum drug levels (APS; *Merck Manuals,* n.d.).

Antidepressants: Tricyclic antidepressants (TCAs) and dual reuptake serotonin and norepinephrine inhibitors (SNRIs) are first-line treatments for neuropathic pain (*Merck Manuals,* n.d.). TCAs relieve pain independently of an antidepressant effect. The doses for analgesic effect often are much lower than the antidepressant doses. TCAs are useful for neuropathic pain related to surgical trauma, postherpetic neuralgia, radiation therapy, chemotherapy, or malignant nerve infiltration. These drugs typically are started at a low dose and then are slowly titrated up until the desired pain relief is achieved (APS, 2005). TCAs are contraindicated in those with coronary disease and can worsen ventricular arrhythmia. Baseline electrocardiogram is recommended to rule out conduction abnormalities, especially in patients receiving anthracycline antitumor agents.

SNRIs: Duloxetine has demonstrated significant pain relief compared to placebo in three randomly controlled trials in patients with diabetic neuropathy and has a favorable side effect profile (*Merck Manuals*, n.d.). Venlafaxine demonstrated inconsistent results in postmastectomy pain but was effective in other painful polyneuropathies (*Merck Manuals*).

Local anesthetics: A topical lidocaine patch may be effective for peripheral neuropathies and for complex regional pain syndromes, mononeuropathy, and stump pain (APS, 2005). Systemic lidocaine is helpful with postherpetic neuralgia. Epidural and IV treatments are effective, but for short-term use (APS; Solassol et al., 2005).

Opioids

Randomized controlled trials have demonstrated consistent efficacy of opioids with a variety of peripheral and central neuropathic pain conditions. For dosing and side effects, nurses should refer to the practice guidelines routinely used in their institution. Opioids, in combination with antidepressants and anticonvulsants, are considered first-line treatment of neuropathic pain, especially in patients who have severe acute neuropathic pain, as the other agents will have a delayed onset of pain relief (Keskinbora, Pekel, & Aydinli, 2007).

Tramadol: This weak mu-opioid agonist has been effective as a second-line medication when stronger opioids are not effective. Side effects are more pronounced when the drug is started at full dose. Side effects include dizziness, nausea, constipation, and somnolence. Tolerance and physical and psychological dependence are rare (Moryl, Kogan, Comfort, & Obbens, 2005).
- Dose should be gradually titrated over weeks/months. The maximum dose of 400 mg/day limits usefulness in severe pain.
- Drug effects are not fully reversible with naloxone.
- Use with caution with concurrent TCAs because of increased risk of central nervous system (CNS) depression, psychomotor impairment, seizures, and serotonin syndrome.
- **Caution:** Tramadol has not been well studied when given simultaneously with transdermal fentanyl. Studies suggest a synergistic effect (Marinangeli et al., 2007).

Likely to Be Effective

Interventions for which effectiveness has been demonstrated by supportive evidence from a single rigorously conducted controlled trial, consistent supportive evidence from well-designed controlled trials using small samples, or guidelines developed from evidence and supported by expert opinion

NOCICEPTIVE PAIN

Coanalgesics

Bisphosphonates: Bisphosphonates (e.g., pamidronate disodium, zoledronate) inhibit osteoclastic bone resorption and have been shown to reduce pain in skeletal complications, such as pathologic fractures in breast cancer and multiple myeloma. Bisphosphonates should be considered when analgesics and/or radiotherapy are inadequate (Auret et al., 2006; Glare, Walsh, & Sheehan, 2006). Bisphosphonates may cause osteoradionecrosis of the jaw (Challapalli, Tremont-Lukats, McNicol, Lau, & Carr, 2005; Novartis, 2007). Zoledronic acid has a more convenient infusion schedule than pamidronate (APS, 2005).

Radionuclides/radioisotopes: Radionuclides/radioisotopes are a useful adjunct for diffuse metastatic bone pain (Baczyk et al., 2007; Liepe & Kotzerke, 2007; Sartor, Reid, Bushnell, Quick, & Ell, 2007). Response can take as long as two to three weeks and depend upon the type of radionuclide used (Sartor et al.); patients must continue analgesic therapy (APS, 2005). Adverse effects, particularly leukocytopenia and thrombocytopenia, can occur (Baczyk et al.; Dworkin et al., 2007; Sartor et al.).

Benefits Balanced With Harms

Interventions for which clinicians and patients should weigh the beneficial and harmful effects according to individual circumstances and priorities

NOCICEPTIVE PAIN

Opioids

Spinal opioids: Long-term use of spinal (intrathecal and epidural) opioids can be complicated by problems with catheters and can be costly (Ross et al., 2005). In selected patients, spinal opioids may improve pain relief while limiting opioid/analgesic side effects (Dunteman, 2005; Mercadante, Arcuri, Ferrera, et al., 2005).

Coanalgesics

Caffeine: Caffeine increases analgesia when given with aspirin-like drugs for uterine cramping, headaches, and other pain symptoms. The optimal dose has not been established. Exercise caution with chronic use. Rebound pain and headache may occur when use is stopped abruptly (APS, 2005).

NEUROPATHIC PAIN

Coanalgesics

Sympatholytic agents: Epidural clonidine may be effective in relieving neuropathic pain. However, bradycardia and hypotension may occur (APS, 2005).

Effectiveness Not Established

Interventions for which insufficient or conflicting data or data of inadequate quality currently exist, with no clear indication of harm

NOCICEPTIVE PAIN

Coanalgesics

Antihistamines: Antihistamines (e.g., hydroxyzine, diphenhydramine) can be used concurrently with analgesia as sleep aids and to reduce itching. As mild CNS depressants, they may increase analgesic effect, but data are lacking (APS, 2005). Hydroxyzine has antiemetic and mild sedative activity. Oral hydroxyzine is used for nausea and anxiety in chronic cancer pain.

Dextroamphetamine: When combined with opioids in the postoperative period, dextroamphetamine may produce additive analgesia. The usual indication is to counteract opioid sedation (APS, 2005).

Ketamine: Ketamine has been studied in two forms, IV and sublingual. A small controlled trial reported effectiveness with nonmalignant neuropathic pain, but intolerable side effects occurred with IV administration (APS, 2005). A case series of three patients reported pain relief with sublingual administration (Mercadante, Arcuri, Ferrera, Villari, & Mangione, 2005).

Skeletal muscle relaxants: Skeletal muscle relaxants have mixed evidence for use in acute muscle injury. They should be used for only a few days as needed (APS, 2005).

Topical agents: Topical agents penetrate the skin and act locally in the peripheral tissues when applied directly on the painful body area. Medications from "compounding pharmacies" should be used cautiously, as the vehicle that allows for skin penetration in the drug formulation is as important as the pharmacologically active agent and can result in either systemic activity or lack of penetration (APS, 2005).

Tetrodotoxin: Tetrodotoxin is a neurotoxin that has been studied in the treatment of nociceptive and neuropathic pain, administered both subcutaneously and intramuscularly (Hagen et al., 2007, 2008). The few studies on tetrodotoxin use in patients with cancer report inconsistent findings, and a minimal efficacious dose has not been established.

Effectiveness Unlikely

Interventions for which lack of effectiveness has been demonstrated by negative evidence from a single rigorously conducted controlled trial, consistent negative evidence from well-designed controlled trials using small samples, or guidelines developed from evidence and supported by expert opinion

NEUROPATHIC PAIN

Antidepressants: Selective serotonergic reuptake inhibitors have had mixed efficacy results. One randomized controlled trial showed fluoxetine to not be effective in treating diabetic neuropathy, whereas many small controlled trials did demonstrate efficacy. Although these drugs are better tolerated than TCAs, the analgesic effect is poor (APS, 2005).

Antiarrhythmics: Studies have found mixed results in treating neuropathic pain (APS, 2005; Solassol et al., 2005). Antiarrhythmics should not be given to those with second- and third-degree heart block, congestive heart failure, or abnormal liver function tests (APS).

Calcitonin: No support exists for the use of calcitonin in treating pain caused by bone metastasis (Wong & Wiffen, 2002).

Dextromethorphan: No evidence of effectiveness has been demonstrated (APS, 2005; Dudgeon et al., 2007).

Capsaicin: Although capsaicin has been used effectively in surgical neuropathic pain and mastectomy patients, it has been inconclusive with postherpetic neuralgia and polyneuropathy. Clinical experience with cancer pain has been disappointing (APS, 2005).

Not Recommended for Practice

Interventions for which lack of effectiveness or harmfulness has been demonstrated by strong evidence from rigorously conducted studies, meta-analyses, or systematic reviews, or interventions for which the costs, burden, or harms associated with the intervention exceed anticipated benefit

Mixed agonists-antagonists (APS, 2005)

Meperidine (APS, 2005; Maltoni et al., 2005)

Propoxyphene (APS, 2005; NCCN, 2008)

Codeine (Maltoni et al., 2005)

Intramuscular route (APS, 2005)

Placebos (APS, 2005)

Phenothiazines (APS, 2005)

Carbamazepine (APS, 2005)

Expert Opinion

Low-risk interventions that are (1) consistent with sound clinical practice, (2) suggested by an expert in a peer-reviewed publication (journal or book chapter), and (3) for which limited evidence exists. An expert is an individual who has published articles in a peer-reviewed journal in the domain of interest.

Equianalgesic dosing charts should be consulted for switching opioids of drugs or routes of administration (APS, 2005). A good example is Table 3 at www.residentandstaff.com/issues/articles/2007-04_06.asp (Yuen, Shelley, Sze, Wilt, & Mason, 2006). Small studies (Roque et al., 2003) and expert opinion recommend opioid switching when a patient's regimen becomes ineffective or when side effects become intolerable (Ballantyne & Carwood, 2005; Bell, Eccleston, & Kalso, 2003; Mercadante, Arcuri, Ferrera, et al., 2005; Mercadante, Ferrera, Villari, & Casuccio, 2005; Stearns et al., 2005).

Definitions of the interventions are available at **www.ons.org/outcomes**.
Literature search completed through May 2008.

References

American Geriatrics Society Panel on Persistent Pain in Older Persons. (2002). Clinical practice guidelines: The management of persistent pain in older persons. *Journal of the American Geriatrics Society, 50*(Suppl. 6), S205–S224.

American Pain Society. (2005). *Guideline for the management of cancer pain in adults and children.* Glenview, IL: Author.

Arbaiza, D., & Vidal, O. (2007). Tramadol in the treatment of neuropathic cancer pain: A double-blind, placebo-controlled study. *Clinical Drug Investigation, 27*(1), 75–83.

Auret, K., Roger Goucke, C., Ilett, K.F., Page-Sharp, M., Boyd, F., & Oh, T.E. (2006). Pharmacokinetics and pharmacodynamics of methadone enantiomers in hospice patients with cancer pain. *Therapeutic Drug Monitoring, 28*(3), 359–366.

Baczyk, M., Czepczynski, R., Milecki, P., Pisarek, M., Oleksa, R., & Sowinski, J. (2007). 89Sr versus 153Sm-EDTMP: Comparison of treatment efficacy of painful bone metastases in prostate and breast carcinoma. *Nuclear Medicine Communications, 28*(4), 245–250.

Ballantyne, J.C., & Carwood, C.M. (2005). Comparative efficacy of epidural, subarachnoid, and intracerebroventricular opioids in patients with pain due to cancer. *Cochrane Database of Systematic Reviews* 2005, Issue 2. Art. No.: CD005178. DOI: 10.1002/14651858.CD005178.

Bell, R., Eccleston, C., & Kalso, E. (2003). Ketamine as an adjuvant to opioids for cancer pain. *Cochrane Database of Systematic Reviews* 2003, Issue 1. Art. No.: CD003351. DOI: 10.1002/14651858.CD003351.

Centeno, C., & Vara, F. (2005). Intermittent subcutaneous methadone administration in the management of cancer pain. *Journal of Pain and Palliative Care Pharmacotherapy, 19*(2), 7–12.

Challapalli, V., Tremont-Lukats, I.W., McNicol, E.D., Lau, J., & Carr, D.B. (2005). Systemic administration of local anesthetic agents to relieve neuropathic pain. *Cochrane Database of Systematic Reviews* 2005, Issue 4. Art. No.: CD003345. DOI: 10.1002/14651858.CD003345.pub2.

Colella, J., Scrofine, S., Galli, B., Knorr-Mulder, C., Gejerman, G., Scheuch, J., et al. (2006). Prostate HDR radiation therapy: A comparative study evaluating the effectiveness of pain management with peripheral PCA vs. PCEA. *Urologic Nursing, 26*(1), 57–61.

Currow, D.C., Plummer, J.L., Cooney, N.J., Gorman, D., & Glare, P.A. (2007). A randomized, double-blind, multi-site, crossover, placebo-controlled equivalence study of morning versus evening once-daily sustained-release morphine sulfate in people with pain from advanced cancer. *Journal of Pain and Symptom Management, 34*(1), 17–23.

Darwish, M., Kirby, M., Robertson, P., Tracewell, W., & Jiang, J.G. (2007). Absorption of fentanyl from fentanyl buccal tablet in cancer patients with or without oral mucositis: A pilot study. *Clinical Drug Investigation, 27*(9), 605–611.

Dudgeon, D.J., Bruera, E., Gagnon, B., Watanabe, S.M., Allan, S.J., Warr, D.G., et al. (2007). A phase III randomized, double-blind, placebo-controlled study evaluating dextromethorphan plus slow-release morphine for chronic cancer pain relief in terminally ill patients. *Journal of Pain and Symptom Management, 33*(4), 365–371.

Dunteman, E.D. (2005). Levetiracetam as an adjunctive analgesic in neoplastic plexopathies: Case series and commentary. *Journal of Pain and Palliative Care Pharmacotherapy, 19*(1), 35–43.

Dworkin, R.H., O'Connor, A.B., Backonja, M., Farrar, J.T., Finnerup, N.B., Jensen, T.S., et al. (2007). Pharmacologic management of neuropathic pain: Evidence-based recommendations. *Pain, 132*(3), 225–226.

Elsner, F., Radbruch, L., Loick, G., Gartner, J., & Sabatowski, R. (2005). Intravenous versus subcutaneous morphine titration in patients with persisting exacerbation of cancer pain. *Journal of Palliative Medicine, 8*(4), 743–750.

Freye, E., Levy, J.V., & Braun, D. (2007). Effervescent morphine results in faster relief of breakthrough pain in patients compared to immediate release morphine sulfate tablet. *Pain Practice, 7*(4), 324–331.

Glare, P., Walsh, D., & Sheehan, D. (2006). The adverse effects of morphine: A prospective survey of common symptoms during repeated dosing for chronic cancer pain. *American Journal of Hospice and Palliative Medicine, 23*(3), 229–235.

Grosset, A.B., Roberts, M.S., Woodson, M.E., Shi, M., Swanton, R.E., Reder, R.F., et al. (2005). Comparative efficacy of oral extended-release hydromorphone and immediate-release hydromorphone in patients with persistent moderate to severe pain: Two randomized controlled trials. *Journal of Pain and Symptom Management, 29*(6), 584–594.

Hagen, N.A., du Souich, P., Lapointe, B., Ong-Lam, M., Dubuc, B., Walde, D., et al. (2008). Tetrodotoxin for moderate to severe cancer pain: A randomized, double blind, parallel design multicenter study. *Journal of Pain and Symptom Management, 35*(4), 420–429.

Hagen, N.A., Fisher, K., Victorino, C., & Farrar, J.T. (2007). A titration strategy is needed to manage breakthrough cancer pain effectively: Observations from data pooled from three clinical trials. *Journal of Palliative Medicine, 10*(1), 47–55.

Hagen, N.A., Fisher, K.M., Lapointe, B., du Souich, P., Chary, S., Moulin, D., et al. (2007). An open-label, multi-dose efficacy and safety study of intramuscular tetrodotoxin in patients with severe cancer-related pain. *Journal of Pain and Symptom Management, 34*(2), 171–182.

Herr, K., Bjoro, K., Steffensmeier, J., & Rakel, B. (2006). *Acute pain management in older adults.* Iowa City, IA: University of Iowa Gerontological Nursing Interventions Research Center, Research Translation and Dissemination Core.

Keskinbora, K., Pekel, A.F., & Aydinli, I. (2007). Gabapentin and an opioid combination versus opioid alone for the management of neuropathic cancer pain: A randomized open trial. *Journal of Pain and Symptom Management, 34*(2), 183–189.

Komurcu, S., Turhal, S., Altundag, K., Atahan, L., Turna, H.S., Manavoglu, O., et al. (2007). Safety and efficacy of transdermal fentanyl in patients with cancer pain: Phase IV, Turkish Oncology Group trial. *European Journal of Cancer Care, 16*(1), 67–73.

Koshy, R.C., Kuriakose, R., Sebastian, P., & Koshy, C. (2005). Continuous morphine infusions for cancer pain in resource-scarce environments: Comparison of the subcutaneous and intravenous routes of administration. *Journal of Pain and Palliative Care Pharmacotherapy, 19*(1), 27–33.

Liepe, K., & Kotzerke, J. (2007). A comparative study of 188Re-HEDP, 186Re-HEDP, 153Sm-EDTMP and 89Sr in the treatment of painful skeletal metastases. *Nuclear Medicine Communications, 28*(8), 623–630.

Maltoni, M., Scarpi, E., Modonesi, C., Passardi, A., Calpona, S., Turriziani, A., et al. (2005). A validation study of the WHO analgesic ladder: A two-step vs three-step strategy. *Supportive Care in Cancer, 13*(11), 888–894.

Marinangeli, F., Ciccozzi, A., Aloisio, L., Colangeli, A., Paladini, A., Bajocco, C., et al. (2007). Improved cancer pain treatment using combined fentanyl-TTS and tramadol. *Pain Practice, 7*(4), 307–312.

McNichol, E., Strassels, S.A., Goudas, L., Lau, J., & Carr, D.B. (2005). NSAIDS or paracetamol, alone or combined with opioids, for cancer pain. *Cochrane Database of Systematic Reviews* 2005, Issue 2. Art. No.: CD005180. DOI: 10.1002/14651858.CD005180.

Mercadante, S., Arcuri, E., Ferrera, P., Villari, P., & Mangione, S. (2005). Alternative treatments of breakthrough pain in patients receiving spinal analgesics for cancer pain. *Journal of Pain and Symptom Management, 30*(5), 485–491.

Mercadante, S., Arcuri, E., Fusco, F., Tirelli, W., Villari, P., Bussolino, C., et al. (2005). Randomized double-blind, double-dummy crossover clinical trial of oral tramadol versus rectal tramadol administration in opioid-naive cancer patients with pain. *Supportive Care in Cancer, 13*(9), 702–707.

Mercadante, S., Ferrera, P., Villari, P., & Casuccio, A. (2005). Rapid switching between transdermal fentanyl and methadone in cancer patients. *Journal of Clinical Oncology, 23*(22), 5229–5234.

Mercadante, S., Intravaia, G., Villari, P., Ferrera, P., Riina, S., & Mangione, S. (2008). Intravenous morphine for breakthrough (episodic-) pain in an acute palliative care unit: A confirmatory study. *Journal of Pain and Symptom Management, 35*(3), 307–313.

Mercadante, S., Villari, P., Ferrera, P., & Casuccio, A. (2006). Opioid-induced or pain relief-reduced symptoms in advanced cancer patients? *European Journal of Pain, 10*(2), 153–159.

Mercadante, S., Villari, P., Ferrera, P., Casuccio, A., Mangione, S., & Intravaia, G. (2007). Transmucosal fentanyl vs intravenous morphine in doses proportional to basal opioid regimen for episodic-breakthrough pain. *British Journal of Cancer, 96*(12), 1828–1833.

Merck manuals, online medical library. (n.d.). Retrieved June 26, 2007, from http://www.merck.com/mmpe/sec16/ch209/ch209a.html?qt=neuropathic%20pain&alt=sh#sec16-ch209-ch209a-240

Moryl, N., Kogan, M., Comfort, C., & Obbens, E. (2005). Methadone in the treatment of pain and terminal delirium in advanced cancer patients. *Palliative and Supportive Care, 3*(4), 311–317.

National Comprehensive Cancer Network. (2008). *NCCN Clinical Practice Guidelines in Oncology™: Adult cancer pain* [v.1.2008]. Retrieved August 24, 2008, from http://www.nccn.org/professionals/physician_gls/PDF/pain.pdf

Nicholson, A.B. (2007). Methadone for cancer pain. *Cochrane Database of Systematic Reviews* 2007, Issue 4. Art. No.: CD003971. DOI: 10.1002/14651858.CD003971.pub3.

Novartis. (2007). Aredia [Package insert]. Retrieved June 26, 2007, from http://www.pharma.us.novartis .com/product/pi/pdf/aredia.pdf

Pan, H., Zhang, Z., Zhang, Y., Xu, N., Lu, L., Dou, C., et al. (2007). Efficacy and tolerability of oxycodone hydrochloride controlled-release tablets in moderate to severe cancer pain. *Clinical Drug Investigation, 27*(4), 259–267.

Pergolizzi, S., Iati, G., Santacaterina, A., Palazzolo, C., Di Pietro, A., Garufi, G., et al. (2006). Treatment planning in patients with bone metastases. Final results of a prospective study using pre-medication with fentanyl to improve irradiation reproducibility. *Supportive and Palliative Cancer Care, 2*(2), 71–75.

Pfizer Inc. (2007, February). Celebrex [Package insert]. Retrieved June 26, 2007, from http://pfizer.com/ pfizer/download/uspi_celebrex.pdf

Reid, C.M., Martin, R.M., Sterne, J.A., Davies, A.N., & Hanks, G.W. (2006). Oxycodone for cancer-related pain: Meta-analysis of randomized controlled trials. *Archives of Internal Medicine, 166*(8), 837–843.

Rodriguez, R.F., Bravo, L.E., Castro, F., Montoya, O., Castillo, J.M., Castillo, M.P., et al. (2007). Incidence of weak opioids adverse events in the management of cancer pain: A double-blind comparative trial. *Journal of Palliative Medicine, 10*(1), 56–60.

Roque, M., Martinez-Zapata, M.J., Alonso-Coello, P., Catala, E., Garcia, J.L., & Ferrandiz, M. (2003). Radioisotopes for metastatic bone pain. *Cochrane Database of Systematic Reviews* 2003, Issue 4. Art. No.: CD003347. DOI: 10.1002/14651858.CD003347.

Ross, J.R., Goller, K., Hardy, J., Riley, J., Broadley, K., A'hern, R., et al. (2005). Gabapentin is effective in the treatment of cancer-related neuropathic pain: A prospective, open-label study. *Journal of Palliative Medicine, 8*(6), 1118–1126.

Sartor, O., Reid, R.H., Bushnell, D.L., Quick, D.P., & Ell, P.J. (2007). Safety and efficacy of repeat administration of samarium Sm-153 lexidronam to patients with metastatic bone pain. *Cancer, 109*(3), 637–643.

Slatkin, N.E., Xie, F., Messina, J., & Segal, T.J. (2007). Fentanyl buccal tablet for relief of breakthrough pain in opioid-tolerant patients with cancer-related chronic pain. *Journal of Supportive Oncology, 5*(7), 327–334.

Smith, T.J., & Coyne, P.J. (2005). Implantable drug delivery systems (IDDS) after failure of comprehensive medical management (CMM) can palliate symptoms in the most refractory cancer pain patients. *Journal of Palliative Medicine, 8*(4), 736–742.

Solassol, I., Caumette, L., Bressolle, F., Garcia, F., Thezenas, S., Astre, C., et al. (2005). Inter- and intra-individual variability in transdermal fentanyl absorption in cancer pain patients. *Oncology Reports, 14*(4), 1029–1036.

Stearns, L., Boortz-Marx, R., Du Pen, S., Friehs, G., Gordon, M., Halyard, M., et al. (2005). Intrathecal drug delivery for the management of cancer pain: A multidisciplinary consensus of best clinical practices. *Journal of Supportive Oncology, 3*(6), 399–408.

Swarm, R., Anghelescu, D.L., Benedetti, C., Boston, B., Cleeland, C., Coyle, N., et al. (2007). Adult cancer pain. *Journal of the National Comprehensive Cancer Network, 5*(8), 726–751.

Tassinari, D., Sartori, S., Tamburini, E., Scarpi, E., Raffaeli, W., Tombesi, P., et al. (2008). Adverse effects of transdermal opiates treating moderate-severe cancer pain in comparison to long-acting morphine: A meta-analysis and systematic review of the literature. *Journal of Palliative Medicine, 11*(3), 492–501.

Wallace, M., Rauck, R.L., Moulin, D., Thipphawong, J., Khanna, S., & Tudor, I.C. (2008). Conversion from standard opioid therapy to once-daily oral extended-release hydromorphone in patients with chronic cancer pain. *Journal of International Medical Research, 36*(2), 343–352.

Weinbroum, A.A. (2005). Superiority of postoperative epidural over intravenous patient-controlled analgesia in orthopedic oncologic patients. *Surgery, 138*(5), 869–876.

Wiffen, P.J., & McQuay, H.J. (2007). Oral morphine for cancer pain. *Cochrane Database of Systematic Reviews* 2007, Issue 4. Art. No.: CD003868. DOI: 10.1002/14651858.CD003868.pub2.

Wong, R., & Wiffen, P.J. (2002). Bisphosphonates for the relief of pain secondary to bone metastases. *Cochrane Database of Systematic Reviews* 2002, Issue 2. Art. No.: CD002068. DOI: 10.1002/14651858 .CD002068.

Wootton, M. (2004). Morphine is not the only analgesic in palliative care: Literature review. *Journal of Advanced Nursing, 45*(5), 527–532.

Yuen, K.K., Shelley, M., Sze, W.M., Wilt, T., & Mason, M.D. (2006). Bisphosphonates for advanced prostate cancer. *Cochrane Database of Systematic Reviews* 2006, Issue 4. Art. No.: CD006250. DOI: 10.1002/14651858.CD006250.

Zeppetella, G., & Ribeiro. M.D. (2006). Opioids for the management of breakthrough (episodic) pain in cancer patients. *Cochrane Database of Systematic Reviews* 2006, Issue 1. Art. No.: CD004311. DOI: 10.1002/14651858.CD004311.pub2.

CHAPTER 15

Peripheral Neuropathy

Problem

Peripheral neuropathy is a dysfunction of peripheral, motor, sensory, and autonomic neurons, resulting in peripheral neuropathic signs and symptoms (Postma & Heimans, 2000).

Incidence

Fifty percent of patients receiving vincristine develop paresthesias of the hands and feet, depending on the doses received. Up to 90% of patients receiving cisplatin and 62% of patients receiving paclitaxel develop chemotherapy-induced peripheral neuropathy (CIPN) (Weiss, 2001). The incidence may be higher in those with preexisting peripheral neuropathy and those receiving higher-dose chemotherapy, or in those receiving combination therapy with overlapping toxicity. CIPN is a major quality-of-life issue for patients, affecting functional ability and comfort and is becoming increasingly common because of the influx of chemotherapy agents that cause peripheral neuropathy.

Assessment

A baseline assessment for peripheral neuropathy is important before beginning chemotherapy. Table 15-1 presents common risk factors for the development of CIPN. Assessing patients for CIPN at regular intervals is important, as comfort and patient safety should be priorities. Clinical manifestations and symptoms include numbness, tingling, weakness, and pain. Patients receiving oxaliplatin should be assessed for cold-induced symptoms, and management strategies should be developed as appropriate. In addition, hypersensitivity reactions can occur with several drugs that cause CIPN. The onset and duration of symptoms, as well as effect on activities of daily living, are relevant to quality of life.

Clinical Measurement Tools

The following clinical measurement tools for CIPN are presented in Table 15-2.
1. Common Terminology Criteria for Adverse Events (CTCAE) (National Cancer Institute Cancer Therapy Evaluation Program [NCI CTEP], 2006) (see Table 15-3)

Table 15-1. Baseline Assessment for Chemotherapy-Induced Peripheral Neuropathy

Assessment	Yes	No
History of diabetes		
Arthritis or other connective tissue disease		
Peripheral vascular disease		
Chronic alcohol use		
History of HIV/AIDS		
History of chemical exposures		
History of previous neurotoxic chemotherapy		
Taxanes (paclitaxel, docetaxel, nanoparticle albumin paclitaxel)		
Epothilones (ixebepilone)		
Vinca alkaloids (vincristine, vinblastine, vinorelbine)		
Platinum compounds (cisplatin, carboplatin, oxaliplatin)		
Angiogenesis agents (thalidomide)		
Proteosome inhibitors (bortezomib)		
Current symptoms of neuropathy: Sensory (numbness and tingling, burning or stabbing pain in hands or feet, diminished reflexes)		
Review medication list (prescription, over-the-counter, and vitamins/herbals)		
Pertinent physical examination findings		
Vibration sense with tuning fork		
Proprioception		
Deep tendon reflexes		
Cutaneous sensation		
Muscle strength		
Gait/balance		

Note. Based on information from Visovsky & Daly, 2004; Wickham, 2007; Wilkes, 2004.

2. Functional Assessment of Cancer Therapy/Gynecologic Oncology Group–Neurotoxicity
3. Peripheral Neuropathy Scale (see Figure 15-1)

References

Almadrones, L., McGuire, D.B., Walczak, J.R., Florio, C.M., & Tian, C. (2004). Psychometric evaluation of two scales assessing functional status and peripheral neuropathy associated with chemotherapy for ovarian cancer: A Gynecologic Oncology Group study. *Oncology Nursing Forum, 31*(3), 615–623.

Table 15-2. Clinical Measurement Tools for Peripheral Neuropathy					
Name of Tool	Number of Items	Domains	Reliability and Validity	Populations	Clinical Utility
Peripheral Neuropathy Scale	11	Peripheral neuropathy	Reliability and validity established	Used most commonly with patients with gynecologic cancers	Brief, easy to use
Functional Assessment of Cancer Therapy/ Gynecologic Oncology Group– Neurotoxicity	11 7 6 7 11	Physical well-being Social well-being Emotional well-being Functional well-being Additional concerns related to neuropathy	Reliability and validity established	Patients with ovarian cancer	Assesses several domains, evaluates quality of life
Common Terminology Criteria for Adverse Events	Grading scale	Sensory and motor alterations, impact on functional ability	Unknown	Unknown	Often used in practice to guide treatment decisions and to compare data in clinical trials Inconsistent in approach to measure toxicity associated with chemotherapy-induced peripheral neuropathy

Note. Based on information from Almadrones et al., 2004; Dunlap & Paice, 2006; National Cancer Institute Cancer Therapy Evaluation Program, 2006; Visovsky, 2005.

Grade	Criteria
Table 15-3. Common Terminology Criteria for Adverse Events Grading Scale for Neuropathy	
1	Motor: Asymptomatic, detected on examination only Sensory: Asymptomatic, loss of deep tendon reflexes or paresthesias, but not interfering with function
2	Motor: Symptomatic weakness interfering with function but not activities of daily living (ADLs) Sensory: Sensory alteration or paresthesia that interferes with function but not ADLs
3	Motor: Weakness interfering with ADLs, bracing, or assistance to walk indicate Sensory: Sensory alteration or paresthesia interfering with ADLs
4	Motor: Life-threatening, disabling Sensory: Disabling

Note. Based on information from National Cancer Institute Cancer Therapy Evaluation Program, 2006.

Calhoun, E.A., Fishman, D.A., Roland, P.Y., Lurain, J.R., Chang, C.H., & Cella, D. (2000). Validity and selectivity of the FACT/GOG-Ntx [Abstract 1751]. *Proceedings of the American Society of Clinical Oncology.* Retrieved April 7, 2008, from http://www.asco.org/ASCO/Abstracts+%26+Virtual+Meeting/Abstracts?&vmview=abst_detail_view&confID=2&abstractID=202320

Cella, D.F. (1997). *FACIT: Functional Assessment of Cancer Therapy.* Retrieved September 24, 2007, from http://www.facit.org/qview/qlist.aspx

Cella, D.F., Tulsky, D.S., Gray, G., Serafian, B., Linn, E., Bonomi, A., et al. (1993). The Functional Assessment of Cancer Therapy Scale: Development and validation of the general measure. *Journal of Clinical Oncology, 11*(3), 570–579.

Dunlap, B., & Paice, J.A. (2006). Chemotherapy-induced peripheral neuropathy: A need for standardization in measurement. *Journal of Supportive Oncology, 4*(8), 398–399.

National Cancer Institute Cancer Therapy Evaluation Program. (2006). *Common terminology criteria for adverse events* (version 3.0). Bethesda, MD: National Cancer Institute. Retrieved August 31, 2008, from http://ctep.cancer.gov/protocolDevelopment/electronic_applications/docs/ctcaev3.pdf

Postma, T.J., & Heimans, J.J. (2000). Grading of chemotherapy-induced peripheral neuropathy. *Annals of Oncology, 11*(5), 509–513.

Visovsky, C. (2005). *Measuring oncology nursing-sensitive patient outcomes: Evidence-based summary: Chemotherapy-induced peripheral neuropathy.* Retrieved August 31, 2008, from http://www.ons.org/outcomes/measures/peripheral.shtml

Visovsky, C., & Daly, B.J. (2004). Clinical evaluation and patterns of chemotherapy-induced peripheral neuropathy. *Journal of the American Academy of Nurse Practitioners, 16*(8), 353–359.

Weiss, R.B. (2001). Miscellaneous toxicity: Neurotoxicity. In V.T. DeVita Jr., S. Hellman, & S.A. Rosenberg (Eds.), *Cancer: Principles and practice of oncology* (6th ed., pp. 2964–2976). Philadelphia: Lippincott Williams & Wilkins.

Wickham, R. (2007). Chemotherapy-induced peripheral neuropathy: A review and implications for oncology nursing practice. *Clinical Journal of Oncology Nursing, 11*(3), 361–376.

Wilkes, G.M. (2004). Peripheral neuropathy. In C.H. Yarbro, M.H. Frogge, & M. Goodman (Eds.), *Cancer symptom management* (3rd ed., pp. 333–358). Sudbury, MA: Jones and Bartlett.

Figure 15-1. Neurotoxicity Assessment Tool

Instructions for Patients

By circling one number per line, please indicate how true each statement has been for you during the past seven days using the following scale.

0 = not at all
1 = a little bit
2 = somewhat
3 = quite a bit
4 = very much

I have numbness or tingling in my hands.	0	1	2	3	4
I have numbness or tingling in my feet.	0	1	2	3	4
I feel discomfort in my hands.	0	1	2	3	4
I feel discomfort in my feet.	0	1	2	3	4
I have joint pain or muscle cramps.	0	1	2	3	4
I feel weak all over.	0	1	2	3	4
I have trouble hearing.	0	1	2	3	4
I get a ringing or buzzing in my ears.	0	1	2	3	4
I have trouble buttoning buttons.	0	1	2	3	4
I have trouble feeling the shape of small objects when they are in my hand.	0	1	2	3	4
I have trouble walking.	0	1	2	3	4

Instructions for Healthcare Professionals

This assessment tool is provided to help you evaluate peripheral neuropathy in patients receiving chemotherapy. Healthcare professionals may find discussion of patients' responses helpful in determining the grade of neuropathy as defined by the National Cancer Institute Common Terminology Criteria for Adverse Events (http://ctep.cancer.gov); however, no direct correlation exists between assessment scores and toxicity grades.

Case Study

R.P. was a 60-year-old man diagnosed with stage IV non-small cell lung cancer. R.P.'s oncologist ordered paclitaxel 175 mg/m² and carboplatin (area under the curve 6) on an every-three-week cycle. During the initial visit, the nurse taught R.P. about the signs and symptoms of peripheral neuropathy and the importance of reporting them to his doctor or nurse. According to the Oncology Nursing Society (ONS) Putting Evidence Into Practice (PEP) resource on peripheral neuropathy, no interventions currently are available in the *Recommended for Practice* or *Likely to Be Effective* categories for preventing or reducing the effects of peripheral neuropathy; however, the *Expert Opinion* section includes information on how to support and preserve patient safety.

After his second cycle of chemotherapy, R.P. started to notice some tingling, numbness, and sensation of pins and needles in his fingertips and toes. He was concerned that the oncologist would stop his chemotherapy if it worsened. R.P. asked if there was anything he could do to alleviate this symptom. Reviewing the ONS PEP resource on peripheral neuropathy with R.P., the nurse explained that although many different interventions have been tried to improve peripheral neuropathy, they often were used on small numbers of patients or on patients who did not have cancer. R.P. looked over the list of interventions and asked about glutamine and vitamin E supplementation. The nurse spoke with the oncologist, who was not opposed to the patient taking normal doses of those supplements during treatment. Currently, the evidence does not support taking these supplements for CIPN, and more research is needed to evaluate their place in therapy.

After the third cycle of chemotherapy, the numbness and tingling extended further into R.P.'s feet (mostly on the bottom) and fingers. He also was having difficulty buttoning his shirt and noted that his signature was becoming illegible (CTCAE grade 2). At this point, the paclitaxel/carboplatin was discontinued and the oncologist started pregabalin 75 mg twice daily.

After a break of several weeks, R.P. was rescanned and found to have stable disease and was started on vinorelbine weekly. At each visit, R.P. focused on the neuropathy, hoping that it would "go away soon now that [he was] not on [paclitaxel]." The nurse explained to R.P. that vinorelbine may also cause neuropathy and gave him an information sheet developed from the *Expert Opinion* section of the ONS PEP resource on peripheral neuropathy, which included important safety measures for patients.

After three doses of vinorelbine, R.P. reported improvement in his ability to button buttons and decreased sensation of pins and needles in his hands. Unfortunately, the effect on his feet had worsened to the point that his sense of joint position in his right foot was impaired. R.P. confided that he had been tripping and fell once getting out of the car, stating, "It's like I couldn't tell if my foot was on the ground or not" (CTCAE grade 3).

The vinorelbine was discontinued, and R.P. was started on pemetrexed. The nurse requested a physical therapy referral for R.P. after consulting with him about his concerns. Although the ONS PEP resource on peripheral neuropathy has categorized assistive devices in the *Benefits Balanced With Harms* category, R.P. stated, "I would have felt better having a walker to help keep my balance when walking a long way—I don't need to fall again."

Patricia Starr, RN, MSN, OCN®
Neuro-Oncology/CyberKnife® Care Coordinator
Waukesha Memorial Hospital
Waukesha, WI

Peripheral Neuropathy

2009 AUTHORS
Constance Visovsky, RN, PhD, ACNP, and Mary L. Collins, RN, MSN, OCN®
ONS STAFF: Heather Belansky, RN, MSN

2007 AUTHORS
Constance Visovsky, PhD, RN, ACNP, Mary L. Collins, RN, MSN, OCN®, Connie Hart, RN, BSN, OCN®,
Linda I. Abbott, RN, MSN, AOCN®, CWON, and Julie A. Aschenbrenner, RN, OCN®
ONS STAFF: Kristen Baileys, RN, MSN, CRNP, AOCNP®

What interventions are used to prevent or reduce the effects of peripheral neuropathy for people with cancer?

Recommended for Practice

Interventions for which effectiveness has been demonstrated by strong evidence from rigorously designed studies, meta-analyses, or systematic reviews and for which expectation of harms is small compared with the benefits

There are no interventions as of May 2008.

Likely to Be Effective

Interventions for which effectiveness has been demonstrated by supportive evidence from a single rigorously conducted controlled trial, consistent supportive evidence from well-designed controlled trials using small samples, or guidelines developed from evidence and supported by expert opinion

There are no interventions as of May 2008.

Benefits Balanced With Harms

Interventions for which clinicians and patients should weigh the beneficial and harmful effects according to individual circumstances and priorities

TREATMENT INTERVENTIONS

Assistive Devices

No studies have been done of assistive device use in the cancer population. However, two small, nonrandomized studies of cane and orthotic use were done in the diabetes population that showed benefits, including prevention of foot drop and improvement in balance and proprioception (Ashton-Miller, Yeh, Richardson, & Galloway, 1996; Richardson, Thies, De-Mott, & Ashton-Miller, 2004).
- Although the use of assistive devices will not directly reduce the effects of peripheral neuropathy, some patients may find them beneficial.

- Healthcare professionals should refer clients to a physical therapist for a cane, orthotic braces, or a splint to assist with lower-extremity alignment and balance.
- Referral to a professional who is familiar with these devices and has the ability to educate patients on their use is recommended.

Effectiveness Not Established

Interventions for which insufficient or conflicting data or data of inadequate quality currently exist, with no clear indication of harm

TREATMENT INTERVENTIONS

Carbamazepine

In a nonrandomized pilot study, 40 pretreated patients who received oxaliplatin were studied (Eckel et al., 2002). Ten of these patients also received carbamazepine 200–600 mg orally daily (titrated to serum levels of 3–6 mg/L) just prior to and throughout treatment of oxaliplatin.

- No grade 2–4 peripheral neuropathy, according to the World Health Organization scale, occurred in any patient (Eckel et al., 2002).

In a multicenter, phase II study of carbamazepine for prevention of oxaliplatin-associated neuropathy in patients with colorectal cancer, 36 patients were randomly assigned to receive folic acid, 5-fluorouracil, and oxaliplatin with carbamazepine 200 mg daily beginning six days prior to chemotherapy (treatment A). Seventeen patients were randomized to receive the same chemotherapy regimen without carbamazepine (treatment B).

- No major differences were reported between both groups in peripheral neuropathy scores or in the incidence of grade 3 or 4 neurotoxicity. Because of methodologic issues, conclusions regarding the efficacy and safety of carbamazepine cannot be drawn regarding prevention of oxaliplatin-associated neuropathy (von Delius et al., 2007).

Lamotrigine

In a phase 3, randomized, double-blind, placebo-controlled trial, 125 patients treated previously with neurotoxic chemotherapy who reported symptomatic chemotherapy-induced peripheral neuropathy (CIPN) for ≥ one month were randomized to either lamotrigine or placebo. The lamotrigine dose was escalated from 25 mg at bedtime to 150 mg BID, which then was continued for two weeks, followed by a drug taper.

- Only 80 patients completed the study. No significant differences were noted between the two groups on pain or efficacy. The researchers concluded that lamotrigine was not effective for relieving CIPN (Rao et al., 2008).

PREVENTION INTERVENTIONS

Acetyl-L-Carnitine

Only two small studies (nonrandomized, one-group design) of patients treated with acetyl-L-carnitine for CIPN were found (Bianchi et al., 2005; Maestri et al., 2005).

Acetyl-L-carnitine administered as 1 g/day IV for 10 consecutive days or 1 g by mouth TID for eight weeks was used for prevention of paclitaxel- or cisplatin-induced peripheral neuropathy (Bianchi et al., 2005; Maestri et al., 2005). Results of these studies showed improvement in motor and sensory neuropathy. However, further randomized clinical trials are necessary before acetyl-L-carnitine can be recommended as a potential treatment for CIPN.

Alpha-Lipoic Acid

No studies have been done using alpha-lipoic acid in the oncology population, but some evidence exists of benefit in diabetic polyneuropathy (Ziegler, Nowak, Kempler, Vargha, & Low, 2004).

A meta-analysis of four trials comprising 1,258 patients with diabetic polyneuropathy demonstrated that treatment with alpha-lipoic acid (600 mg/day IV) Monday through Friday for three weeks improved the chief symptoms of diabetic polyneuropathy to a clinically meaningful degree (Ziegler et al., 2004). Further study is needed to determine the safety and efficacy of alpha lipoic acid in the prevention or treatment of CIPN.

Amifostine

Three studies have tested amifostine in prevention of chemotherapy-induced neurotoxicity (Hilpert et al., 2005; Moore et al., 2003; Openshaw et al., 2004).
- Two of these studies have not shown amifostine to be effective in preventing or reducing symptoms of peripheral neuropathy (Hilpert et al., 2005; Moore et al., 2003).

A prospective, double-blind, randomized, placebo-controlled trial was performed (Openshaw et al., 2004). Patients with advanced ovarian cancer received carboplatin/paclitaxel-based chemotherapy and were pretreated with amifostine 740 mg/m² versus placebo. Assessments included a questionnaire, the National Cancer Institute Cancer Therapy Evaluation Program's Common Terminology Criteria for Adverse Events (CTCAE), vibration threshold measurements, and quality of life. In all three studies, no differences were found in sensory or motor neurotoxic symptoms in patients treated with amifostine. Amifostine was also found to be ineffective in preventing or reducing the neurotoxic effects of high-dose paclitaxel.

Calcium and Magnesium

One nonrandomized, retrospective study suggested that calcium and magnesium given IV over 15 minutes before and after administration of oxaliplatin may decrease the incidence and intensity of peripheral neuropathy in patients (Gamelin et al., 2004).
- Results indicated that only 4% of patients who received calcium and magnesium withdrew from treatment because of the neurotoxic effects of oxaliplatin, whereas 31% of patients withdrew in the control group. At the end of treatment, 20% of the patients who received calcium and magnesium had neuropathy, whereas 45% of patients who did not receive calcium/magnesium infusions developed neuropathy (Gamelin et al., 2004).
- The researchers stated that a prospective, multicenter, double-blind, randomized, placebo-controlled trial is under way to determine the impact of calcium/magnesium on the neurotoxic effects of oxaliplatin (Gamelin et al., 2004).

In a letter to the editor of the *Journal of Clinical Oncology*, the termination of the Combined Oxaliplatin Neuropathy Prevention Trial was reported (Hochster, Grothey, & Childs, 2007). The trial randomly assigned 140 patients to receive calcium gluconate and magnesium sulfate or placebo before and after oxaliplatin to potentially reduce neurotoxicity. However, preliminary data showed those patients who received calcium and magnesium infusions had a significantly lower response rate as compared to the placebo group, and the study was closed. A subsequent review of computed tomography scans from the trial showed the antitumor response rate to be numerically higher in the group that received the calcium and magnesium infusions as compared to patients who received placebo. Further data analysis and findings are pending (Hochster et al., 2007; Hochster, Grothey, Shpilsky, & Childs, 2008).

Gabapentin

In a phase 3, randomized, double-blind, placebo-controlled crossover trial, 115 patients with symptomatic CIPN were randomized to receive either gabapentin (300 mg capsules incrementally escalated over three weeks to a target dose of 2,700 mg per day) or placebo over the course of two six-week phases separated by a two-week "washout" period.

- No significant differences were reported in primary or secondary end points between the groups on scores of pain, symptom distress, or mood states. The only significant difference between the groups was in the McGill Pain Rating Index, which showed lower levels of pain in the gabapentin group at the end of the first six-week treatment period. The study failed to demonstrate the benefit of gabapentin to treat CIPN symptoms (Rao et al., 2007).

Glutamine

Glutamine 10 g by mouth TID beginning 24 hours after chemotherapy and continuing for four days has been reviewed as a neuroprotective agent in CIPN (Stubblefield et al., 2005; Vahdat et al., 2001).

- Results of two small, nonrandomized, nonplacebo-controlled studies indicate that some signs and symptoms of CIPN may be reduced by glutamine with paclitaxel-containing regimens. The neurologic assessments seemed to be a better indicator of signs and symptoms than nerve conduction studies (Stubblefield et al., 2005; Vahdat et al., 2001).

Eighty-six patients with colorectal cancer were enrolled in a nonrandomized pilot study to evaluate oral glutamine for reducing the incidence and severity of peripheral neuropathy in patients receiving oxaliplatin. Patients received glutamine 15 g BID for seven days every two weeks, starting on the day of treatment.

- Glutamine supplementation significantly reduced the incidence and severity of oxaliplatin-induced neuropathy. After two cycles of treatment, grade 1–2 sensory neuropathy was significantly lower in the intervention group versus the control group. The percentage of grade 3–4 sensory neuropathy was lower in the glutamine group after four cycles of treatment and remained that way for six cycles.
- Glutamine supplementation appeared to reduce the need for oxaliplatin dose reduction without affecting response to chemotherapy and survival.
- Glutamine is a potential neuroprotective agent but needs to be studied in larger populations in a randomized, placebo-controlled trial. Concern still exists regarding glutamine supplements possibly protecting tumor cells from the cytotoxic effects of chemotherapy (Wang et al., 2007).

Glutathione

Studies investigating glutathione as a neuroprotective agent in the oncology population are dated and do not demonstrate a clear benefit with its use (Cascinu, Cordella, Del Ferro, Fronzoni, & Catalana, 1995; Cascinu et al., 2002; Smyth et al., 1997).

- The studies question whether glutathione actually prevents toxicities or only delays them (Cascinu et al., 1995, 2002; Smyth et al., 1997).
- According to one study, glutathione may have some benefit in reducing signs and symptoms of peripheral neuropathy (Cascinu et al., 2002).

Nortriptyline

One small study revealed modest improvement at best with nortriptyline over placebo for preventing cisplatin neurotoxicity (Hammack et al., 2002).

Recombinant Human Leukemia Inhibitory Factor

One study in patients receiving carboplatin/paclitaxel and recombinant human leukemia inhibitory factor (rhuLIF) (2–4 mcg/kg) concluded that no evidence supported that rhuLIF prevented, delayed, or diminished peripheral neuropathy (Davis et al., 2005). There are no future plans to continue development of rhuLIF for the prevention or treatment of peripheral neuropathy (Davis et al.).

Vitamin E

Two pilot studies (Argyriou et al., 2005; Bove, Picardo, Maresca, Jaredolo, & Pace, 2001) and one small randomized study (Pace et al., 2003) showed some benefit to using oral vitamin E with cisplatin regimens. However, standard doses have not been determined, and more randomized controlled clinical trials are needed to further evaluate the neuroprotective effects of vitamin E.

TREATMENT INTERVENTIONS

Acupuncture

Only one small case series study has been done on the use of acupuncture for CIPN (Wong & Sagar, 2006).
- Acupuncture improved sensation and movement and resulted in decreased analgesic dosages for the five patients involved. Gait also was improved, and no adverse effects were noted. Control of symptoms persisted for six months for four of the five patients treated.
- Acupuncture also has been studied in the diabetic and HIV populations, with some mixed results (Abuaisha, Costanzi, & Boulton, 1998; Jiang, Shi, Li, Zhou, & Cao, 2006; Phillips, Skelton, & Hand, 2004; Shlay et al., 1998).
- None of the studies employing acupuncture identified any risks or hazards associated with the treatment.

Capsaicin

This therapy has not been studied in the oncology population. Capsaicin has been studied for the treatment of peripheral neuropathy in the diabetic population, with inconclusive results that prevent recommendation at this time (Forst et al., 2004).
- Ten patients completed the study, with significant decreases found in the total symptom score of the capsaicin-treated arm and no significant changes occurring in the control feet. Two patients in this study, discontinued treatment because of adverse events related to the treatment (Forst et al., 2004).

Physical Activity/Exercise

Physical activity/exercise interventions have not been studied in the prevention or treatment of peripheral neuropathy in patients with cancer.
- Three studies with small sample sizes have examined progressive resistance exercise, aerobic exercise, and stretching exercises in the treatment of diabetic peripheral neuropathy and myotonic dystrophy (Balducci et al., 2006; Lindeman et al., 1995; Richardson et al., 2004; Richardson, Sandman, & Vela, 2001).
- All three studies found significant improvement in stance, functional reach, and peroneal and sural motor nerve conduction velocity. These studies contain findings that need to be interpreted with caution, as these studies have not been replicated in patients with cancer (Balducci et al., 2006; Linderman et al., 1995; Richardson et al., 2001, 2004).

Pulsed Infrared Light Therapy (Also Called Anodyne® Therapy)

Pulsed infrared light therapy (PILT) has not been studied in the oncology population. Three studies in the diabetic population were reviewed (Arnall et al., 2006; Leonard, Farooqi, & Myers, 2004; Prendergast, Miranda, & Sanchez, 2004). Only one study was a randomized clinical trial (Leonard et al.).

- One study identified an improvement in sensation, neuropathy symptoms, and pain (Leonard et al., 2004). Those with the most severe neuropathy scores on entry into the study, however, did not show significant improvement in these symptoms.
- Two other studies also found improvement in sensation when using Anodyne therapy in diabetic patients with peripheral neuropathy (Arnall et al., 2004; Prendergast et al., 2004).
- None of the studies using PILT demonstrated any risks associated with the treatment.

Spinal Cord Stimulation

Use of spinal cord stimulation in two patients with CIPN was reported in one case study (Arnall et al., 2006).

- Improvement in pain scores, gait, flexibility, and sensation scores and reduction in the use of analgesic medications were found with the use of the stimulator for 6–18 hours a day (Cata et al., 2006).

Because surgical risks and costs are associated with this intervention, it is not recommended for practice at this time (Cata et al., 2006).

Transcutaneous Electrical Nerve Stimulation and High-Frequency External Muscle Stimulation

Transcutaneous electrical nerve stimulation (TENS) and high-frequency external muscle stimulation have not been investigated in the oncology population, but limited studies have been done in the diabetic population with peripheral neuropathy. TENS has demonstrated some benefit in the treatment of diabetic peripheral neuropathy (Forst et al., 2004; Reichstein, Labrenz, Ziegler, & Martin, 2005).

- One study demonstrated improvement in numbness, lancinating pain, and allodynia with no changes in vibration, temperature, and pain perception thresholds with TENS therapy (Forst et al., 2004).
- Another study found that high-frequency muscle stimulation was more effective than TENS in improving pain rating scores and peripheral neuropathic symptom reports, but both were effective in decreasing symptoms (Reichstein et al., 2005).
- No risks were reported with the use of TENS.

Effectiveness Unlikely

Interventions for which lack of effectiveness has been demonstrated by negative evidence from a single rigorously conducted controlled trial, consistent negative evidence from well-designed controlled trials using small samples, or guidelines developed from evidence and supported by expert opinion

There are no interventions as of May 2008.

Not Recommended for Practice

Interventions for which lack of effectiveness or harmfulness has been demonstrated by strong evidence from rigorously conducted studies, meta-analyses, or systematic reviews, or interventions where the costs, burden, or harms associated with the intervention exceed anticipated benefit

There are no interventions as of May 2008.

Expert Opinion

Low-risk interventions that are (1) consistent with sound clinical practice, (2) suggested by an expert in a peer-reviewed publication (journal or book chapter), and (3) for which limited evidence exists. An expert is an individual who has authored articles published in a peer-reviewed journal in the domain of interest.

Important nursing practice includes education and support to preserve patient safety (Armstrong, Almadrones, & Gilbert, 2005; Marrs & Newton, 2003; Paice, 2007; Reichstein et al., 2005).

- Teach patients the signs and symptoms of peripheral neuropathy, and instruct patients to report them to their healthcare providers as soon as they or their families notice them.
- Teach patients strategies for managing personal safety, such as using visual input to compensate for loss of lower-extremity sensation in navigating changing terrain, removing throw rugs, clearing walkways of clutter, using skid-free shower and bathroom mats, or using a cane or walker if gait is unsteady.
- Teach patients the principles of foot care, including inspection of the feet and the importance of wearing properly fitted shoes.
- Teach patients about preventing the risk for ischemic or thermal injury resulting from loss of sensation in extremities, such as lowering water temperature in the home water heater to avoid burns, using a bath thermometer to make sure the temperature of water in the shower or tub is 120°F or below, and inspecting the hands and feet every day for sores or blisters.
- Teach strategies to prevent symptoms of autonomic dysfunction (postural hypotension, constipation, urinary retention), such as dangling the legs prior to arising and consuming a high-fiber diet and adequate fluid intake.

For information on pharmacologic interventions for neuropathic pain, please refer to the ONS PEP resource on pain.

Definitions of the interventions are available at **www.ons.org/outcomes**.
Literature search completed through May 2008.

References

Abuaisha, B.B., Costanzi, J.B., & Boulton, A.J. (1998). Acupuncture for the treatment of chronic painful peripheral diabetic neuropathy: A long-term study. *Diabetes Research and Clinical Practice, 39*(2), 115–121.

Argyriou, A.A., Chroni, E., Koutras, A., Ellul, J., Papapetropoulos, S., Katsoulas, G., et al. (2005). Vitamin E for prophylaxis against chemotherapy-induced neuropathy. *Neurology, 64*(1), 26–31.

Armstrong, T., Almadrones, L., & Gilbert, M. (2005). Chemotherapy-induced peripheral neuropathy. *Oncology Nursing Forum, 32*(2), 305–311.

Arnall, D.A., Nelson, A.G., Lopez, L., Sanz, M., Iversen, L., Sanz, I., et al. (2006). The restorative effects of pulsed infrared light therapy on significant loss of peripheral protective sensation in patients with long-term type 1 and type 2 diabetes mellitus. *Acta Diabetologica, 43*(1), 26–33.

Ashton-Miller, J., Yeh, M., Richardson, J.K., & Galloway, T. (1996). A cane reduces loss of balance in patients with peripheral neuropathy: Results from a challenging unipedal balance test. *Archives of Physical Medicine and Rehabilitation, 77*(5), 446–452.

Balducci, S., Iacobellis, G., Parisi, L., Di Biase, N., Calandriello, E., Leonetti, F., et al. (2006). Exercise training can modify the natural history of diabetic peripheral neuropathy. *Journal of Diabetes and Its Complications, 20*(4), 216–223.

Bianchi, G., Vitali, A., Ravaglia, S., Capri, G., Cundari, S., Zanna, C., et al. (2005). Symptomatic and neurophysiological responses of paclitaxel or cisplatin induced neuropathy to oral acetyl-L-carnitine. *European Journal of Cancer, 41*(12), 1746–1750.

Bove, L., Picardo, M., Maresca, V., Jaredolo, B., & Pace, A. (2001). A pilot study on the relation between cisplatin neuropathy and vitamin E. *Journal of Experimental and Clinical Cancer Research, 20*(2), 277–280.

Cascinu, S., Catalano, V., Cordella, L., Labiance, R., Giordani, P., Baldelli, A.M., et al. (2002). Neuroprotective effect of reduced glutathione on oxaliplatin-based chemotherapy in advanced colorectal cancer: A randomized, double-blind, placebo-controlled trial. *Journal of Clinical Oncology, 20*(16), 3478–3483.

Cascinu, S., Cordella, L., Del Ferro, E., Fronzoni, M., & Catalana, G. (1995). Neuroprotective effect of reduced glutathione on cisplatin-based chemotherapy in advanced gastric cancer: A randomized double-blind placebo-controlled trial. *Journal of Clinical Oncology, 13*(1), 26–32.

Cata, J.P., Cordella, J.V., Burton, A.W., Hassenbusch, S.J., Weng, H.R., & Dougherty, P.M. (2004). Spinal cord stimulation relieves chemotherapy-induced pain: A clinical case report. *Journal of Pain and Symptom Management, 27*(1), 72–78.

Davis, I.D., Kiers, L., MacGregor, L., Quinn, M., Arezo, J., Green, M., et al. (2005). A randomized, double-blinded, placebo-controlled phase II trial of recombinant human leukemia inhibitory factor (rhuLIF, emfilermin, AMg424) to prevent chemotherapy-induced peripheral neuropathy. *Clinical Cancer Research, 11*(5), 1890–1898.

Eckel, F., Schmelz, R., Adelsberger, H., Erdmann, J., Quasthoff, F., & Lersch, C. (2002). [Prevention of oxaliplatin-induced neuropathy by carbamazepine. A pilot study]. *Deutsche Medizinische Wochenschrift, 127*(3), 78–82.

Forst, T., Nguyen, M., Forst, S., Disselhoff, B., Pohlmann, T., & Pfutzner, A. (2004). Impact of low frequency transcutaneous electrical nerve stimulation on symptomatic diabetic neuropathy using the new Salutaris device. *Diabetes, Nutrition and Metabolism, 17*(3), 163–168.

Gamelin, L., Boisdron-Celle, M., Delva, R., Geurin-Meyer, V., Ifrah, N., Morel, A., et al. (2004). Prevention of oxaliplatin-related neurotoxicity by calcium and magnesium infusions: A retrospective study of 161 patients receiving oxaliplatin combined with 5-fluourouracil and leucovorin for advanced colorectal cancer. *Clinical Cancer Research, 10*(12, Pt. 1), 4055–4061.

Hammack, J., Michalak, J., Loprinzi, C., Sloan, J., Novotny, P., Soori, G., et al. (2002). Phase III evaluation of nortriptyline for alleviation of symptoms of cis-platinum–induced peripheral neuropathy. *Pain, 98*(1–2), 195–203.

Hilpert, F., Stahle, A., Tome, O., Burges, A., Rossner, D., Spatke, K., et al. (2005). Neuroprotection with amifostine in the first-line treatment of advanced ovarian cancer with carboplatin/paclitaxel-based chemotherapy—A double-blind, placebo-controlled, randomized phase II study from the Arbeitsgemeinschaft Gynäkologische Onkologoie (AGO) Ovarian Cancer Study Group. *Supportive Care in Cancer, 13*(10), 797–805.

Hochster, H.S., Grothey, A., & Childs, B.H. (2007). Use of calcium and magnesium salts to reduce oxaliplatin-related neurotoxicity. *Journal of Clinical Oncology, 25*(25), 4028–4029.

Hochster, H.S., Grothey, A., Shpilsky, A., & Childs, B.H. (2008, January). *Effect of intravenous (IV) calcium and magnesium (CA/Mg) versus placebo on response to FOLFOX + bevacizumab (BEV) in the CONcePT trial* [Abstract 280]. Abstract presented at the 2008 Gastrointestinal Cancers Symposium, Orlando, FL. Retrieved May 5, 2008, from http://www.asco.org/ASCO/Abstracts+&+Virtual+Meeting/Abstracts?&vmview=abst_detail_view&confID=53&abstractID=10402

Jiang, H., Shi, K., Li, X., Zhou, W., & Cao, Y. (2006). Clinical study on the wrist-ankle acupuncture treatment for 30 cases of diabetic peripheral neuritis. *Journal of Traditional Chinese Medicine, 26*(1), 8–12.

Leonard, D.R., Farooqi, M.H., & Myers, S. (2004). Restoration of sensation, reduced pain, and improved balance in subjects with diabetic peripheral neuropathy. *Diabetes Care, 27*(1), 168–172.

Lindeman, E., Leffers, P., Spaans, F., Drukker, J., Kerckhoffs, M., & Koke, A. (1995). Strength training in patients with myotonic dystrophy and hereditary motor and sensory neuropathy: A randomized clinical trial. *Archives of Physical Medicine and Rehabilitation, 76*(7), 612–620.

Maestri, A., De Pasquale Ceratti, A., Cundari, S., Zanna, C., Cortesi, E., & Crino, L. (2005). A pilot study on the effect of acetyl-L-carnitine in paclitaxel- and cisplatin-induced peripheral neuropathy. *Tumori, 91*(2), 135–138.

Marrs, J., & Newton, S. (2003). Updating your peripheral neuropathy "know-how." *Clinical Journal of Oncology Nursing, 7*(3), 299–303.

Moore, D., Donnelly, J., McGuire, W.P., Almadrones, L., Cella, D.F., Herzog, T.J., et al. (2003). Limited access trial using amifostine for protection against cisplatin and three hour paclitaxel-induced neurotoxicity: A phase II study of the Gynecologic Oncology Group. *Journal of Clinical Oncology, 21*(22), 4207–4213.

Openshaw, H., Beamon, K., Synold, T.W., Lougmate, J., Slatkin, N.E., Doroshaw, J.H., et al. (2004). Neurophysiological study of peripheral neuropathy after high-dose paclitaxel: Lack of neuroprotective effect of amifostine. *Clinical Cancer Research, 10*(2), 461–467.

Pace, A., Savarese, A., Picardo, M., Maresca, V., Pacetti, U., Del Monte, G., et al. (2003). Neuroprotective effect of vitamin E supplementation in patients treated with cisplatin chemotherapy. *Journal of Clinical Oncology, 21*(5), 927–931.

Paice, J.A. (2007). Peripheral neuropathy: Experimental findings, clinical approaches. *Journal of Supportive Oncology, 5*(2), 61–63.

Phillips, K.D., Skelton, W.D., & Hand, G.A. (2004). Effect of acupuncture administered in a group setting on pain and subjective peripheral neuropathy in persons with human immunodeficiency virus disease. *Journal of Alternative and Complementary Medicine, 10*(3), 449–455.

Prendergast, J.J., Miranda, G., & Sanchez, M. (2004). Improvement of sensory impairment in patients with peripheral neuropathy. *Endocrine Practice, 10*(1), 24–30.

Rao, R.D., Flynn, P.J., Sloan, J.A., Wong, G.Y., Novotny, P., Johnson, D.B., et al. (2008). Efficacy of lamotrigine in the management of chemotherapy-induced peripheral neuropathy: A phase 3 randomized, double blind, placebo-controlled trial, N01C3. *Cancer, 112*(12), 2802–2808.

Reichstein, L., Labrenz, S., Ziegler, D., & Martin, S. (2005). Effective treatment of symptomatic diabetic polyneuropathy by high-frequency external muscle stimulation. *Diabetologia, 48*(5), 824–828.

Richardson, J.K., Sandman, D., & Vela, S. (2001). A focused exercise regimen improves clinical measures of balance in patients with peripheral neuropathy. *Archives of Physical Medicine and Rehabilitation, 82*(2), 205–209.

Richardson, J.K., Thies, S., DeMott, T., & Ashton-Miller, J.A. (2004). Interventions improve gait regularity in patients with peripheral neuropathy while walking on an irregular surface under low light. *Journal of the American Geriatrics Society, 52*(4), 510–515.

Shlay, J.D., Chaloner, K., Max, M.B., Flaws, B., Reichelderfer, P., Wentworth, D., et al. (1998). Acupuncture and amitriptyline for pain due to HIV-related peripheral neuropathy. *JAMA, 280*(18), 1590–1595.

Smyth, J.F., Bowman, A., Perren, T., Wilkinson, P., Prescott, R.J., Quinn, K.J., et al. (1997). Glutathione reduces the toxicity and improves quality of life of women diagnosed with ovarian cancer treated with cisplatin: Results of a double-blind, randomized trial. *Annals of Oncology, 8*(6), 569–573.

Stubblefield, M.D., Vahdat, L.T., Balmaceda, C.M., Troxel, A.B., Hesdorffer, C.S., & Gooch, C.L. (2005). Glutamine as a neuroprotective agent in high-dose paclitaxel-induced peripheral neuropathy: A clinical and electrophysiologic study. *Clinical Oncology, 17*(4), 271–276.

Vahdat, L., Papadopoulos, K., Lange, D., Leuin, S., Kaufman, E., Donovan, D., et al. (2001). Reduction of paclitaxel-induced peripheral neuropathy with glutamine. *Clinical Cancer Research, 7*(5), 1192–1197.

von Delius, S., Eckel, F., Wagenpfeil, S., Mayr, M., Stock, K., Kullmann, F., et al. (2007). Carbamazepine for prevention of oxaliplatin-related neurotoxicity in patients with advanced colorectal cancer: Final results of a randomized, controlled, multicenter phase II study. *Investigational New Drugs, 25*(2), 173–180.

Wang, W., Lin, J., Lin, T., Chen, W., Jiang, J., Wang, H., et al. (2007). Oral glutamine is effective for preventing oxaliplatin-induced neuropathy in colorectal cancer patients. *Oncologist, 12*(3), 312–319.

White, C.M., Pritchard, J., & Turner-Stokes, L. (2004). Exercise for people with peripheral neuropathy. *Cochrane Database of Systematic Reviews* 2004, Issue 4. Art. No.: CD003904. DOI: 10.1002/14651858. CD003904.pub2.

Wong, R., & Sagar, S. (2006). Acupuncture treatment for chemotherapy-induced peripheral neuropathy—A case series. *Acupuncture in Medicine, 24*(2), 87–91.

Ziegler, D., Nowak, H., Kempler, P., Vargha, P., & Low, P.A. (2004). Treatment of symptomatic diabetic polyneuropathy with the antioxidant alpha-lipoic acid: A meta-analysis. *Diabetic Medicine, 21*(2), 114–121.

CHAPTER 16

Prevention of Bleeding

Problem

Bleeding in the patient with cancer results from a complex interplay of disease- and treatment-related factors. Bleeding may be the result of a reduction in the quantity or functional quality of platelets, an alteration in clotting factors, a paraneoplastic syndrome, or a combination of such factors. Only interventions that prevent, ameliorate, or manage bleeding directly related to cancer and/or its treatment are addressed in this chapter. Interventions that prevent or treat the consequences of bleeding or those that are associated with comorbidity are not addressed.

Incidence

Certain malignancies, such as leukemia, particularly acute promyelocytic leukemia (APL), have a higher probability of bleeding. Up to 90% of patients with APL will develop a hemorrhagic complication (DeSancho & Rand, 2001). In addition, mucin-producing adenocarcinomas are solid tumors that have a tendency to cause bleeding. Ongoing bleeding can affect quality of life, increasing fatigue and weakness. Bleeding can become an issue of safety, and more serious forms of bleeding with hemorrhage can be dramatic and life-threatening. Thrombocytopenia may be caused by treatment, such as chemotherapy or radiation therapy. Other causes include infection, disseminated intravascular coagulation, liver disease, and platelet dysfunction secondary to medications (Kwaan & Vicuna, 2007). The dose intensity of chemotherapy may improve response for many types of cancer; however, prolonged thrombocytopenia may compromise subsequent dose and clinical benefit. Bleeding may also occur in up to 10% of patients with advanced cancer (Pereira & Phan, 2004). This can be distressing to patients and caregivers, particularly when it is visible.

Assessment

Prior to initiating therapy, a thorough assessment of bleeding tendency is important in a patient with cancer. Table 16-1 provides an assessment for patients at risk for bleeding.

Table 16-1. Assessment of Risk Factors for Bleeding		
Assessment	**Yes**	**No**
Patient History		
Bleeding or clotting disorders		
Bleeding tendencies		
Petechiae		
Easy bruising		
Pain		
Headaches		
Nosebleeds		
Poor nutritional status		
Medication history (prescription, over the counter, vitamins/herbals)		
History of transfusions		
History of liver disease		
History of renal disease		
History of allergic reactions		
Known infections		
Type of malignancy		
Types of treatment		
Physical Assessment		
Body system review		
Performance status		
Diagnostic workup		
Laboratory data		
Note. Based on information from Friend & Pruett, 2004.		

Clinical Measurement Tools

There is little in the way of measurement tools for the prevention of bleeding. Most tools available are for grading of toxicity and quality-of-life measurements. Further development and testing of clinical measurement tools is needed.

1. Common Terminology Criteria for Adverse Events (CTCAE) (National Cancer Institute Cancer Therapy Evaluation Program [NCI CTEP], 2006): Used to grade degree of thrombocytopenia and toxicity in clinical trials; no reliability and validity data are available (see Table 16-2).
2. Functional Assessment of Cancer Therapy–Thrombocytopenia: This 18-item scale has shown reliability and validity and is a useful measure for self-reported symptoms related to thrombocytopenia (Cella, Beaumont, Webster, Lai, & Eiting, 2006).

Table 16-2. Common Terminology Criteria for Adverse Events Grading Criteria for Thrombocytopenia	
Grade	**Criteria (Platelet Count)**
1	< LLN–75,000/mm^3; < LLN – 75 × 10^9/L
2	< 75,000–50,000/mm^3; < 75–50 × 10^9/L
3	< 50,000–25,000/mm^3; < 50–25 × 10^9/L
4	< 25,000/mm^3; < 25 × 10^9/L
5	Death

LLN—lower limit of normal

Note. Based on information from National Cancer Institute Cancer Therapy Evaluation Program, 2006.

References

Cella, D., Beaumont, J.L., Webster, K.A., Lai, J., & Eiting, L. (2006). Measuring the concerns of cancer patients with low platelet counts: The Functional Assessment of Cancer Therapy–Thrombocytopenia (FACT-Th) questionnaire. *Supportive Care in Cancer, 14*(12), 1220–1231.

DeSancho, M.T., & Rand, J.H. (2001). Bleeding and thrombotic complications in critically ill patients with cancer. *Critical Care Clinics, 17*(3), 599–622.

Friend, P.H., & Pruett, J. (2004). Bleeding and thrombotic complications. In C.H. Yarbro, M.H. Frogge, & M. Goodman (Eds.), *Cancer symptom management* (3rd ed., pp. 233–251). Sudbury, MA: Jones and Bartlett.

Kwaan, H.C., & Vicuna, B. (2007). Thrombosis and bleeding in cancer patients. *Oncology Reviews, 1*(1), 14–27.

National Cancer Institute Cancer Therapy Evaluation Program. (2006). *Common terminology criteria for adverse events* (version 3.0). Bethesda, MD: National Cancer Institute. Retrieved August 31, 2008, from http://ctep.cancer.gov/protocolDevelopment/electronic_applications/docs/ctcaev3.pdf

Pereira, J., & Phan, T. (2004). Management of bleeding in patients with advanced cancer. *Oncologist, 9*(5), 561–570.

Case Study

   T.S. was a 32-year-old female who was recently diagnosed with acute myeloid leukemia. She was admitted to the hospital for induction therapy with cytarabine and daunorubicin. During her nadir, her platelet count fell to 6,000 (6 × 10^3/microliter). As per the *Recommended for Practice* section of the Oncology Nursing Society (ONS) Putting Evidence Into Practice (PEP) resource on prevention of bleeding, platelet transfusions should be initiated once platelet counts fall below 10,000 (10 × 10^3/microliter). T.S., however, continued to bleed at this level, and as outlined on the ONS PEP resource, her platelet transfusion threshold was pushed up to 20,000 (20 × 10³/microliter) as she was actively bleeding. Keeping her platelet count at this higher level did slow her menstrual bleeding, which finally resolved once her platelet count recovered to above 50,000 (50 × 10³/microliter).

T.S.'s next step was to prepare for bone marrow transplantation (BMT). The nursing staff was concerned about her previous menorrhagia, which started when her platelets dropped below 10,000 (10 × 10³/microliter). Her hemoglobin also dropped, both in response to the marrow-toxic chemotherapy and to her menorrhagia. She did require a number of packed red blood cell transfusions.

The nurses consulted the ONS PEP resource for ideas to minimize T.S.'s menstrual bleeding with her upcoming BMT. Few studies have been done in cancer populations, but the ONS PEP resource cited one small study using leuprolide (Lupron®, TAP Pharmaceuticals) at a dose of 3.75 mg subcutaneous (SC) given at least one month before transplant to prevent menstrual bleeding during the expected prolonged nadir. This was brought to the attention of the physician, and a dose of leuprolide 3.75 mg SC was given prior to T.S.'s discharge from the hospital. She had a few weeks of slight spotting after the leuprolide. She then had another dose 28 days later, which was directly prior to her admission for transplant. She completed the BMT with no further menstrual bleeding. Her platelet transfusion threshold was able to be kept at 10,000 (10 ×10³/microliter), which minimized the number of transfusions required. She ultimately went on to a full remission, with no lasting effects of previous menorrhagia.

Anna D. Schaal, RN, BScN, MS, ARNP
Hematology Nurse Practitioner
Norris Cotton Cancer Center at Dartmouth-Hitchcock Medical Center
Lebanon, NH

Prevention of Bleeding

2009 AUTHORS
Barbara I. Damron, PhD, RN, and Susan M. Samsonow, RN, OCN®
ONS STAFF: Heather Belansky, RN, MSN

2007 AUTHORS
Jeannine M. Brant, RN, MS, AOCN®, Barbara I. Damron, PhD, RN, Patricia J. Friend, PhD, RN, AOCN®,
Michele Lacher, RN, OCN®, Anna D. Schaal, RN, BScN, MS, ARNP, and Susan M. Samsonow, RN
RESEARCH CONSULTANT: Sandra Mitchell, CRNP, MScN, AOCN®
ONS STAFF: Heather Belansky, RN, MSN, and Annette Parry Bush, RN, BSN, MBA, OCN®

What interventions are available to prevent and manage bleeding in patients with cancer?

Recommended for Practice

Interventions for which effectiveness has been demonstrated by strong evidence from rigorously conducted studies, meta-analyses, or systematic reviews and for which expectation of harms is small compared with the benefits

PLATELET THRESHOLDS

Guidelines developed by an expert panel, a Cochrane review, and others (Callow, Swindell, Randall, & Chopra, 2002; Heddle et al., 2006; Stanworth et al., 2004) support the following guidelines for platelet thresholds.
Maintain platelet threshold at 10,000 (10×10^3/microliter) for the majority of patients (e.g., acute leukemia, solid tumors, those undergoing stem cell transplantation).
* Maintain threshold at 20,000 (20×10^3/microliter) for patients undergoing minor procedures and those with bladder tumors, necrotic tumors, and highly vascular tumors that are more likely to bleed.
* Maintain prophylactic threshold at 40,000–50,000 ($40–50 \times 10^3$/microliter) for patients undergoing invasive procedures (e.g., major surgery).

Nurses should assess all patients with thrombocytopenia for frank or occult bleeding and recognize that platelet thresholds may need to be individualized, for example, in patients at risk for hemorrhage and in those with fever, a rapidly declining platelet count, or coagulation abnormalities.

PLATELET TRANSFUSIONS TO CONTROL ACTIVE BLEEDING

Platelet transfusion should be considered in patients with thrombocytopenia who are actively bleeding (Callow et al., 2002; Heddle et al., 2006; Schiffer et al., 2001; Stanworth et al., 2004).

MESNA FOR THE PREVENTION OF HEMORRHAGIC CYSTITIS

Mesna commonly is used in conjunction with ifosfamide to decrease the incidence of urothelial toxicity associated with ifosfamide. The American Society of Clinical Oncology recommends the use of mesna as follows (Schuchter, Hensley, Meropol, & Winer, 2002).

- For ifosfamide doses < 2.5 g/m^2/day administered as a short infusion, the IV dose of mesna is recommended at 60% of the ifosfamide dose and should be given 15 minutes before chemotherapy and then at four and eight hours following each dose of ifosfamide.
- If ifosfamide is given via continuous infusion, then mesna should be given prior to chemotherapy as a bolus dose at 20% of the ifosfamide dose followed by a continuous infusion of mesna at 40% of the ifosfamide dose and continuing for 12–24 hours after the completion of the ifosfamide infusion.
- Evidence is insufficient to recommend a specific dosing regimen for the use of mesna with high-dose ifosfamide in excess of 2.5 g/m^2/day. More frequent and/or prolonged mesna dosing regimens may be necessary to achieve urothelial protection, given the longer half-life of ifosfamide at higher doses.
- Oral mesna may be used as a substitute for the second and third doses of IV mesna when the ifosfamide dose is < 2 g/m^2/day (Mace et al., 2003). When using oral mesna, the first dose should be given via IV at 20% of the ifosfamide dose followed by oral doses of mesna at 40% of the ifosfamide dose two and six hours after chemotherapy administration. The total daily dose of mesna is 100% of the ifosfamide dose. Patients who vomit within two hours of taking oral mesna should have the oral dose repeated or should receive IV mesna. This dosing schedule is repeated on each day that ifosfamide is given.
- Mesna plus saline diuresis or forced saline diuresis commonly is used with cyclophosphamide administration in the stem cell transplantation setting (Schuchter et al., 2002).

Likely to Be Effective

Interventions for which effectiveness has been demonstrated by supportive evidence from a single rigorously conducted controlled trial, consistent supportive evidence from well-designed controlled trials using small samples, or guidelines developed from evidence and supported by expert opinion

There are no interventions as of May 2008.

Benefits Balanced With Harms

Interventions for which clinicians and patients should weigh the beneficial and harmful effects according to individual circumstances and priorities

There are no interventions as of May 2008.

Effectiveness Not Established

Interventions for which insufficient or conflicting data or data of inadequate quality currently exist, with no clear indication of harm

PROHEMOSTATIC AGENTS

Several single-arm trials and small case series reports have described the results of using prohemostatic agents to prevent and manage bleeding in patients with cancer.

- **Desmopressin (DDAVP, 1-desamino-8-D-arginine vasopressin):** A small single-arm pilot study suggested that desmopressin can be a safe and immediately effective option in the treatment and/or prevention of episodes of bleeding in patients experiencing thrombocytopenia associated with hematologic malignancies (Castaman et al., 1997).
- **Epsilon amino-caproic acid (EACA):** In three trials of EACA in different cancer populations, varying outcomes have occurred. In a randomized trial comparing EACA, aprotinin, and a placebo in patients undergoing surgery for a malignancy, blood loss and red blood cell (RBC) transfusion requirements in the two intervention groups were not significantly better compared with those who received the placebo (Amar et al., 2003). The two intervention groups did have significantly lower D-dimer levels than the placebo control group, and the study may not have been sufficiently powered to detect a difference in blood loss or transfusion requirements. In contrast, two small case series reports suggested that EACA was effective in reducing bleeding and decreasing RBC transfusion requirements in patients with thrombocytopenic hemorrhage (Kalmadi, Tiu, Lowe, Jin, & Kalaycio, 2006) and diffuse alveolar hemorrhage (Wanko, Broadwater, Folz, & Chao, 2006).
- **EACA together with tranexamic acid (TA):** In a pilot study (N = 16), the use of EACA together with TA in patients with tumor-associated hemorrhage resulted in cessation of bleeding in 14 of the 16 participants (Dean & Tuffin, 1997).
- **Recombinant activated factor VII (rFVIIa):** Several reports have suggested that rFVIIa may be helpful in preventing or managing bleeding. These reports include a small case series of patients with thrombocytopenia and experiencing uncontrolled hemorrhage (Dean & Tuffin, 1997), a Web-based study of patients from an international database (Brenner et al., 2005), a case study of a patient with acute myeloid leukemia and alveolar hemorrhage (Hicks, Peng, & Gajewski, 2002), and a randomized controlled trial (RCT) of prophylactic administration of rFVIIa in patients undergoing hepatectomy for malignancy (Lodge et al., 2005).
- **TA alone:** A small RCT in patients (N = 38) with acute myeloid leukemia found that the use of TA during consolidation chemotherapy was associated with significantly less bleeding and fewer requirements for platelet transfusion (Shpilberg et al., 1995). However, no difference was reported in the number of bleeding episodes or platelet transfusion requirements when TA was used during the induction phase of therapy.

PLATELET GROWTH FACTORS

Recombinant Interleukin-11 (rhIL-11, Neumega® [Wyeth Pharmaceuticals], Oprelvekin)

rhIL-11 is a megakaryopoietic cytokine that directly stimulates the proliferation and maturation of megakaryocyte progenitors. This results in increased platelet production, decreased need for platelet transfusions (Isaacs et al., 1997; Teplar et al., 1996), higher platelet nadirs (thus avoiding delays between myelosuppressive chemotherapy cycles) (Tsimberidou et al., 2005), and a shorter median time for platelets to reach a threshold of > 100,000 (100×10^3/microliter) (Teplar et al.). Although platelet growth factors may reduce the requirements for platelet transfusions after myelosuppressive chemotherapy in patients who have previously experienced thrombocytopenia, their role in the prevention of bleeding has not been established.

When rhIL-11 is used in practice, the following dosages and guidelines should be followed in accordance with the literature.

- Adult dosage of 50 mcg/kg/day subcutaneous (SC) should be administered 6–24 hours after completion of myelosuppressive chemotherapy and continued for 14–21 days or until the platelet count is ≥ 100,000 (100×10^3/microliter) (Isaacs et al., 1997; Teplar et al., 1996).

- To date, no controlled clinical studies have established a safe and effective dose of rhIL-11 in children. Significant side effects were observed in children at dosages > 50 mcg/kg/day SC (Cairo et al., 2004). Therefore, the administration of Neumega in children, particularly those < 12 years of age, should be restricted to controlled clinical trial settings with closely monitored safety assessments.

The beneficial effects of rhIL-11 should be balanced with its potential side effects and costs (Cantor, Elting, Hudson, & Rubenstein, 2003). Fatigue, cardiac arrhythmias, syncope, transient ischemic attack, mild peripheral edema, conjunctival injection, dyspnea, and pleural effusion have occurred in trials of this agent in adults (Isaacs et al., 1997; Kurzrock et al., 2001; Teplar et al., 1996; Tsimberidou et al., 2005). In children, tachycardia, conjunctival injection, edema, pain, rhinitis, diarrhea, cardiomegaly, papilledema, and periosteal bone changes also have occurred (Cairo et al., 2004).

INTERVENTIONS TO PREVENT OR ATTENUATE MENSTRUAL BLEEDING

Measures to attenuate menstrual bleeding are common in patients receiving cancer treatments expected to induce thrombocytopenia, as defined by World Health Organization guidelines (Amsterdam et al., 2004; Meirow, Rabinovici, Katz, Or, & Ben-Yehuda, 2006). Although the use of hormonal agents prevents menstrual bleeding, few studies have tested these agents in women with cancer who are at high risk for bleeding. In addition, dosages and specific treatment regimens have not been thoroughly investigated. One small study supported using a low dose of Lupron® (TAP Pharmaceuticals) in thrombocytopenic hematopoietic stem cell transplant (HSCT) recipients (Chiusolo et al., 1998). A 3.75 mg SC dose given at least one month before transplantation and again 28 days later prevented menstrual bleeding. Common methods to suppress menstrual bleeding identified in the literature include oral contraceptives, progesterone, progestin intrauterine device, gonadotropin-releasing hormone analogs, and danazol.

INTERVENTIONS TO MANAGE HEMORRHAGIC CYSTITIS

Recombinant Epidermal Growth Hormone (rhEGF) for Urothelial Cytoprotection

rhEGF is a cytoprotective agent that acts as a potent stimulant for cellular repair. One case report described the successful use of rhEGF as a continuous bladder irrigant to treat hemorrhagic cystitis in a patient following HSCT (Dorticus et al., 2003).

Tetrachlorodecaoxygen (TCDO) Anion Complex IV Solution/WF 10 (Oxoferin®, Immunokine™, Macrokine™ [OXO Chemie]) for Radiation-Induced Hemorrhagic Cystitis and/or Proctitis

Three studies have investigated the use of WF 10 (a chlorite-containing agent) to manage radiation-induced hemorrhagic cystitis and proctitis. One RCT (Veerasarn et al., 2004) in patients with cervical cancer and two single-arm studies (Srisupundit et al., 1999; Veerasarn, Boonnuch, & Kakanaporn, 2006) have administered TCDO anion complex 0.5 ml/kg IV over two hours on five consecutive days every three weeks for up to four cycles to treat radiation-induced hemorrhagic cystitis and proctitis. In a single-arm study of patients with endoscopically confirmed late hemorrhagic cystitis and proctitis (Common Terminology Criteria for Adverse Events grades III–IV), 88%–100% had improvement to grade 0–I within three months (Veerasarn, Boonnuch, et al.). Although in the RCT the TCDO anion complex and control groups demonstrated comparable improvement after two cycles of treatment, the TCDO anion complex group experienced significantly fewer late recurrences of hematuria ($p = 0.01$) and used fewer antibiotics and antispasmodics ($p < 0.002$) (Veerasarn, Khorprasert, et al.; Veerasarn, Boonnuch, et al.).

PROCEDURES TO ATTENUATE BLEEDING

Endoscopic Procedures

Several small, descriptive studies described the use of self-expandable metallic stents (SEMS) for patients with esophageal cancer (Iraha et al., 2006; Johnsson, Lundell, & Liedman, 2005; Siersema, 2006; Wenger et al., 2005). Few addressed the use of SEMS in the prevention or management of bleeding directly. One of the studies used SEMS to alleviate dysphagia (Iraha et al.). Another used SEMS to treat esophageal perforations, thereby preventing bleeding (Johnsson et al.). In a different study, researchers performed a meta-analysis examining therapeutic intervention for bleeding esophageal varices, concluding that endoscopic band ligation was the optimal technique for the treatment of varices (Siersema).

ENDOVASCULAR EMBOLIZATION PROCEDURES

One study examined embolization procedures using gelatin sponge particles, steel and/or platinum coils, or a combination of these embolization devices and materials in 10 patients with head and neck tumors who were experiencing oral hemorrhage (Kakizawa, Toyota, Naito, & Ito, 2005). Because open surgical exploration with ligation of the hemorrhaging vessels is difficult and dangerous, in this small study, superselective embolization of the affected arteries with the use of a microcatheter system was shown to be an effective, safe, and repeatable treatment for the control of oral hemorrhage caused by malignant head and neck tumors.

In a retrospective review describing two cases of patients with head and neck cancer presenting with a carotid blowout, the authors noted that management of the carotid blowout with endovascular placement of a covered stent and preliminary endovascular coiling can be successful (Desuter et al., 2005). Bleeding was stopped effectively by the procedure, although both patients developed a postprocedure thromboembolism that necessitated immediate treatment with anticoagulation therapy.

The use of microcoils and microparticles for embolization also has been reported in a retrospective review of seven patients with advanced head and neck cancer (Sesterhenn, Iwinska-Zelder, Dalchow, Bien, & Werner, 2006). The authors reported that all seven patients experienced a decrease in bleeding as a result of the superselective endovascular embolization procedure.

Ultrasonic-Activated Surgical Instruments

Several small case series reports described the application of ultrasonically activated surgical instruments to improve surgical outcomes and reduce bleeding complications and the need for electrocoagulation or suture ligature in patients undergoing breast, head and neck, or hepatic resections for malignancy. Although ultrasound cutting devices may reduce the risk of seroma formation in women with breast cancer undergoing axillary dissection (Lumachi et al., 2004), an uncontrolled study comparing ultrasound dissection with scissors and electrocautery in women undergoing mastectomy with axillary dissection suggested comparable bleeding outcomes (Galatius, Okholm, & Hoffmann, 2003). For patients undergoing hepatic resection for malignancy, one study found that the surgical time and intraoperative blood loss were significantly reduced with the use of an ultrasonically activated scalpel as compared to ultrasonic cavitational aspirator for these patients (Ouchi et al., 2000). Authors in another study reported favorable bleeding outcomes in their small case series examining the use of ultrasonic scissors in 13 consecutive patients undergoing glossectomy for carcinoma of the tongue (Yuen & Wong, 2005).

Effectiveness Unlikely

Interventions for which lack of effectiveness has been demonstrated by negative evidence from a single rigorously conducted controlled trial, consistent negative evidence from well-designed controlled trials using small samples, or guidelines developed from evidence and supported by expert opinion

There are no interventions as of May 2008.

Not Recommended for Practice

Interventions for which lack of effectiveness or harmfulness has been demonstrated by strong evidence from rigorously conducted studies, meta-analyses, or systematic reviews, or interventions where the costs, burden, or harms associated with the intervention exceed anticipated benefit

There are no interventions as of May 2008.

Expert Opinion

Low-risk interventions that are (1) consistent with sound clinical practice, (2) suggested by an expert in a peer-reviewed publication (journal or book chapter), and (3) for which limited evidence exists. An expert is an individual who has published articles in a peer-reviewed journal in the domain of interest.

AMERICAN RED CROSS RECOMMENDATIONS

The American Red Cross integrated new first aid and cardiopulmonary resuscitation guidelines into its training and educational programs in 2006. Control of bleeding is one of the few actions by which a person can critically influence the outcome in a first aid situation. The former recommendation for control of bleeding was to use a combination of direct pressure, elevation, and pressure points to stop the bleeding (American Red Cross, 2005). The guidelines now recommend the application of direct pressure firmly over the bleeding area until bleeding stops or emergency medical service rescuers arrive. The methods of pressure include the following.

- Use manual pressure on gauze or other cloth placed over the source of bleeding, adding more gauze/cloth and pressure if bleeding persists.
- Use an elastic bandage firmly wrapped over gauze to hold it in place with pressure.

INTERVENTIONS TO PREVENT AND MANAGE WOUND AND ORIFICIAL BLEEDING

The following interventions to manage wound and orificial bleeding are supported by expert opinion (Gabay, 2006; McMurray, 2006; Pereira & Phan, 2004; Seaman, 2006).

Wound Care Interventions

- Gentle dressing removal using saline if the dressing adheres to the wound
- Nonadherent or amorphous dressings or moist wound products
- Multiple-layer dressings to prevent wound trauma

- Direct pressure for 10–15 minutes when bleeding does occur
- Packing the wound (nose, vagina, rectum)
- Minimizing the frequency of dressing changes to prevent trauma

Hemostasis Interventions (Gabay, 2006; McMurray, 2006; Pereira & Phan, 2004; Seaman, 2006)

- Gauze saturated with topical vasoconstrictors (epinephrine to control profuse bleeding) or sucralfate paste
- Packing swabs containing hemostatic agents (acetone-soaked packing in vagina or co-caine-soaked packing in nose)
- Topical dressings, including the use of thromboplastin, absorbable gelatin (in nose, rectum, vagina), fibrin sealants, collagen, or alginate
- Vasoconstricting or cauterizing agents (epinephrine, silver nitrate, formalin, alum)

Definitions of the interventions are available at **www.ons.org/outcomes**.
Literature search completed through May 2008.

References

Amar, D., Grant, F.M., Zhang, H., Boland, P.J., Leung, D.H., & Healey, J.A. (2003). Antifibrinolytic therapy and perioperative blood loss in cancer patients undergoing major orthopedic surgery. *Anesthesiology, 98*(2), 337–342.

American Red Cross. (2005). *First aid and CPR guideline changes.* Retrieved December 14, 2006, from http://www.redcross.org/article/0,1072,0_332_4975,00.html

Amsterdam, A., Jakubowski, A., Castro-Malaspina, H., Baxi, E., Kauff, N., Krychman, M., et al. (2004). Treatment of menorrhagia in women undergoing hematopoietic stem cell transplantation. *Bone Marrow Transplantation, 34*(4), 363–366.

Brenner, B., Hoffman, R., Balashov, D., Shutluko, E., Culic, S.D., & Nizamoutdinova, E. (2005). Control of bleeding caused by thrombocytopenia associated with hematologic malignancy: An audit of the clinical use of recombinant activated factor VII. *Clinical and Applied Thrombosis/Hemostasis, 11*(4), 401–410.

Cairo, M.S., Davenport, V., Bessmertny, O., Goldman, S.C., Berg, S.L., Kreissman, S.G., et al. (2004). Phase I/II dose escalation study of recombinant human interleukin-11 following ifosfamide, carboplatin and etoposide in children, adolescents and young adults with solid tumours or lymphoma: A clinical, haematological and biological study. *British Journal of Haematology, 128*(1), 49–58.

Callow, C.R., Swindell, R., Randall, W., & Chopra, R. (2002). The frequency of bleeding complications in patients with haematological malignancy following the introduction of a stringent prophylactic platelet transfusion policy. *British Journal of Haematology, 118*(2), 677–682.

Cantor, S.B., Elting, L.S., Hudson, D.V., Jr., & Rubenstein, E.B. (2003). Pharmacoeconomic analysis of oprelvekin (recombinant human interleukin-11) for secondary prophylaxis of thrombocytopenia in solid tumor patients receiving chemotherapy. *Cancer, 97*(12), 3099–3106.

Castaman, G., Bona, E.D., Schiavotto, C., Trentin, L., D'Emilio, A., & Rodeghiero, F. (1997). Pilot study on the safety and efficacy of desmopressin for the treatment or prevention of bleeding in patients with hematologic malignancies. *Haematologica, 82*(5), 584–587.

Chiusolo, P., Salutari, P., Sica, S., Scirpa, P., Laurenti, L., Piccirillo, N., et al. (1998). Luteinizing hormone-releasing hormone analogue: Leuprorelin acetate for the prevention of menstrual bleeding in premenopausal women undergoing stem cell transplantation. *Bone Marrow Transplantation, 21*(8), 821–823.

Dean, A., & Tuffin, P. (1997). Fibrinolytic inhibitors for cancer-associated bleeding problems. *Journal of Pain and Symptom Management, 13*(1), 20–24.

Desuter, G., Hammer, F., Gerdiner, Q., Gregoire, V., Machiels, J.P., Hamoir, M., et al. (2005). Carotid stenting for impending carotid blowout: Suitable supportive care for head and neck cancer patients. *Palliative Medicine, 19*(5), 427–429.

Dorticus, E., Pavon, V., Jaime, J.C., Reboredo, M., Lopez Saura, P., Berlanga, J., et al. (2003). Successful application of epidermal growth factor for treatment of hemorrhagic cystitis after bone marrow transplantation. *Bone Marrow Transplantation, 31*(7), 615–616.

Gabay, M. (2006). Absorbable hemostatic agents. *American Journal of Health-System Pharmacy, 63*(13), 1244–1253.

Galatius, H., Okholm, M., & Hoffmann, J. (2003). Mastectomy using ultrasonic dissection: Effect on seroma formation. *Breast, 12*(5), 338–341.

Heddle, N.M., Cook, R.J., Sigouin, C., Slichter, S.J., Murphy, M., & Rebulla, P. (2006). A descriptive analysis of international transfusion practice and bleeding outcomes in patients with acute leukemia. *Transfusion, 46*(6), 903–911.

Hicks, K., Peng, D., & Gajewski, J.L. (2002). Treatment of diffuse alveolar hemorrhage after allogeneic bone marrow transplant with recombinant factor VIIa. *Bone Marrow Transplantation, 30*(12), 975–978.

Iraha, Y., Murayama, S., Toita, T., Utsunomiya, T., Nagata, O., Akamine, T., et al. (2006). Self-expandable metallic stent placement for patients with inoperable esophageal carcinoma: Investigation of the influence of prior radiotherapy and chemotherapy. *Radiation Medicine, 24*(4), 247–252.

Isaacs, C., Robert, N.J., Bailey, F.A., Schuster, M.W., Overmoyer, B., Graham, M., et al. (1997). Randomized placebo-controlled study of recombinant human interleukin-11 to prevent chemotherapy-induced thrombocytopenia in patients with breast cancer receiving dose-intensive cyclophosphamide and doxorubicin. *Journal of Clinical Oncology, 15*(11), 3368–3377.

Johnsson, E., Lundell, L., & Liedman, B. (2005). Sealing of esophageal perforation or ruptures with expandable metallic stent prospective controlled study on treatment efficacy and limitations. *Diseases of the Esophagus, 18*(4), 262–266.

Kakizawa, H., Toyota, N., Naito, A., & Ito, K. (2005). Endovascular therapy for management of oral hemorrhage in malignant head and neck tumors. *Cardiovascular and Interventional Radiology, 28*(6), 722–729.

Kalmadi, S., Tiu, R., Lowe, C., Jin, T., & Kalaycio, M. (2006). Epsilon aminocaproic acid reduces transfusion requirements in patients with thrombocytopenic hemorrhage. *Cancer, 107*(1), 136–140.

Kurzrock, R., Cortes, J., Thomas, D.A., Jeha, S., Pilat, S., & Talpaz, M. (2001). Pilot study of low-dose interleukin-11 in patients with bone marrow failure. *Journal of Clinical Oncology, 19*(21), 4165–4172.

Lodge, J.P., Jonas, S., Oussoultzoglou, E., Malago, M., Jayr, C., Cherqui, D., et al. (2005). Recombinant coagulation factor VIIa in major liver resection: A randomized placebo-controlled, double-blind clinical trial. *Anesthesiology, 102*(2), 269–275.

Lumachi, F., Brandes, A.A., Burellin, P., Basso, S.M., Iacobone, M., & Ermani, M. (2004). Seroma prevention following axillary dissection in patients with breast cancer by using ultrasound scissors: A prospective study. *Journal of Cancer Surgery, 30*(5), 526–530.

Mace, J.R., Keohan, M.L., Bernardy, H., Junge, K., Niebch, G., Romeis, P., et al. (2003). Crossover randomized comparison of intravenous versus intravenous/oral mesna in soft tissue sarcoma treated with high-dose ifosfamide. *Clinical Cancer Research, 9*(16, Pt. 1), 5829–5834.

McMurray, V. (2006). Managing bleeding malignant skin lesions. *Nursing Times, 102*(5), 58–60.

Meirow, D., Rabinovici, J., Katz, D., Or, R., & Ben-Yehuda, D. (2006). Prevention of severe menorrhagia in oncology patients with treatment-induced thrombocytopenia by luteinizing hormone-releasing hormone agonist and depo-medroxyprogesterone acetate. *Cancer, 107*(7), 1634–1641.

Ouchi, K., Mikuni, J., Sugawara, T., Ono, H., Fujiya, T., Kamiyama, Y., et al. (2000). Hepatectomy using an ultrasonically activated scalpel for hepatocellular carcinoma. *Digestive Surgery, 17*(2), 138–142.

Pereira, J., & Phan, T. (2004). Management of bleeding in patients with advanced cancer. *Oncologist, 9*(5), 561–570.

Schiffer, C.A., Anderson, K.C., Bennett, C.L., Bernstein, S., Elting, L.S., Goldsmith, M., et al. (2001). Platelet transfusion for patients with cancer: Clinical practice guidelines of the American Society of Clinical Oncology. *Journal of Clinical Oncology, 19*(5), 1519–1538.

Schuchter, L.M., Hensley, M.L., Meropol, N.J., & Winer, E.P. (2002). 2002 update of recommendations for the use of chemotherapy and radiotherapy protectants: Clinical practice guidelines of the American Society of Clinical Oncology. *Journal of Clinical Oncology, 20*(12), 2895–2903.

Seaman, S. (2006). Management of malignant fungating wounds in advanced cancer. *Seminars in Oncology Nursing, 22*(3), 185–193.

Sesterhenn, A.M., Iwinska-Zelder, J., Dalchow, C.V., Bien, S., & Werner, J.A. (2006). Acute haemorrhage in patients with advanced head and neck cancer: Value of endovascular therapy as palliative treatment option. *Journal of Laryngology and Otology, 120*(2), 117–124.

Shpilberg, O., Blumenthal, R., Sofer, O., Katz, Y., Chetrit, A., Ramot, B., et al. (1995). A controlled trial of tranexamic acid therapy for the reduction of bleeding during treatment of acute myeloid leukemia. *Leukemia and Lymphoma, 19*(1–2), 141–144.

Siersema, P.D. (2006). Therapeutic esophageal interventions for dysphagia and bleeding. *Current Opinion in Gastroenterology, 22*(4), 442–447.

Srisupundit, S., Kraiphibul, P., Sangruchi, S., Linasmita, V., Chinmgskol, K., & Veerasarn, V. (1999). The efficacy of chemically-stabilized chlorite-matrix (TCDO) in the management of late post radiation cystitis. *Journal of the Medical Association of Thailand, 82*(8), 798–802.

Stanworth, S.J., Hyde, C., Heddle, N., Rebulla, P., Brunskill, S., & Murphy, M.F. (2004). Prophylactic platelet transfusion for haemorrhage after chemotherapy and stem cell transplantation. *Cochrane Database of Systematic Reviews* 2004, Issue 4. Art. No.: CD004269. DOI: 10.1002/14651858.CD004269.pub2.

Teplar, I., Elias, L., Smith, J.W., Hussein, M., Rosen, G., Chang, A.Y., et al. (1996). A randomized placebo-controlled trial of recombinant human interleukin-11 in cancer patients with severe thrombocytopenia due to chemotherapy. *Blood, 87*(9), 3607–3614.

Tsimberidou, A.M., Giles, F.J., Khouri, I., Bueso-Ramos, C., Pilat, S., Thomas, D.A., et al. (2005). Low-dose interleukin-11 in patients with bone marrow failure: Update of the M.D. Anderson Cancer Center experience. *Annals of Oncology, 16*(1), 139–145.

Veerasarn, V., Boonnuch, W., & Kakanaporn, C. (2006). A phase II study to evaluate WF10 in patients with late hemorrhagic radiation cystitis and proctitis. *Gynecologic Oncology, 100*(1), 179–184.

Veerasarn, V., Khorprasert, C., Lorvidhaya, V., Sangruchi, S., Tantivatana, T., Narkwong, L., et al. (2004). Reduced recurrence of late hemorrhagic radiation cystitis by WF10 therapy in cervical cancer patients: A multicenter, randomized, two-arm, open-label trial. *Radiotherapy and Oncology, 73*(2), 179–185.

Wanko, S.O., Broadwater, G., Folz, R.J., & Chao, N.J. (2006). Diffuse alveolar hemorrhage: Retrospective review of clinical outcome in allogeneic transplant recipients treated with aminocaproic acid. *Biology of Blood and Marrow Transplantation, 12*(9), 949–953.

Wenger, U., Johnsson, E., Bergquist, H., Nyman, J., Ejnell, H., Lagergren, J., et al. (2005). Health economic evaluation of stent or endoluminal brachytherapy as a palliative strategy in patients with incurable cancer of the oesophagus or gastro-oesophageal junction: Results of a randomized clinical trial. *European Journal of Gastroenterology and Hepatology, 17*(12), 1369–1377.

Yuen, A.P.-W., & Wong, B.Y.-H. (2005). Ultrasonic glossectomy—Simple and bloodless. *Head and Neck, 27*(8), 690–695.

CHAPTER 17

Prevention of Infection

Problem

Patients with cancer may be immunocompromised because of their malignancy or the treatment of their malignancy, resulting in susceptibility to specific pathogens. The prevention of infection in patients with cancer focuses on interventions to prevent infections related to neutropenia or other immune deficiency related to malignancy or the treatment of malignancy. Literature specific to hematopoietic stem cell transplant (HSCT) recipients was excluded from the review, as this population has a unique profile of immunodeficiency, and interventions specific to HSCT recipients are well described elsewhere. Select references to HSCT recipients were included if they were cited in general guidelines for patients with cancer.

Incidence

Many treatments for cancer, including chemotherapy, radiation therapy, surgery, and biologic therapy, are known to put patients at risk for significant infection. The compromised immune function caused by these treatments can affect morbidity and mortality. Febrile neutropenia, in particular, is a recognized entity that requires attention to risk assessment to provide the best evidence-based management. Fever in patients with cancer can be due to infection (80%) or tumor (20%). The risk of infection is associated with the degree of neutropenia and for the length of the neutropenic period. More than 60% of neutropenic patients will become infected. Bacterial infections are the most common type of infection in febrile neutropenic patients, whereas fungal infections are the most common cause of fatal infections (Segal, Walsh, & Holland, 2001).

Infectious complications can affect overall quality of life and have an economic impact on patients, families, and hospital systems. Infection is a preventable adverse event that has significant safety concerns. It is a common and challenging clinical problem that is a high-priority nursing-sensitive area in which to affect patient outcomes.

Assessment

Assessment of patients who are likely to become immunocompromised includes a thorough review of risk factors, physical examination, and diagnostic evaluation. Table

17-1 identifies common risk factors for patients who will be susceptible to infection and neutropenia. Patients should be assessed prior to therapy and at regular intervals during therapy. Clinical evaluations are best done in person, although often patients with cancer are initially assessed by telephone.

Table 17-1. Risk Factors to Be Assessed for Neutropenia		
Risk Factor	**Yes**	**No**
Comorbidities		
Chronic obstructive pulmonary disease		
Cardiovascular disease		
Liver disease		
Renal insufficiency		
Diabetes mellitus		
Baseline anemia		
Patient Related		
Increased age (> 65 years)		
Female sex		
Poor performance status (Eastern Cooperative Oncology Group ≥ 2)		
Poor nutritional status		
Decreased immune function		
Decreased body surface area		
Inpatient versus outpatient		
Cancer Related		
Bone marrow involvement of tumor		
Advanced cancer		
Type of malignancy: leukemia, lymphoma, lung cancer		
Elevated lactate dehydrogenase level (especially with non-Hodgkin lymphoma)		
Treatment Related		
Previous chemotherapy and type (specify)_____		
Planned relative dose intensity		
Concurrent or prior irradiation to marrow		
Preexisting neutropenia (prolonged)		

(Continued on next page)

Table 17-1. Risk Factors to Be Assessed for Neutropenia *(Continued)*		
Risk Factor	**Yes**	**No**
History of severe neutropenia with chemotherapy		
Conditions With Increased Risk		
Open wounds		
Active infection		
Mucositis (Common Terminology Criteria for Adverse Events grades 3–4)		
Physical Examination		
Head to toe assessment, with high-risk areas for infection, perirectal area, oral mucosa, sinuses, lung, skin, and indwelling catheter sites		
Diagnostic Evaluation		
Complete blood count/differential, blood and other cultures, chemistry profile, chest x-ray		
Note. Based on information from Klastersky et al., 2000; Maxwell & Stein, 2006; Wujcik, 2004.		

Clinical Measurement Tools

Dilemmas exist when considering measurement tools for the prevention of infection. Data regarding measurement techniques of infection are scant. This is partly because of the heterogenicity of infection; however, very little empirical evidence exists on how clinicians and scientists should measure infection from a quality perspective and the frequency of measurement (Friese, 2004, 2007). In the past, the National Quality Forum (NQF) has endorsed performance measures for cancer care at the institutional level (i.e., hospital, health plan) but not at the clinician level. In 2003, NQF endorsed a set of 15 consensus-based nursing-sensitive standards for inpatient care. Although not specific to cancer care, preliminary data exist regarding catheter-related infections per 1,000 days and urinary catheter-related infections to support measurement, education, and standards of care (NQF, 2007).

The Multinational Association of Supportive Care in Cancer (MASCC) risk index is an internationally validated scoring system to stratify patients with febrile neutropenia into low-risk and high-risk groups. A number of variables such as age, outpatient status, comorbid conditions, burden of illness, and tumor type are assigned weighted numerical values. A risk index score ≤ 21 identifies low-risk individuals, and a score > 21 identifies high-risk patients. Additional research is contributing to data that are necessary to determine low-risk patients and treatment strategies (Baskaran, Gran, & Adeeba, 2008; De Souza, Serufo, Rocha, Costa, & Duarte, 2008; Klastersky et al., 2000).

The National Comprehensive Cancer Network (NCCN) has developed guidelines to assist clinicians in the management of fever and neutropenia for infection in patients with cancer (NCCN, 2009) and for use of myeloid growth factors (NCCN, 2008). Although the primary focus is on management of infection, attention to stratification of risk and assessment in both guidelines is helpful in practice. The identification of risk factors that have been associated with poorer clinical outcomes is critical in assessment and selection of interventions to prevent and manage infection.

The Patient Care Monitor–Neutropenia Index and the Functional Assessment of Cancer Therapy–Neutropenia are examples of quality-of-life instruments that are reliable and sensitive related to febrile neutropenia in limited studies. Further data are needed to determine the clinical utility of these tools for use as outcome measures, risk assessment, and documentation tools (Moore, Johnson, Fortner, & Houts, 2008; Padilla & Ropka, 2005).

Although not a measurement of infection, the Common Terminology Criteria for Adverse Events (National Cancer Institute Cancer Therapy Evaluation Program, 2006) often is used as a tool for grading white blood cell count and absolute neutrophil count (see Table 17-2). The tool is used in clinical trials and daily oncology practice but does not correlate directly with the incidence of infection. Therefore, it is not a tool that is suitable for clinical management of febrile neutropenia.

Table 17-2. Common Terminology Criteria for Adverse Events for Neutropenia	
Grade	**Criteria (Neutrophil Count)**
1	$< LLN–1,500/mm^3$; $< LLN– 1.5 \times 10^9/L$
2	$< 1,500–1,000/mm^3$; $< 1.5–1.0 \times 10^9/L$
3	$< 1,000–500/mm^3$; $< 1.0–0.5 \times 10^9/L$
4	$< 500/mm^3$; $< 0.5 \times 10^9/L$
5	Death

LLN—lower limit of normal

Note. Based on information from National Cancer Institute Cancer Therapy Evaluation Program, 2006.

References

Baskaran, N.D., Gan, G.G., & Adeeba, K. (2008). Applying the Multinational Association for Supportive Care in Cancer risk scoring in predicting outcome of febrile neutropenia patients in a cohort of patients. *Annals of Hematology, 87*(7), 563–569.

De Souza, L., Serufo, J.C., Rocha, M.O., Costa, R.N., & Duarte, R.C. (2008). Performance of a modified MASCC index score for identifying low-risk febrile neutropenic cancer patients. *Supportive Care in Cancer, 16*(7), 841–846.

Friese, C.R. (2004). *Measuring oncology nursing-sensitive patient outcomes: Evidence-based summary: Prevention of infection.* Retrieved August 31, 2008, from http://www.ons.org/outcomes/measures/prevention.shtml

Friese, C.R. (2007). Prevention of infection in patients with cancer. *Seminars in Oncology Nursing, 23*(3), 174–183.

Klastersky, J., Paesmans, M., Rubenstein, E.J., Boyer, M., Elting, L., Feld, R., et al. (2000). The Multinational Association for Supportive Care in Cancer risk index: A multinational scoring system for identifying low-risk febrile neutropenic cancer patients. *Journal of Clinical Oncology, 18*(16), 3038–3051.

Maxwell, C., & Stein, A. (2006). Implementing evidence-based guidelines for preventing chemotherapy-induced neutropenia: From paper to clinical practice. *Community Oncology, 3*(8), 530–536.

Moore, K., Johnson, G., Fortner, B.V., & Houts, A.C. (2008). The AIM Higher Initiative: New procedures implemented for assessment, information, and management of chemotherapy toxicities in community oncology clinics. *Clinical Journal of Oncology Nursing, 12*(2), 229–238.

National Cancer Institute Cancer Therapy Evaluation Program. (2006). *Common terminology criteria for adverse events* (version 3.0). Bethesda, MD: National Cancer Institute. Retrieved August 31, 2008, from http://ctep.cancer.gov/protocolDevelopment/electronic_applications/docs/ctcaev3.pdf

National Comprehensive Cancer Network. (2009). *Clinical Practice Guidelines in Oncology™: Myeloid growth factors* [v.1.2009]. Retrieved December 21, 2008, from http://www.nccn.org/professionals/physician/PDF/myeloid_growth.pdf

National Comprehensive Cancer Network. (2008). *Clinical Practice Guidelines in Oncology™: Prevention and treatment of cancer-related infections* [v.1.2008]. Retrieved August 31, 2008, from http://www.nccn.org/professionals/physician_gls/PDF/infections.pdf

National Quality Forum. (2007). *Nursing performance measurement and reporting: A status report*. Retrieved August 31, 2008, from http://www.qualityforum.org/pdf/Issue_Brief_Nursing_Performance.pdf

Padilla, G., & Ropka, M.E. (2005). Quality of life and chemotherapy-induced neutropenia. *Cancer Nursing, 28*(3), 167–171.

Segal, B.H., Walsh, T.J., & Holland, S.M. (2001). Infections in the cancer patient. In V.T. DeVita Jr., S. Hellman, & S.A. Rosenberg (Eds.), *Cancer: Principles and practice of oncology* (6th ed., pp. 2815–2868). Philadelphia: Lippincott Williams & Wilkins.

Wujcik, D. (2004). Infection. In C.H. Yarbro, M.H. Frogge, & M. Goodman (Eds.), *Cancer symptom management* (3rd ed., pp. 252–275). Sudbury, MA: Jones and Bartlett.

Clinical Example

Prevention of Infection: How Strict Is Too Strict?

Precautions to prevent infection are instrumental to prevent infection-related morbidity and mortality in neutropenic patients. But how strict is too strict? This question was continually raised by nurses at Northwestern Memorial Hospital (NMH) in Chicago, IL. In particular, the nurses were concerned that patients' diets were restricted during a time when nutrition was of the utmost importance. After chemotherapy, patients often lose taste for many of their favorite foods, and all they want instead is a nice salad or some fruit. However, the neutropenic diet restrictions prevented patients with neutropenia from eating uncooked fruits or vegetables. The nurses questioned the evidence supporting the effectiveness of this restriction, thus leading to an evidence-based practice review.

First, a journal club was convened that included nurses, dietitians, and infection control staff. The Oncology Nursing Society (ONS) Putting Evidence Into Practice (PEP) resource on prevention of infection was invaluable to guide the discussion. Using the information and references cited on the resource, the group reviewed the current research surrounding dietary restrictions for patients with neutropenia. The 2006 version of the ONS PEP information categorizes diet modification for neutropenic patients as *Effectiveness Not Established*, which indicates that insufficient data or inadequate quality of data exist to recommend the intervention. Several studies showed that no link existed between dietary restrictions and risk of infection for neutropenic patients. However, as stated on the ONS PEP resource, taking general precautions such as avoiding uncooked meats, seafood, and eggs may be wise. Teaching patients to wash any fresh fruits and vegetables once they are home also is advisable. At NMH, as in most hospitals, all fresh fruits and vegetables are cleaned with a chlorination system, rendering them safe for consumption.

The next step was to attempt to change the policy, which was not an easy task at such a large institution. The proposal was presented to practice committees, infection control committees, and physician groups. There was resistance to change from some members of these groups who were concerned that reducing the level of restrictions would increase the incidence of infection from foods consumed. Armed with the information from the journal club and the references cited on the ONS PEP resource, solid evidence was presented, not simply opinion. During the discussion of the evidence, one physician presented an article that showed the meat of Roma tomatoes may increase risk of infection. By generally accepted standards to assess the quality of research studies, the study design and results did not provide high-level or high-quality evidence. However, a compromise was necessary to achieve consensus among the physicians, and after much discussion and several revisions, the neutropenic policy at NMH was changed. Now patients can enjoy fresh fruits and vegetables, other than tomatoes, whenever they choose. This was the first of many times that nurses would have a question, pull out their arsenal of evidence included in the ONS PEP resources, and decide what the best practice truly was based on the research.

Colleen O'Leary, RN, MSN, OCN®, AOCNS®
Registered Nurse, Staff Educator, Medical Oncology
Northwestern Memorial Hospital
Chicago, IL

Prevention of Infection

2009 AUTHORS
Laura Zitella, RN, MS, NP, AOCN®, Barbara Holmes Gobel, MS, RN, AOCN®,
and Colleen O'Leary, RN, MSN, AOCNS®
ONS STAFF: Heather Belansky, RN, MSN

2006 AUTHORS
Laura Zitella, RN, MS, NP, AOCN®, Christopher R. Friese, PhD, MS, RN, AOCN®,
Barbara Holmes Gobel, MS, RN, AOCN®, Myra Woolery, RN, MN,
Colleen O'Leary, RN, BSN, OCN®, Jody Hauser, RN, MS, NP, and Felicia Andrews, RN, BSN
ONS STAFF: Barbara G. Lubejko, MS, RN

What interventions are effective in preventing infection in people with cancer?

Recommended for Practice

Interventions for which effectiveness has been demonstrated by strong evidence from rigorously conducted studies, meta-analyses, or systematic reviews and for which expectation of harms is small compared with the benefits

Hand hygiene using soap and water or an antiseptic hand rub for all patients with cancer and their caregivers (Boyce, Pittet, & Healthcare Infection Control Practices Advisory Committee, 2002; Hilburn, Hammond, Fendler, & Groziak, 2003; Mank & van der Lelie, 2003; Sehulster & Chinn, 2003; Shelton, 2003; Siegel, Rhinehart, Jackson, Chiarello, & Healthcare Infection Control Practices Advisory Committee, 2007; Tablan, Anderson, Besser, Bridges, & Hajjeh, 2004; Wilson, 2002)

- Wash hands with soap and water, especially if hands are visibly soiled or contaminated with proteinaceous material.
- Use either soap and water or alcohol-based hand rubs when hands are not visibly soiled or contaminated.
- Hands may remain colonized with microorganisms after hand washing if hands are not dried properly.
- Spore-forming bacteria are not killed by alcohol, so the most effective way to remove them from hands is by washing with soap and water. Therefore, when caring for patients with spore-forming bacterial infections, such as *Clostridium difficile* or *Bacillus* species, perform hand hygiene with soap and water rather than with alcohol-based hand rubs.
- Do not wear artificial fingernails.

Colony-stimulating factors (CSFs) for all patients with cancer undergoing chemotherapy with ≥ 20% risk of febrile neutropenia (Aapro et al., 2006; Bohlius, Herbst, Reiser, Schwarzer, & Engert, 2008; Kuderer, Dale, Crawford, & Lyman, 2007; Lyman, Kuderer, Agboola, & Balducci, 2003; Lyman, Kuderer, & Djulbegovic, 2002; National Comprehensive Cancer Network [NCCN], 2007, 2008; Shelton, 2003; Sung, Nathan, Alibhai, Tomlinson, & Beyene, 2007; Sung, Nathan, Lange, Beyene, & Buchanan, 2004)

- CSFs may be considered in patients with cancer undergoing chemotherapy with a 10%–20% risk of febrile neutropenia if the patient has other risk factors such as age, comorbidities, previous history of febrile neutropenia, disease factors, or treatment variables that increase the risk of febrile neutropenia or other complications from neutropenia.
- CSFs have been shown to decrease the risk of neutropenia, febrile neutropenia, infection, and duration of hospitalization in adult and pediatric patients with cancer who are undergoing chemotherapy, but there is conflicting evidence as to whether CSFs impact infection-related mortality or overall survival. Four large meta-analyses showed that CSFs did not decrease infection-related mortality or overall mortality (Bohlius et al., 2008; Lyman et al., 2002; Sung et al., 2004, 2007), whereas one small meta-analysis showed decreased infection-related mortality and overall mortality with the use of prophylactic CSFs (Kuderer et al., 2007).

Influenza vaccine annually for all patients with cancer (NCCN, 2007; Ring, Marx, Steer, & Harper, 2002; Tablan et al., 2004)

- Although influenza infection is a potential cause of serious infection in patients with cancer, the rate of influenza vaccination among the oncology population is low. Several studies have suggested similar immune responses in patients with cancer and healthy controls, whereas other studies have suggested that serologic responses may be lower in immunocompromised patients, especially if they are undergoing chemotherapy. Because a percentage of patients will achieve protection from the vaccination and the risk for adverse effects is low, all patients with cancer and their household contacts should receive annual vaccination. The timing and efficacy of influenza vaccination has not been clearly established; however, NCCN recommends vaccination at least two weeks prior to cytotoxic or immunosuppressive therapy. If this is not possible, patients can be vaccinated during treatment and revaccinated at least three months after therapy is discontinued.

23-valent pneumococcal polysaccharide vaccine for all patients with cancer older than five years of age and 7-valent pneumococcal polysaccharide protein-conjugate vaccine for all patients with cancer younger than five years of age (NCCN, 2007; Tablan et al., 2004)

- Patients should be revaccinated five years after initial vaccination.
- NCCN recommends vaccination at least two weeks before cytotoxic or immunosuppressive therapy. If this is not possible, patients can be vaccinated during treatment and revaccinated at least three months after therapy is discontinued.
- Pneumococcal vaccination, in addition to meningococcal and *Haemophilus influenzae* type b vaccination, should occur at least two weeks prior to elective splenectomy.

Trimethoprim-sulfamethoxazole (TMP-SMZ) to prevent Pneumocystis carinii *pneumonia (PCP) for all patients at risk* (Hughes et al., 2002; NCCN, 2007)

- High-risk patients include patients receiving prolonged steroid treatment ($\geq$ 20 mg prednisone or equivalent daily for $\geq$ four weeks), patients with acute leukemia, patients receiving alemtuzumab or T-cell–depleting agents, patients receiving temozolomide and radiation therapy, and hematopoietic stem cell transplant (HSCT) recipients.
- Consider TMP-SMZ desensitization, atovaquone, dapsone, or aerosolized pentamidine when PCP (recently renamed as *Pneumocystis jiroveci*) prophylaxis is required and patients are allergic to or intolerant of TMP-SMZ.

Antifungal drugs absorbed or partially absorbed from the gastrointestinal (GI) tract to prevent oral candidiasis in patients with cancer undergoing chemotherapy (Clarkson, Worthington, & Eden, 2007)

- Antifungal drugs absorbed from the GI tract (fluconazole, ketoconazole, and itraconazole) or partially absorbed from the GI tract (miconazole and clotrimazole) prevented oral candidiasis.
- Antifungal drugs not absorbed from the GI tract (amphotericin B, nystatin, nystatin plus chlorhexidine, thymostimulin, amphotericin B plus nystatin, polyenes, natamycin, and norfloxacin plus amphotericin B) did not prevent oral candidiasis.
- No clear consensus exists regarding the population of patients that require prophylaxis for oral candidiasis; however, it may be considered for patients who are at risk for mucositis, patients receiving prolonged steroid treatment (≥ 20 mg prednisone or equivalent daily for ≥ four weeks), patients with acute leukemia, patients receiving alemtuzumab or T-cell–depleting agents, patients receiving temozolomide and radiation therapy, and HSCT recipients.

Antifungal prophylaxis to prevent fungal infections in high-risk patients

- In general, antifungal prophylaxis is not recommended for all neutropenic patients with cancer; however, it is recommended for high-risk patients such as those with acute leukemia, patients with myelodysplastic syndromes, patients undergoing HSCT, or patients with graft-versus-host disease (GVHD) (Bow et al., 2002; Cornely, Ullmann, & Karthaus, 2003; Glasmacher et al., 2003; Gotzsche & Johansen, 2002; Hughes et al., 2002; Kanda et al., 2000; NCCN, 2007).
- Effective agents include fluconazole (Bow et al., 2002; Cornely et al., 2003; Gotzsche & Johansen, 2002; Kanda et al., 2000; NCCN, 2007), posaconazole (Cornely et al., 2007; NCCN, 2007), voriconazole (NCCN, 2007), echinocandins (NCCN, 2007), oral itraconazole suspension (Cornely et al., 2003; Glasmacher et al., 2003; Gotzsche & Johansen; NCCN, 2007), itraconazole IV (Bow et al.; Cornely et al., 2003; Glasmacher et al.; Gotzsche & Johansen), or IV amphotericin B (Bow et al.; Cornely et al., 2003; Gotzsche & Johansen; Johansen & Gotzsche, 2000, 2002; NCCN, 2007). Lipid-based formulations of IV amphotericin B may increase efficacy of amphotericin because of increased patient tolerability (Johansen & Gotzsche, 2000). Itraconazole capsules are not effective (Glasmacher et al.).
- Meta-analyses indicate that IV amphotericin B is the only antifungal agent proven to significantly decrease overall mortality when used as prophylactic or empirical antifungal therapy in high-risk neutropenic patients with cancer (Gotzsche & Johansen, 2002; Johansen & Gotzsche, 2002).

Antibacterial prophylaxis with quinolones for patients at high risk for infection

- Quinolones (e.g., ciprofloxacin 500–750 mg BID for 7 days or levofloxacin 500 mg QD for 7 days) are recommended for the prevention of infection in high-risk afebrile neutropenic patients after chemotherapy (Bucaneve et al., 2005; Cruciani et al., 1996; Cullen, Billingham, Gaunt, & Steven, 2007; Cullen et al., 2005; Engels, Lau, & Barza, 1998; Gafter-Gvili, Fraser, Paul, & Leibovici, 2005; Gafter-Gvili, Fraser, Paul, van de Wetering, et al., 2005; NCCN, 2007; Shelton, 2003; van de Wetering et al., 2005). Patients at high risk for infection include patients with hematologic malignancies, HSCT recipients, patients receiving purine analogs, or patients expected to have neutropenia for more than seven days. Most of the patients evaluated in clinical trials had hematologic malignancies or were undergoing HSCT, although one recent randomized controlled trial demonstrated a decreased rate of infection in patients with solid tumors undergoing chemotherapy (Cullen et al., 2005). Nonetheless, controversy exists regarding its use in low-risk patients, such as those with solid tumors, because of concerns about antibiotic resistance (Bucaneve et al.; Cruciani et al., 1996; Cullen et al., 2005; Engels et al.; Gafter-Gvili, Fraser, Paul, & Leibovici, 2005; Gafter-Gvili, Fraser, Paul, van de Wetering, et al., 2005; Gafter-Gvili, Paul, Fraser, & Leibovici, 2007; Hughes et al., 2002; NCCN, 2007; van de Wetering et al.). The benefit of antibiotic prophylaxis if patients are receiving CSFs requires further study (Lalami et al., 2004).

Penicillin prophylaxis to prevent pneumococcal infection for patients who have undergone splenectomy or who are functionally asplenic, allogeneic HSCT recipients, and patients with chronic GVHD (NCCN, 2007)

- Penicillin prophylaxis should continue for at least five years after splenectomy, at least one year after allogeneic HSCT, and until immunosuppressive therapy is discontinued in patients with chronic GVHD.
- Daily double-strength TMP-SMZ also may be used for prophylaxis.

Herpes viral prophylaxis for selected seropositive patients with cancer (NCCN, 2007)

- During cytotoxic therapy–induced neutropenia in patients with cancer who have had prior reactivations requiring treatment
- During cytotoxic therapy–induced neutropenia in patients with lymphoma, multiple myeloma, or chronic lymphocytic leukemia
- Patients receiving T-cell–depleting agents (i.e., fludarabine, 2-CdA)
- During autologous or allogeneic HSCT until day 30 post-transplant
- During induction or reinduction therapy for acute leukemia through the neutropenic period
- During treatment with alemtuzumab for a minimum of two months after treatment and until CD4 count ≥ 200 cells/microliter.

Cytomegalovirus prophylaxis for patients at high risk for disease (NCCN, 2007)

- Allogeneic HSCT recipients
- Patients treated with alemtuzumab

Hepatitis B prophylaxis with lamivudine is indicated for immunocompromised patients with positive hepatitis B surface antigen (NCCN, 2007).

Protective gowns should be worn if contamination of clothing with blood, body fluids, secretions, or excretions is anticipated (Siegel et al., 2007; Tablan et al., 2004).

Gloves should be worn for direct patient care or if contamination of hands with blood, body fluids, secretions, or excretions is anticipated (Siegel et al., 2007).

Do not allow visitors with symptoms of respiratory infections (Siegel et al., 2007; Tablan et al., 2004).

Environmental interventions (Sehulster & Chinn, 2003; Siegel et al., 2007)

- Keep windows closed.
- Patients with airborne respiratory viruses (e.g., varicella, tuberculosis) should be placed in rooms equipped with an anteroom to maintain proper air balance. High-efficiency particulate air (HEPA) filters should be used for air recirculation. Portable HEPA filters should be used when anterooms are not available.

- Negative-pressure rooms should be used for patients with documented or suspected airborne infections or viral hemorrhagic fever.

Contact precautions for all patients known to be colonized or infected with multidrug-resistant organisms (Montecalvo et al., 1999; Shaikh et al., 2002; Siegel, Rhinehart, Jackson, Chiarello, & Healthcare Infection Control Practices Advisory Committee, 2006; Siegel et al., 2007; Srinivasan et al., 2002)

- In addition to contact precautions, nonrandomized single-institution studies have suggested that enhanced infection control measures may decrease the transmission of vancomycin-resistant enterococci. Interventions evaluated included contact isolation, limiting the use of empiric vancomycin, spatial separation of patients based on vancomycin-resistant enterococci status, infection control surveillance, and staff and patient education. Multiple interventions were implemented simultaneously, so the effect of each intervention is unknown (Montecalvo et al., 1999; Shaikh et al., 2002; Srinivasan et al., 2002).

Likely to Be Effective

Interventions for which effectiveness has been demonstrated by supportive evidence from a single rigorously conducted controlled trial, consistent supportive evidence from well-designed controlled trials using small samples, or guidelines developed from evidence and supported by expert opinion

Private rooms to decrease the transmission of infection (Chaudhury, Mahmood, & Valente, 2003; Siegel et al., 2007)

Oxygen and respiratory care (Tablan et al., 2004)

- Oxygen humidifiers: Change the humidifier tubing, nasal prongs, and/or mask when it malfunctions or becomes visibly contaminated.
- Small-volume medication nebulizers: (1) Disinfect, rinse with sterile water, and dry between uses on the same patient; (2) use only sterile fluid for nebulization, and dispense fluid aseptically; (3) single-dose dispensing is preferred.
- Mist tent: (1) Replace mist tents and their nebulizers, reservoirs, and tubing with those that have undergone sterilization or high-level disinfection between uses on different patients; (2) mist tent nebulizers and tubing that are used on the same patient should undergo daily low-level disinfection or pasteurization followed by air drying.

HEPA filters and HEPA filter masks for patients with prolonged neutropenia (NCCN, 2007; Sehulster & Chinn, 2003; Shelton, 2003)

- It is reasonable to use HEPA filters in nontransplant patients with prolonged neutropenia. Immunocompromised patients placed in protective environments should have mask protection when traveling outside of their protected area.

Flower and plant guidelines

- Patients with cancer should avoid fresh or dried flowers and plants because of the risk of *Aspergillus* infection (Sehulster & Chinn, 2003; Shelton, 2003; Smith & Kagan, 2005).

- Limit plant care to staff not directly caring for patients (Sehulster & Chinn, 2003).
- If plant care by patient care staff is unavoidable, staff should wear gloves while handling plants and flowers and perform hand hygiene after glove removal (Sehulster & Chinn, 2003).
- Change vase water every two days; discharge water outside the patient's room (Sehulster & Chinn, 2003).
- Clean and disinfect vases after use (Sehulster & Chinn, 2003).

Ice handling (Sehulster & Chinn, 2003)

- Automated ice-dispensing systems are preferred to ice bins, but adherence to cleaning procedures and schedules is essential.
- Do not handle ice by hand, and wash hands prior to obtaining ice.

Animal encounters (Sehulster & Chinn, 2003)

- Advise patients to avoid contact with animal feces, saliva, urine, or solid litter box material.
- Promptly clean and treat scratches, bites, or other wounds that break the skin.
- Advise patients to avoid direct and indirect contact with reptiles.
- Practice hand hygiene after any animal contact.

Preconstruction planning (Kidd, Buttner, & Kressel, 2007; Sehulster & Chinn, 2003; Siegel et al., 2007)

- Planning should include risk assessment, documentation and monitoring of the construction barrier, and education to the clinical staff about appropriate precautionary measures.
- High-risk patients should wear HEPA filter masks when not in a functioning protective environment room during construction and renovation activities.

Benefits Balanced With Harms

Interventions for which clinicians and patients should weigh the beneficial and harmful effects according to individual circumstances and priorities

There are no interventions as of May 2008.

Effectiveness Not Established

Interventions for which insufficient or conflicting data or data of inadequate quality currently exist, with no clear indication of harm

Immune globulin for respiratory syncytial virus (Tablan et al., 2004)

Protective isolation (Larson & Nirenberg, 2004; Mank & van der Lelie, 2003; Nauseef & Maki, 1981; Shelton, 2003; Siegel et al., 2007)

- Recommended only for allogeneic HSCT recipients to minimize fungal spore counts in the air and to reduce the risk of invasive environmental fungal infections. In this setting, protective isolation includes a private room with HEPA filtration, positive pressure airflow, and adequate ventilation. Gowns, gloves, and/or masks are not indicated for healthcare workers or visitors for routine entry into the room but should be used according to standard precautions and when indicated because of transmission-based precautions (e.g., contact precautions).

Effectiveness Unlikely

Interventions for which lack of effectiveness has been demonstrated by negative evidence from a single rigorously conducted controlled trial, consistent negative evidence from well-designed controlled trials using small samples, or guidelines developed from evidence and supported by expert opinion

Low microbial diet for neutropenic patients (DeMille, Deming, Lupinacci, & Jacobs, 2006; Gardner et al., 2008; Larson & Nirenberg, 2004; Mank & Davies, 2008; Moody, Charlson, & Finlay, 2002; Moody, Finlay, Mancuso, & Charlson, 2006; Shelton, 2003; Smith & Kagan, 2005; Smith & Besser, 2000; Somerville, 1986; Van Tiel et al., 2007; Wilson, 2002)
- Three recent randomized studies demonstrated no significant difference in the rate of infections between patients allowed a regular diet including raw fruits and vegetables compared with patients restricted to a low microbial diet (Gardner et al., 2008; Moody et al., 2006; Van Tiel et al., 2007).
- Basic food safety principles, such as avoiding uncooked meats, seafood, and eggs and unwashed fruits and vegetables, are prudent.
- Multivitamin supplementation for patients with cancer anticipating neutropenia requires further study (Branda, Naud, Brooks, Chen, & Muss, 2004).

Laminar air flow (NCCN, 2007; Sehulster & Chinn, 2003)

Routine donning of gowns upon entrance into a high-risk unit (e.g., HSCT unit) (Siegel et al., 2007)

Not Recommended for Practice

Interventions for which lack of effectiveness or harmfulness has been demonstrated by strong evidence from rigorously conducted studies, meta-analyses, or systematic reviews, or interventions where the costs, burden, or harms associated with the intervention exceed anticipated benefit

Antifungal prophylaxis for neutropenic patients with cancer with solid tumors (Bow et al., 2002; Cornely et al., 2003; Glasmacher et al., 2003; Gotzsche & Johansen, 2002; Hughes et al., 2002; Johansen & Gotzsche, 2002; Kanda et al., 2000; NCCN, 2007)
- Antifungal prophylaxis is not recommended for all neutropenic patients with cancer. It is only recommended for high-risk patients such as those with acute leukemia and those undergoing HSCT.

Itraconazole capsules are not effective for any cancer population (Glasmacher et al., 2003).

Nonabsorbable topical antifungal drugs to prevent oral candidiasis (Clarkson et al., 2007)

- Antifungal drugs not absorbed from the GI tract (amphotericin B, nystatin, nystatin plus chlorhexidine, thymostimulin, amphotericin B plus nystatin, polyenes, natamycin, and norfloxacin plus amphotericin B) did not have significant benefit in preventing oral candidiasis.

Gram-positive prophylaxis and fluoroquinolone in combination for antibacterial prophylaxis in afebrile neutropenic patients with cancer (Cruciani et al., 2003)

Live attenuated vaccines (NCCN, 2007)

- Patients with cancer receiving chemotherapy should not receive live attenuated vaccines for at least three months after discontinuation of therapy.
- Examples of live attenuated vaccines include FluMist® (MedImmune) (intranasal attenuated influenza vaccine), varicella (chicken pox) vaccine, oral polio vaccine, and measles, mumps, and rubella vaccine.

Expert Opinion

Low-risk interventions that are (1) consistent with sound clinical practice, (2) suggested by an expert in a peer-reviewed publication (journal or book chapter), and (3) for which limited evidence exists. An expert is an individual with peer-reviewed journal publications in the domain of interest.

There are no interventions as of May 2008.

Definitions of the interventions are available at **www.ons.org/outcomes**.
Literature search completed through May 2008.

References

Aapro, M.S., Cameron, D.A., Pettengell, R., Bohlius, J., Crawford, J., Ellis, M., et al. (2006). EORTC guidelines for the use of granulocyte-colony stimulating factor to reduce the incidence of chemotherapy-induced febrile neutropenia in adult patients with lymphomas and solid tumours. *European Journal of Cancer, 42*(15), 2433–2453.

Bohlius, J., Herbst, C., Reiser, M., Schwarzer, G., & Engert, A. (2008). Granulopoiesis-stimulating factors to prevent adverse effects in the treatment of malignant lymphoma. *Cochrane Database of Systematic Reviews* 2008, Issue 4. Art. No.: CD003189. DOI: 10.1002/14651858.CD003189.pub4.

Bow, E.J., Laverdiere, M., Lussier, N., Rotstein, C., Cheang, M.S., & Ioannou, S. (2002). Antifungal prophylaxis for severely neutropenic chemotherapy recipients: A meta analysis of randomized-controlled clinical trials. *Cancer, 94*(12), 3230–3246.

Boyce, J.M., Pittet, D., & Healthcare Infection Control Practices Advisory Committee/Society for Healthcare Epidemiology of America/Association for Professionals in Infection Control/Infectious Diseases Society of America Hand Hygiene Task Force. (2002). Guideline for hand hygiene in health-care settings: Recommendations of the Healthcare Infection Control Practices Advisory Committee and the HICPAC/SHEA/APIC/IDSA Hand Hygiene Task Force. *Infection Control and Hospital Epidemiology, 23*(Suppl. 12), S3–S40.

Branda, R.F., Naud, S.J., Brooks, E.M., Chen, Z., & Muss, H. (2004). Effect of vitamin B12, folate, and dietary supplements on breast carcinoma chemotherapy-induced mucositis and neutropenia. *Cancer, 101*(5), 1058–1064.

Bucaneve, G., Micozzi, A., Menichetti, F., Martino, P., Dionisi, M.S., Martinelli, G., et al. (2005). Levofloxacin to prevent bacterial infection in patients with cancer and neutropenia. *New England Journal of Medicine, 353*(10), 977–987.

Chaudhury, H., Mahmood, A., & Valente, M. (2003). *The use of single patient rooms vs. multiple occupancy rooms in acute care environments: A review and analysis of the literature. American Institute of Architects Guidelines for design and construction of health care facilities.* Retrieved June 8, 2008, from http://www.aia.org/SiteObjects/files/04_Review_and_Anal_Literature.pdf

Clarkson, J.E., Worthington, H.V., & Eden, O.B. (2007). Interventions for preventing oral candidiasis for patients with cancer receiving treatment. *Cochrane Database of Systematic Reviews* 2007, Issue 1. Art. No.: CD003807. DOI: 10.1002/14651858.CD003807.pub3.

Cornely, O.A., Maertens, J., Winston, D.J., Perfect, J., Ullmann, A.J., Walsh, T.J., et al. (2007). Posaconazole vs. fluconazole or itraconazole prophylaxis in patients with neutropenia. *New England Journal of Medicine, 356*(4), 348–359.

Cornely, O.A., Ullmann, A.J., & Karthaus, M. (2003). Evidence-based assessment of primary antifungal prophylaxis in patients with hematologic malignancies. *Blood, 101*(9), 3365–3372.

Cruciani, M., Malena, M., Bosco, O., Nardi, S., Serpelloni, G., & Mengoli, C. (2003). Reappraisal with meta-analysis of the addition of gram-positive prophylaxis to fluoroquinolone in neutropenic patients. *Journal of Clinical Oncology, 21*(22), 4127–4137.

Cruciani, M., Rampazzo, R., Malena, M., Lazzarini, L., Todeschini, G., Messori, A., et al. (1996). Prophylaxis with fluoroquinolones for bacterial infections in neutropenic patients: A meta-analysis. *Clinical Infectious Diseases, 23*(4), 795–805.

Cullen, M., Steven, N., Billingham, L., Gaunt, C., Hastings, M., Simmonds, P., et al. (2005). Antibacterial prophylaxis after chemotherapy for solid tumors and lymphomas. *New England Journal of Medicine, 353*(10), 988–998.

Cullen, M.H., Billingham, L.J., Gaunt, C.H., & Steven, N.M. (2007). Rational selection of patients for antibacterial prophylaxis after chemotherapy. *Journal of Clinical Oncology, 25*(30), 4821–4828.

DeMille, D., Deming, P., Lupinacci, P., & Jacobs, L. (2006). The effect of the neutropenic diet in the outpatient setting: A pilot study. *Oncology Nursing Forum, 33*(2), 337–343.

Engels, E.A., Lau, J., & Barza, M. (1998). Efficacy of quinolone prophylaxis in neutropenic cancer patients: A meta-analysis. *Journal of Clinical Oncology, 16*(3), 1179–1187.

Gafter-Gvili, A., Fraser, A., Paul, M., & Leibovici, L. (2005). Meta-analysis: Antibiotic prophylaxis reduces mortality in neutropenic patients. *Annals of Internal Medicine, 142*(12, Pt. 1), 979–995.

Gafter-Gvili, A., Fraser, A., Paul, M., van de Wetering, M., Kremer, L., & Leibovici, L. (2005). Antibiotic prophylaxis for bacterial infections in afebrile neutropenic patients following chemotherapy. *Cochrane Database of Systematic Reviews* 2005, Issue 4. Art. No.: CD004386. DOI: 10.1002/14651858. CD004386.pub2.

Gafter-Gvili, A., Paul, M., Fraser, A., & Leibovici, L. (2007). Effect of quinolone prophylaxis in afebrile neutropenic patients on microbial resistance: Systematic review and meta-analysis. *Journal of Antimicrobial Chemotherapy, 59*(1), 5–22.

Gardner, A., Mattiuzzi, G., Faderl, S., Borthakur, G., Garcia-Manero, G., Pierce, S., et al. (2008). Randomized comparison of cooked and noncooked diets in patients undergoing remission induction therapy for acute myeloid leukemia. *Journal of Clinical Oncology, 26*(35), 5684–5688.

Glasmacher, A., Prentice, A., Gorschluter, M., Engelhart, S., Hahn, C., Djulbegovic, B., et al. (2003). Itraconazole prevents invasive fungal infections in neutropenic patients treated for hematologic malignancies: Evidence from a meta-analysis of 3,597 patients. *Journal of Clinical Oncology, 21*(24), 4615–4626.

Gotzsche, P.C., & Johansen, H.K. (2002). Routine versus selective antifungal administration for control of fungal infections in patients with cancer. *Cochrane Database of Systematic Reviews* 2002, Issue 2. Art. No.: CD000026. DOI: 10.1002/14651858.CD000026.

Hilburn, J., Hammond, B.S., Fendler, E.J., & Groziak, P.A. (2003). Use of alcohol hand sanitizer as an infection control strategy in an acute care facility. *American Journal of Infection Control, 31*(2), 109–116.

Hughes, W.T., Armstrong, D., Bodey, G.P., Bow, E.J., Brown, A.E., Calandra, T., et al. (2002). 2002 guidelines for the use of antimicrobial agents in neutropenic patients with cancer. *Clinical Infectious Diseases, 34*(6), 730–751.

Johansen, H.K., & Gotzsche, P.C. (2000). Amphotericin B lipid soluble formulations vs amphotericin B in cancer patients with neutropenia. *Cochrane Database of Systematic Reviews* 2000, Issue 3. Art. No.: CD000969. DOI: 10.1002/14651858.CD000969.

Johansen, H.K., & Gotzsche, P.C. (2002). Amphotericin B vs fluconazole for controlling fungal infections in neutropenic cancer patients. *Cochrane Database of Systematic Reviews* 2002, Issue 2. Art. No.: CD000239. DOI: 10.1002/14651858.CD000239.

Kanda, Y., Yamamoto, R., Chizuka, A., Hamaki, T., Suguro, M., Arai, C., et al. (2000). Prophylactic action of oral fluconazole against fungal infection in neutropenic patients. A meta-analysis of 16 randomized, controlled trials. *Cancer, 89*(7), 1611–1625.

Kidd, F., Buttner, C., & Kressel, A.B. (2007). Construction: A model program for infection control compliance. *American Journal of Infection Control, 35*(5), 347–350.

Kuderer, N.M., Dale, D.C., Crawford, J., & Lyman, G.H. (2007). Impact of primary prophylaxis with granulocyte colony-stimulating factor on febrile neutropenia and mortality in adult cancer patients receiving chemotherapy: A systematic review. *Journal of Clinical Oncology, 25*(21), 3158–3167.

Lalami, Y., Paesmans, M., Aoun, M., Munoz-Bermeo, R., Reuss, K., Cherifi, S., et al. (2004). A prospective randomised evaluation of G-CSF or G-CSF plus oral antibiotics in chemotherapy-treated patients at high risk of developing febrile neutropenia. *Supportive Care in Cancer, 12*(10), 725–730.

Larson, E., & Nirenberg, A. (2004). Evidence-based nursing practice to prevent infection in hospitalized neutropenic patients with cancer. *Oncology Nursing Forum, 31*(4), 717–725.

Lyman, G.H., Kuderer, N., Agboola, O., & Balducci, L. (2003). Evidence-based use of colony-stimulating factors in elderly cancer patients. *Cancer Control, 10*(6), 487–499.

Lyman, G.H., Kuderer, N.M., & Djulbegovic, B. (2002). Prophylactic granulocyte colony-stimulating factor in patients receiving dose-intensive cancer chemotherapy: A meta-analysis. *American Journal of Medicine, 112*(5), 406–411.

Mank, A., & van der Lelie, H. (2003). Is there still an indication for nursing patients with prolonged neutropenia in protective isolation? An evidence-based nursing and medical study of 4 years experience for nursing patients with neutropenia without isolation. *European Journal of Oncology Nursing, 7*(1), 17–23.

Mank, A.P., & Davies, M. (2008). Examining low bacterial dietary practice: A survey on low bacterial food. *European Journal of Oncology Nursing, 12*(4), 342–348.

Montecalvo, M.A., Jarvis, W.R., Uman, J., Shay, D.K., Petrullo, C., Rodney, K., et al. (1999). Infection-control measures reduce transmission of vancomycin-resistant enterococci in an endemic setting. *Annals of Internal Medicine, 131*(4), 269–272.

Moody, K., Charlson, M.E., & Finlay, J. (2002). The neutropenic diet: What's the evidence? *Journal of Pediatric Hematology/Oncology, 24*(9), 717–721.

Moody, K., Finlay, J., Mancuso, C., & Charlson, M. (2006). Feasibility and safety of a pilot randomized trial of infection rate: Neutropenic diet versus standard food safety guidelines. *Journal of Pediatric Hematology/Oncology, 28*(3), 126–133.

National Comprehensive Cancer Network. (2008). *NCCN Clinical Practice Guidelines in Oncology™: Myeloid growth factors* [v.1.2008]. Retrieved May 31, 2008, from http://www.nccn.org/professionals/physician_gls/PDF/myeloid_growth.pdf

National Comprehensive Cancer Network. (2007). *NCCN Clinical Practice Guidelines in Oncology™: Prevention and treatment of cancer-related infection* [v.1.2007]. Retrieved May 31, 2008, from http://www.nccn.org/professionals/physician_gls/PDF/fever.pdf

Nauseef, W.M., & Maki, D.G. (1981). A study of the value of simple protective isolation in patients with granulocytopenia. *New England Journal of Medicine, 304*(8), 448–453.

Ring, A., Marx, G., Steer, C., & Harper, P. (2002). Influenza vaccination and chemotherapy: A shot in the dark? *Supportive Care in Cancer, 10*(6), 462–465.

Sehulster, L., & Chinn, R.Y. (2003). Guidelines for environmental infection control in health-care facilities: Recommendations of CDC and the Healthcare Infection Control Practices Advisory Committee (HICPAC). *Morbidity and Mortality Weekly Report, 52*(RR-10), 1–42.

Shaikh, Z.H., Osting, C.A., Hanna, H.A., Arbuckle, R.B., Tarr, J.J., & Raad, I.I. (2002). Effectiveness of a multifaceted infection control policy in reducing vancomycin usage and vancomycin-resistant enterococci at a tertiary care cancer centre. *Journal of Hospital Infection, 51*(1), 52–58.

Shelton, B.K. (2003). Evidence-based care for the neutropenic patient with leukemia. *Seminars in Oncology Nursing, 19*(2), 133–141.

Siegel, J.D., Rhinehart, E., Jackson, M., Chiarello, L., & Healthcare Infection Control Practices Advisory Committee. (2006). *Management of multidrug-resistant organisms in healthcare settings, 2006.* Retrieved May 31, 2008, from http://www.cdc.gov/ncidod/dhqp/pdf/ar/mdroguideline2006.pdf

Siegel, J.D., Rhinehart, E., Jackson, M., Chiarello, L., & Healthcare Infection Control Practices Advisory Committee. (2007). *Guideline for isolation precautions: Preventing transmission of infectious agents in healthcare settings, 2007.* Retrieved May 31, 2008, from http://www.cdc.gov/ncidod/dhqp/pdf/guidelines/Isolation2007.pdf

Smith, C.M., & Kagan, S.H. (2005). Prevention of systemic mycoses by reducing exposure to fungal pathogens in hospitalized and ambulatory neutropenic patients. *Oncology Nursing Forum, 32*(3), 565–579.

Smith, L.H., & Besser, S.G. (2000). Dietary restrictions for patients with neutropenia: A survey of institutional practices. *Oncology Nursing Forum, 27*(3), 515–520.

Somerville, E.T. (1986). Special diets for neutropenic patients: Do they make a difference? *Seminars in Oncology Nursing, 2*(1), 55–58.

Srinivasan, A., Song, X., Ross, T., Merz, W., Brower, R., & Perl, T.M. (2002). A prospective study to determine whether cover gowns in addition to gloves decrease nosocomial transmission of vancomycin-resistant enterococci in an intensive care unit. *Infection Control and Hospital Epidemiology, 23*(8), 424–428.

Sung, L., Nathan, P.C., Alibhai, S.M.H., Tomlinson, G.A., & Beyene, J. (2007). Meta-analysis: Effect of prophylactic hematopoietic colony-stimulating factors on mortality and outcomes of infection. *Annals of Internal Medicine, 147*(6), 400–411.

Sung, L., Nathan, P.C., Lange, B., Beyene, J., & Buchanan, G.R. (2004). Prophylactic granulocyte colony-stimulating factor and granulocyte-macrophage colony-stimulating factor decrease febrile neutropenia after chemotherapy in children with cancer: A meta-analysis of randomized controlled trials. *Journal of Clinical Oncology, 22*(16), 3350–3356.

Tablan, O.C., Anderson, L.J., Besser, R., Bridges, C., & Hajjeh, R. (2004). Guidelines for preventing healthcare associated pneumonia, 2003: Recommendations of CDC and the Healthcare Infection Control Practices Advisory Committee. *Morbidity and Mortality Weekly Report, 53*(RR-3), 1–36.

van de Wetering, M.D., de Witte, M.A., Kremer, L.C., Offringa, M., Scholten, R.J., & Caron, H.N. (2005). Efficacy of oral prophylactic antibiotics in neutropenic afebrile oncology patients: A systematic review of randomised controlled trials. *European Journal of Cancer, 41*(10), 1372–1382.

van Tiel, F.H., Harbers, M.M., Terporten, P.H.W., van Boxtel, R.T.C., Kessels, A.G., Voss, G.B.W.E., et al. (2007). Normal hospital and low-bacterial diet in patients with cytopenia after intensive chemotherapy for hematologic malignancy: A study of safety. *Annals of Oncology, 18*(6), 1080–1084.

Wilson, B.J. (2002). Dietary recommendations for neutropenic patients. *Seminars in Oncology Nursing, 18*(1), 44–49.

CHAPTER **18**

Sleep-Wake Disturbances

Problem

Sleep-wake disturbances are perceived or actual alterations in night sleep with resultant daytime impairment. Among the most common sleep disturbances are insomnia, sleep-related breathing disorders, and sleep-related movement disorders (e.g., restless legs syndrome, periodic limb movement disorder). General criteria for insomnia include difficulty initiating sleep, difficulty maintaining sleep, waking too early, or sleep that is chronically unrestorative or poor in quality that occurs despite adequate opportunity and circumstances for falling asleep (Berger et al., 2005).

Characteristics of sleep-wake disturbances are measured by the following nine parameters (Perlis, Jungquist, Smith, & Posner, 2005).

- **Total sleep time while in bed:** the number of minutes of sleep while in bed
- **Sleep latency:** the number of minutes between lying down in bed to actually falling asleep
- **Frequency of nocturnal awakenings:** the number of awakenings during sleep period
- **Wake time after sleep onset:** the number of minutes awake or percentage of time awake after sleep onset during the sleep period
- **Sleep efficiency:** the number of minutes of sleep divided by the total number of minutes in bed multiplied by 100
- **Napping during the day:** the total number of minutes of sleep during the daytime; can be intentional or unintentional
- **Excessive daytime sleepiness:** subjective or objective episodes of lapses into sleep of short duration, usually in situations in which the person is inactive for even brief periods; can result from acute or chronic sleep deprivation or loss or other pathophysiologic causes
- **Nonrestorative sleep:** multidimensional perceptions of length and depth of sleep and feelings of being rested on awakening; subjective assessment of sufficiency of sleep for daytime functioning

- **Circadian rhythms:** biobehavioral phenomenon associated with fluctuations in light, hormones, eating, and/or socializing that repeat every 24 hours

Incidence

Sleep-wake disturbances are reported in 30%–75% of people with cancer and have a negative impact on other symptoms and quality of life (Berger et al., 2005; Lee, Cho, Miaskowski, & Dodd, 2004). Data suggest that people with cancer have twice the incidence of sleep disturbances compared to the general population (Savard, Laroche, Simard, Ivers, & Morin, 2003). The majority of people with cancer report insomnia with several awakenings during the night (Davidson, MacLean, Brundage, & Schulze, 2002; Lee, 2003).

Assessment

Determining the characteristics of an individual's sleep-wake disturbance, in addition to its onset and duration, is important (Vogel, 2008). Risk and contributing factors should be considered (see Table 18-1) when screening for sleep-wake disturbances. The Adult and Child Sleep Assessment Tools by Lee and Ward (2005) are examples of a brief screening tool designed for completion by patients, parent and child, or caregiver.

Table 18-1. Risk and Contributing Factors for Sleep-Wake Disturbances		
Risk and Contributing Factors	**Yes**	**No**
Female sex		
Older age		
Personal or family history of sleep disorder		
Personal or family history of mood disorder, anxiety, or depression		
Current diagnosis of mood or anxiety or depression disorder		
Psychological distress in response to cancer diagnosis or treatment		
Immunologic and thermoregulatory changes		
Pain		
Gastrointestinal distress		
Respiratory distress		
Chemotherapy		
Medications for treatment of side effects		
Radiation therapy		
Environmental factors (noise, light, exogenous sleep disturbance)		
Menopausal symptoms (night sweats)		
Note. Based on information from Mills & Graci, 2004.		

Clinical Measurement Tools

When a sleep-wake disturbance is identified and nursing interventions are implemented, a clinical measurement tool should be used to evaluate the effectiveness of the interventions on the sleep-wake disturbance. Measurement of sleep-wake disturbances can be divided into several categories: self-report (diary, questionnaire), behavioral (observation, actigraphy), and physiologic (polysomnography) (Berger, 2005). The following three examples of self-report tools are presented in Table 18-2.

1. Insomnia Severity Index (ISI) (see Figure 18-1)
2. Epworth Sleepiness Scale
3. Pittsburgh Sleep Quality Index

Table 18-2. Clinical Measurement Tools for Sleep-Wake Disturbances					
Name of Tool	Number of Items	Domains	Reliability and Validity	Populations	Clinical Utility
Insomnia Severity Index	7	Insomnia	Adequate reliability and validity established	Mixed cancers	Brief screening of insomnia only
Epworth Sleepiness Scale	8	Tendency to doze in particular situations; daytime sleepiness	Adequate reliability and validity established	Prostate cancer	Simple to measure general level of sleepiness; easy to score
Pittsburgh Sleep Quality Index	19 basic and 5 roommate-related	Global score of sleep quality, seven subscales: sleep quality, sleep latency, sleep duration, habitual sleep efficiency, sleep disturbance, use of sleeping medication, daytime functioning	Adequate reliability and validity established	Breast cancer, caregivers of patients with advanced cancer	Gold standard but scoring rather cumbersome

Note. Based on information from Berger, 2005.

Figure 18-1. Insomnia Severity Index

For each question, please *CIRCLE* the number that best describes your answer.
Please rate the *CURRENT (i.e., LAST 2 WEEKS) SEVERITY* of your insomnia problem(s).

Insomnia Problem	None	Mild	Moderate	Severe	Very severe
1. Difficulty falling asleep	0	1	2	3	4
2. Difficulty staying asleep	0	1	2	3	4
3. Problem waking up too early	0	1	2	3	4

4. How SATISFIED/DISSATISFIED are you with your CURRENT sleep pattern?

Very Satisfied	Satisfied	Moderately Satisfied	Dissatisfied	Very Dissatisfied
0	1	2	3	4

5. How NOTICEABLE to others do you think your sleep problem is in terms of impairing the quality of your life?

Not at All Noticeable	A Little	Somewhat	Much	Very Much Noticeable
0	1	2	3	4

6. How WORRIED/DISTRESSED are you about your current sleep problem?

Not at All Worried	A Little	Somewhat	Much	Very Much Worried
0	1	2	3	4

7. To what extent do you consider your sleep problem to INTERFERE with your daily functioning (e.g. daytime fatigue, mood, ability to function at work/daily chores, concentration, memory, mood, etc.) CURRENTLY?

Not at All Interfering	A Little	Somewhat	Much	Very Much Interfering
0	1	2	3	4

Guidelines for Scoring/Interpretation:
Add the scores for all seven items (questions 1 + 2 + 3 + 4 + 5 +6 + 7) = your total score

Total score categories:
0–7 = No clinically significant insomnia
8–14 = Subthreshold insomnia
15–21 = Clinical insomnia (moderate severity)
22–28 = Clinical insomnia (severe)

Note. Copyright by Charles M. Morin, PhD, Université Laval. Available at https://www.myhealth.va.gov/mhv-portal-web/resources/jsp/help.jsp?helpDirectRequest=sleep_insomnia_indexprint.htm. Used with permission.

References

Berger, A. (2005). *Evidence-based outcomes measurement summaries—Sleep/wake disturbances.* Retrieved May 25, 2008, from http://www.ons.org/outcomes/measures/sleep.shtml

Berger, A.M., Parker, K.P., Young-McCaughan, S., Mallory, G.A., Barsevick, A.M., Beck, S.L., et al. (2005). Sleep/wake disturbances in people with cancer and their caregivers: State of the science [Online exclusive]. *Oncology Nursing Forum, 32*(6), E98–E126. Retrieved August 14, 2008, from http://ons.metapress.com/content/7244v4525u2j6408/fulltext.pdf

Davidson, J.R., MacLean, A.W., Brundage, M.D., & Schulze, K. (2002). Sleep disturbance in cancer patients. *Social Science and Medicine, 54*(9), 1309–1321.

Lee, K.A. (2003). Impaired sleep. In V. Carrieri-Kohlman, A. Lindsey, & C. West (Eds.), *Pathophysiological phenomena in nursing* (3rd ed., pp. 363–385). St. Louis, MO: Saunders.

Lee, K.A., Cho, M., Miaskowski, C., & Dodd, M. (2004). Impaired sleep and rhythms in persons with cancer. *Sleep Medicine Reviews, 8*(3), 199–212.

Lee, K.A., & Ward, T.M. (2005). Critical components of a sleep assessment for clinical practice settings. *Issues in Mental Health Nursing, 26*(7), 739–750.

Mills, M., & Graci, G.M. (2004). Sleep disturbances. In C.H. Yarbro, M.H. Frogge, & M. Goodman (Eds.), *Cancer symptom management* (3rd ed., pp. 111–134). Sudbury, MA: Jones and Bartlett.

Perlis, M.L., Jungquist, C., Smith, M., & Posner, D. (2005). *Cognitive behavioral treatment of insomnia: A session-by-session guide.* New York: Springer.

Savard, J., Laroche, L., Simard, S., Ivers, H., & Morin, C.M. (2003). Chronic insomnia and immune functioning. *Psychosomatic Medicine, 65*(2), 211–221.

Vogel, W.H. (2008). Sleep disturbances. In S. Newton, M. Hickey, & J. Marrs (Eds.), *Mosby's oncology nursing advisor* (pp. 389–391). St. Louis, MO: Elsevier Mosby.

Case Study

B.R. was a 45-year-old woman who had been diagnosed with stage IIIA infiltrating breast cancer. She was recovering from surgery and about to start treatment, which included doxorubicin/cyclophosphamide plus paclitaxel, four treatments every two weeks and trastuzumab weekly for one year. She was frantic in explaining to the nurse that she had pain (rated 4 out of 10) and fatigue (rated 5 out of 10) and that she just could not get enough sleep. She was worried that if she did not sleep well, she would not have the reserves to fight the breast cancer because her immune system would be jeopardized and the cancer would come back. She reported that not only did she have difficulty falling asleep but she also woke up in the middle of the night and was unable to go back to sleep. She wondered if she needed a strong sleeping pill.

The nurse used the ISI to measure the level of B.R.'s insomnia. She also learned that B.R. went to bed at a regular time each night. Lately, to help achieve this, she had been drinking a glass of wine before bed. She then woke up at about 2 or 3 am and got frustrated because she knew she had to get back to sleep. The more she tried to go back to sleep, the more futile were her attempts. She was sleepy during the day and took several naps. Because she was sleepy and fatigued during the day, she had given up regular exercise. She also reported being anxious about keeping the house running and helping her husband with chores. She usually helped with clean-up and paying the bills after dinner. She also was concerned about being available to her two daughters, helping them with homework and other plans in the evening.

The nurse reassured B.R. that having sleep disturbances in this setting was not uncommon and that making some simple changes could help her sleep. Using the Oncology Nursing Society Putting Evidence Into Practice resource on sleep-wake disturbances, the nurse reviewed the following points with B.R.

• Go to bed only when sleepy and at approximately the same time each night.
• Get out of bed and go to another room whenever unable to fall asleep. Return to bed only when sleepy again.
• Use the bedroom for sleep and sex only.
• Maintain a regular rising time each day.
• Avoid daytime napping; if needed, limit to around 30 minutes.

The nurse suggested that B.R. use a preferred relaxation technique prior to bed, such as taking a warm bath or shower, reading, listening to soft music, or receiving a massage. In addition, the nurse reviewed sleep hygiene techniques. B.R. should avoid caffeine after noon and alcohol prior to bedtime, which disrupts sleep architecture, and finish dinner three hours before bedtime. She should not go to bed hungry. B.R. also should optimize her sleep environment by keeping the bedroom dark, cool, and quiet, not using night-lights, and using light covers. She should not watch television in the bedroom. The nurse also suggested that B.R. join a support group, choose a relaxation therapy that she would like to learn, resume her exercise routine, and choose concrete areas in which she can make changes. Together they decided to check in weekly to see how things are going. By B.R.'s third visit, the nurse was pleased to learn that the patient's sleep-wake disturbances were decreasing as indicated by her improved score on the ISI.

Margaretta S. Page, RN, MS
Neuro-Oncology Clinical Nurse Specialist
University of California, San Francisco
San Francisco, CA

Sleep-Wake Disturbances

2009 AUTHORS
Margaretta S. Page, RN, MS, and Ann M. Berger, PhD, RN, AOCN®, FAAN
ONS STAFF: Linda H. Eaton, MN, RN, AOCN®

2006 AUTHORS
Margaretta S. Page, RN, MS, Ann M. Berger, PhD, RN, AOCN®, FAAN, and Lauran B. Johnson, RN, MSN
ONS STAFF: Linda H. Eaton, MN, RN, AOCN®

What can nurses do to assist people with cancer with sleep-wake disturbances?

Recommended for Practice

Interventions for which effectiveness has been demonstrated by strong evidence from rigorously conducted studies, meta-analyses, or systematic reviews, and for which expectation of harms is small compared with the benefits

No interventions are available as of May 2008.

Likely to Be Effective

Interventions for which effectiveness has been demonstrated by supportive evidence from a single rigorously conducted controlled trial, consistent supportive evidence from well-designed controlled trials using small samples, or guidelines developed from evidence and supported by expert opinion

COGNITIVE BEHAVIORAL THERAPY

Cognitive behavioral therapy (CBT) involves changing negative thought processes and attitudes about one's ability to fall asleep, stay asleep, get enough sleep, and function during the day (Morin, Culbert, & Schwartz, 1994).

Instruct patients in the following stimulus control and sleep restriction techniques.
- Go to bed only when sleepy and at approximately the same time each night.
- Get out of bed and go to another room whenever unable to fall asleep; return to bed only when sleepy again.
- Use the bedroom for sleep and sex only.
- Maintain a regular rising time each day.
- Avoid daytime napping. If needed, limit to 20–30 minutes and complete four hours before bedtime.

Sleep hygiene techniques include behaviors to promote a good night's sleep and optimal functioning the next day (Morin et al., 1994).

- Create a bedtime routine. Start by winding down one to two hours before bedtime. Use a preferred relaxation technique, such as taking a warm bath or shower, reading, listening to soft music, or receiving a massage.
- Avoid stimulants such as caffeine after noon and nicotine or alcohol prior to bedtime; complete dinner three hours before bedtime; do not go to bed hungry (a protein snack is preferred).
- Create a comfortable sleep environment. Replace mattress every 10–12 years and pillows more frequently; keep the bedroom dark, cool, and quiet, and use light covers; do not watch television in the bedroom.
- Ensure at least 20 minutes of exposure to bright natural light, preferably in the morning.

Three randomized controlled trials (RCTs) and nine quasi-experimental studies have tested CBT in patients with a variety of cancer diagnoses at various times along the continuum of care (Allison, Edgar, et al., 2004; Allison, Nicolau, et al., 2004; Arving et al., 2007; Berger et al., 2002, 2003; Carpenter, Neal, Payne, Kimmick, & Storniolo, 2007; Cohen & Fried, 2007; Davidson, Waisberg, Brundage, & MacLean, 2001; Epstein & Dirksen, 2007; Espie et al., 2008; Quesnel, Savard, Simard, Ivers, & Morin, 2003; Savard et al., 2006; Savard, Simard, Ivers, & Morin, 2005). Studies varied in content, length, and frequency of the CBT intervention and the measured outcomes. Most studies' results included improvement in several sleep outcomes, most commonly perceived sleep quality. Two RCTs tested four to five weekly CBT sessions versus a control group in breast cancer survivors and reported improvement in self-reported sleep latency, awake after sleep onset, and sleep efficiency (Epstein & Dirksen; Espie et al.).

Benefits Balanced With Harms

Interventions for which clinicians and patients should weigh the beneficial and harmful effects according to individual circumstances and priorities

PHARMACOLOGIC

In spite of widespread use, no published meta-analyses or recent experimental design studies examining the efficacy of hypnotic drugs in patients with cancer were found. Nurses must systematically evaluate how patients with cancer respond to a pharmacologic intervention, particularly the efficacy, side effects, and potential interactions with other over-the-counter and prescription medications they are taking (Berger et al., 2005; Clark, Cunningham, McMillan, Vena, & Parker, 2004).

Although the drugs have not been studied in patients with cancer, hypnotics are commonly prescribed for short-term use. Benzodiazepines and nonbenzodiazepine drugs vary in their half-lives. Those with longer half-lives can cause daytime sleepiness and impair functioning; those with shorter half-lives may wear off in the middle of the night. Agents included in the National Cancer Institute's (NCI's) PDQ® Sleep Disorders Web site (NCI, 2008) that are commonly prescribed but must be individually evaluated for side-effect profile include

- Benzodiazepines: diazepam 5–10 mg, triazolam 0.125–0.5 mg, and clonazepam 0.5–2 mg
- Nonbenzodiazepine hypnotics: zolpidem tartrate 5–20 mg, zaleplon 10–20 mg, and eszopiclone 1–3 mg

- Other classes of drugs: Tricyclic antidepressants, second-generation antidepressants, anti-histamines, chloral derivatives, and neuroleptics are used less commonly but may be considered to improve sleep.
  - Venlafaxine 75 mg PO resulted in modest decrease in hot flash perception. However, only women with > 50% reduction in physiologic hot flashes experienced improved sleep (Carpenter, Storniolo, et al., 2007).

HERBAL SUPPLEMENTS

No published meta-analyses or experimental design studies were found specific to the efficacy of herbal therapy in patients with cancer. Studies describe potential interactions between herbal agents with chemotherapy and other common drugs, making herbal agents potentially dangerous for use in people with cancer (Block, Gyllenhaal, & Mead, 2004).

Effectiveness Not Established

Interventions for which insufficient or conflicting data or data of inadequate quality currently exist, with no clear indication of harm

COMPLEMENTARY THERAPIES: EXPRESSIVE THERAPY, EXPRESSIVE WRITING, HEALING, AUTOGENIC TRAINING, MASSAGE, MUSCLE RELAXATION, MINDFULNESS-BASED STRESS REDUCTION (MBSR), YOGA, AROMATHERAPY, MUSIC THERAPY, HAPTOTHERAPY, AND GUIDED IMAGERY

- Encourage patients to decrease stress by selecting relaxation techniques that suit them, including massage, individual muscle relaxation, meditation, MBSR, yoga, guided imagery, and autogenic training.
- Encourage patients to keep a journal in which they document their deepest thoughts and feelings about their illness and treatment.
- Encourage patients to decrease stress by focusing on and isolating various muscle groups while moving progressively up and down the body. Encourage focused breathing, with all attention centered on the sensations of breathing, including the rhythm and rise and fall of the chest.
- Provide referral to appropriate practitioners as needed for expressive therapy, guided imagery instruction, aromatherapy instruction, healing, autogenic training, massage, MBSR, yoga, music therapy, and haptotherapy.

To date, results of five RCTs and 10 quasi-experimental studies using complementary therapies in adult patients with cancer have been reported. One RCT and two quasi-experimental trials looked at MBSR, a combination therapy of relaxation techniques, meditative techniques, and yoga, in breast cancer, early prostate cancer, and a mixed group of cancer populations and found improved sleep quality with the therapy (Carlson & Garland, 2005; Carlson, Speca, Patel, & Goodey, 2003, 2004; Shapiro, Bootzin, Figueredo, Lopez, & Schwartz, 2003). Another large RCT in patients with breast cancer comparing cognitive therapy versus relaxation and guided imagery showed that means of fatigue symptoms and sleep difficulties fell in both intervention groups but were only significant in the relaxation and guided imagery group (Cohen & Fried, 2007).

Two studies using mixed cancer populations found autogenic training to have favorable sleep outcomes (Simeit, Deck, & Conta-Marx, 2004; Wright, Courtney, & Crowther, 2002). Patients with lymphoma showed significant decreases in sleep disturbances with Tibetan yoga (Cohen, Warneke, Fouladi, Rodriguez, & Chaoul-Reich, 2004). Supportive-expressive group therapy intervention resulted in decreased wake-after-sleep-onset time in patients with breast cancer (Fobair et al., 2002). One RCT with subjects with newly diagnosed stage IV metastatic renal cell cancer showed improvement in four measured areas of sleep disturbance when using expressive writing (de Moor et al., 2002). One RCT with a group of patients with a variety of cancer diagnoses showed a reduction in sleep latency, and two feasibility studies in breast cancer survivors demonstrated improved sleep quality when using progressive muscle relaxation (Cannici, Malcolm, & Peek, 1983; Rabin, Pinto, Dunsiger, Nash, & Trask, 2008; Simeit et al.). Patients with a variety of cancer diagnoses showed improvement on self-reported sleep disturbances with the use of healing touch (Weze, Leathard, Grange, Tiplady, & Stevens, 2004). Two studies looked at the use of massage, one of which added aromatherapy to the massage on a group of patients with a variety of cancers undergoing therapy and in palliative care. These two studies showed mixed results (Smith, Richardson, Hoffman, & Pilkington, 2005; Soden, Vincent, Craske, Lucas, & Ashley, 2004).

EDUCATION/INFORMATION

- Provide patients with information regarding specifics of treatment and expected side effects, including sleep-wake disturbances.
- Repeat this information throughout the treatment.
- Teach patients basic information about sleep hygiene (see "Cognitive Behavioral Therapy").

One RCT showed favorable sleep outcomes using an informational tape as an educational intervention with men receiving radiation for localized prostate cancer (Kim, Roscoe, & Morrow, 2002). Another RCT using informational audiotapes with women with breast cancer undergoing chemotherapy showed no change in sleep disturbances (Williams et al., 2006).

EXERCISE

- Rule out bone metastasis or exercise contraindications.
- Have patients complete moderate exercise (e.g., brisk walking 20–30 minutes four to five times per week) at least three hours before bedtime.
- Encourage patients to perform strength and resistance training.

Three quasi-experimental studies showed favorable sleep outcomes using aerobic exercise, two with patients with breast cancer and another with patients with a variety of cancers (Mock et al., 1997; Rabin et al., 2008; Young-McCaughan et al., 2003). A small pilot RCT looking at exercise and sleep in people with multiple myeloma was inconclusive because of a high (42%) attrition rate (Coleman et al., 2003).

Effectiveness Unlikely

Interventions for which lack of effectiveness has been demonstrated by negative evidence from a single rigorously conducted controlled trial, consistent negative evidence from well-designed controlled trials using small samples, or guidelines developed from evidence and supported by expert opinion

No interventions are available as of May 2008.

Not Recommended for Practice

Interventions for which lack of effectiveness or harmfulness has been demonstrated by strong evidence from rigorously conducted studies, meta-analyses, or systematic reviews, or interventions where the costs, burden, or harms associated with the intervention exceed anticipated benefit

No interventions are available as of May 2008.

Expert Opinion

Low-risk interventions that are (1) consistent with sound clinical practice, (2) suggested by an expert in a peer-reviewed publication (journal or book chapter), and (3) for which limited evidence exists. An expert is an individual with peer-reviewed journal publications in the domain of interest.

REFERRAL TO SLEEP SPECIALIST

If therapies employed are not producing subjective improvement in sleep parameters, referral to a sleep specialist is warranted.

Definitions of the interventions are available at **www.ons.org/outcomes**. Literature search completed through May 2008.

References

Allison, P.J., Edgar, L., Nicolau, B., Archer, J., Black, M., & Hier, M. (2004). Results of a feasibility study for a psycho-educational intervention in head and neck cancer. *Psycho-Oncology, 13*(7), 482–485.

Allison, P.J., Nicolau, B., Edgar, L., Archer, J., Black, M., & Hier, M. (2004). Teaching head and neck cancer patients coping strategies: Results of a feasibility study. *Oral Oncology, 40*(5), 538–544.

Arving, C., Sjoden, P.O., Bergh, J., Hellbom, M., Johansson, B., Glimelius, B., et al. (2007). Individual psychosocial support for breast cancer patients: A randomized study of nurse versus psychologist interventions and standard care. *Cancer Nursing, 30*(3), E10–E19.

Berger, A.M., Parker, K.P., Young-McCaughan, S., Mallory, G.A., Barsevick, A.M., Beck, S.L., et al. (2005). Sleep/wake disturbances in people with cancer and their caregivers: State of the science [Online exclusive]. *Oncology Nursing Forum, 32*(6), E98–E126.

Berger, A.M., VonEssen, S., Kuhn, B.R., Piper, B.F., Agrawal, S., Lynch, J.C., et al. (2003). Adherence, sleep, and fatigue outcomes after adjuvant breast cancer chemotherapy: Results of a feasibility intervention study. *Oncology Nursing Forum, 30*(3), 513–522.

Berger, A.M., VonEssen, S., Kuhn, B.R., Piper, B.F., Farr, L., Agrawal, S., et al. (2002). Feasibilty of a sleep intervention during adjuvant breast cancer chemotherapy. *Oncology Nursing Forum, 29*(10), 1431–1441.

Block, K.I., Gyllenhaal, C., & Mead, M.N. (2004). Safety and efficacy of herbal sedatives in cancer care. *Integrative Cancer Therapies, 3*(2), 128–148.

Cannici, J., Malcolm, R., & Peek, L.A. (1983). Treatment of insomnia in cancer patients using muscle relaxation training. *Journal of Behavior Therapy and Experimental Psychiatry, 14*(3), 251–256.

Carlson, L.E., & Garland, S.N. (2005). Impact of mindfulness-based stress reduction (MBSR) on sleep, mood, stress and fatigue symptoms in cancer outpatients. *International Journal of Behavioral Medicine, 12*(4), 278–285.

Carlson, L.E., Speca, M., Patel, K.D., & Goodey, E. (2003). Mindfulness-based stress reduction in relation to quality of life, mood, symptoms of stress, and immune parameters in breast and prostate cancer outpatients. *Psychosomatic Medicine, 65*(4), 571–581.

Carlson, L.E., Speca, M., Patel, K.D., & Goodey, E. (2004). Mindfulness-based stress reduction in relation to quality of life, mood, symptoms of stress and levels of cortisol, dehydroepiandrosterone sulfate (DHEAS) and melatonin in breast and prostate cancer outpatients. *Psychoneuroendocrinology, 29*(4), 448–474.

Carpenter, J.S., Neal, J.G., Payne, J., Kimmick, G., & Storniolo, A.M. (2007). Cognitive-behavioral intervention for hot flashes. *Oncology Nursing Forum, 34*(1), 37.

Carpenter, J.S., Storniolo, A.M., Johns, S., Monahan, P.O., Azzouz, F., Elam, J.L., et al. (2007). Randomized, double-blind, placebo-controlled crossover trials of venlafaxine for hot flashes after breast cancer. *Oncologist, 12*(1), 124–135.

Clark, J., Cunningham, M., McMillan, S., Vena, C., & Parker, K. (2004). Sleep-wake disturbances in people with cancer part II: Evaluating the evidence for clinical decision making. *Oncology Nursing Forum, 31*(4), 747–771.

Cohen, L., Warneke, C., Fouladi, R.T., Rodriguez, M.A., & Chaoul-Reich, A. (2004). Psychological adjustment and sleep quality in a randomized trial of the effects of a Tibetan yoga intervention in patients with lymphoma. *Cancer, 100*(10), 2253–2260.

Cohen, M., & Fried, G. (2007). Comparing relaxation training and cognitive-behavioral group therapy for women with breast cancer. *Research on Social Work Practice, 17*(3), 313–323.

Coleman, E.A., Coon, S., Hall-Barrow, J., Richards, K., Gaylor, D., & Stewart, B. (2003). Feasibility of exercise during treatment for multiple myeloma. *Cancer Nursing, 26*(5), 410–419.

Davidson, J.R., Waisberg, J.L., Brundage, M.D., & MacLean, A.W. (2001). Nonpharmacologic group treatment of insomnia: A preliminary study with cancer survivors. *Psycho-Oncology, 10*(5), 389–397.

de Moor, C., Sterner, J., Hall, M., Warneke, C., Gilani, Z., Amato, R., et al. (2002). A pilot study of the effects of expressive writing on psychological and behavioral adjustment in patients enrolled in a phase II trial of vaccine therapy for metastatic renal cell carcinoma. *Health Psychology, 21*(6), 615–619.

Epstein, D.R., & Dirksen, S.R. (2007). Randomized trial of a cognitive-behavioral intervention for insomnia in breast cancer survivors [Online exclusive]. *Oncology Nursing Forum, 34*(5), E51–E59. Retrieved May 31, 2008, from http://ons.metapress.com/content/l13681kwjk712374/fulltext.pdf

Espie, C.A., Fleming, L., Cassidy, J., Samuel, L., Taylor, L.M., White, C.A., et al. (2008). Randomized controlled clinical trial of cognitive behavior therapy compared with treatment as usual for persistent insomnia in patients with cancer. *Journal of Clinical Oncology, 26*(28), 4651–4658.

Fobair, P., Koopman, C., DiMiceli, S., O'Hanlan, K., Butler, L.D., Classen, C., et al. (2002). Psychosocial intervention for lesbians with primary breast cancer. *Psycho-Oncology, 11*(5), 427–438.

Kim, Y., Roscoe, J.A., & Morrow, G.R. (2002). The effects of information and negative affect on severity of side effects from radiation therapy for prostate cancer. *Supportive Care in Cancer, 10*(5), 416–421.

Mock, V., Dow, K.H., Meares, C.J., Grimm, P.M., Dienemann, J.A., Haisfield-Wolfe, M.E., et al. (1997). Effects of exercise on fatigue, physical functioning, and emotional distress during radiation therapy for breast cancer. *Oncology Nursing Forum, 24*(6), 991–1000.

Morin, C.M., Culbert, J.P., & Schwartz, S.M. (1994). Nonpharmacological interventions for insomnia: A meta-analysis of treatment efficacy. *American Journal of Psychiatry, 151*(8), 1172–1180.

National Cancer Institute. (2008). *Medications commonly used to promote sleep.* Retrieved May 27, 2008, from http://www.cancer.gov/cancertopics/pdq/supportivecare/sleepdisorders/healthprofessional/allpages#Section_75

Quesnel, C., Savard, J., Simard, S., Ivers, H., & Morin, C.M. (2003). Efficacy of cognitive-behavioral therapy for insomnia in women treated for nonmetastatic breast cancer. *Journal of Consulting and Clinical Psychology, 71*(1), 189–200.

Rabin, C., Pinto, B., Dunsiger, S., Nash, J., & Trask, P. (2008, May 13). Exercise and relaxation intervention for breast cancer survivors: Feasibility, acceptability and effects. *Psycho-Oncology* [Epub ahead of print]. Retrieved December 10, 2008, from http://www3.interscience.wiley.com/cgi-bin/fulltext/119138549/PDFSTART

Savard, J., Simard, S., Giguere, I., Ivers, H., Morin, C.M., Maunsell, E., et al. (2006). Randomized clinical trial on cognitive therapy for depression in women with metastatic breast cancer: Psychological and immunological effects. *Palliative and Supportive Care, 4*(3), 219–237.

Savard, J., Simard, S., Ivers, H., & Morin, C.M. (2005). Randomized study on the efficacy of cognitive-behavioral therapy for insomnia secondary to breast cancer, part I: Sleep and psychological effects. *Journal of Clinical Oncology, 23*(25), 6083–6096.

Shapiro, S.L., Bootzin, R.R., Figueredo, A.J., Lopez, A.M., & Schwartz, G.E. (2003). The efficacy of mindfulness-based stress reduction in the treatment of sleep disturbance in women with breast cancer: An exploratory study. *Journal of Psychosomatic Research, 54*(1), 85–91.

Simeit, R., Deck, R., & Conta-Marx, B. (2004). Sleep management training for cancer patients with insomnia. *Supportive Care in Cancer, 12*(3), 176–183.

Smith, J.E., Richardson, J., Hoffman, C., & Pilkington, K. (2005). Mindfulness-based stress reduction as supportive therapy in cancer care: Systematic review. *Journal of Advanced Nursing, 52*(3), 315–327.

Soden, K., Vincent, K., Craske, S., Lucas, C., & Ashley, S. (2004). A randomized controlled trial of aromatherapy massage in a hospice setting. *Palliative Medicine, 18*(2), 87–92.

Weze, C., Leathard, H.L., Grange, J., Tiplady, P., & Stevens, G. (2004). Evaluation of healing by gentle touch in 35 clients with cancer. *European Journal of Oncology Nursing, 8*(1), 40–49.

Williams, P.D., Piamjariyakul, U., Ducey, K., Badura, J., Boltz, K.D., Olberding, K., et al. (2006). Cancer treatment, symptom monitoring, and self-care in adults: Pilot study. *Cancer Nursing, 29*(5), 347–355.

Wright, S., Courtney, U., & Crowther, D. (2002). A quantitative and qualitative pilot study of the perceived benefits of autogenic training for a group of people with cancer. *European Journal of Cancer Care, 11*(2), 122–130.

Young-McCaughan, S., Mays, M.Z., Arzola, S.M., Yoder, L.H., Dramiga, S.A., Leclerc, K.M., et al. (2003). Research and commentary: Change in exercise tolerance, activity and sleep patterns, and quality of life in patients with cancer participating in a structured exercise program. *Oncology Nursing Forum, 30*(3), 441–454.

CHAPTER **19**

Evidence-Based Practice: Its Role in Quality Improvement

Linda Eaton, MN, RN, AOCN®,
and Janelle M. Tipton, MSN, RN, AOCN®

The term *quality improvement* has been around for some time. Previously called *quality assurance* and now referred to as *performance improvement*, many healthcare professionals are challenged to provide evidence of quality care. The Joint Commission (www.jointcommission.org) is an accrediting body that has concern for patient safety and demands accountability for the delivery of quality patient care in various practice settings. The 2001 Institute of Medicine (IOM) report *Crossing the Quality Chasm: A New Health System for the 21st Century* states that healthcare organizations can improve performance only by applying care process and outcome measures to daily work. The use of measures helps to articulate the level at which performance is consistent with best practices and the extent to which patients are being helped (IOM, 2001).

When embarking on quality improvement activities, a good starting point is to be familiar with the scope and standards of nursing care provided to patients with cancer. Tools to assist in developing quality assurance programs are available in the Oncology Nursing Society (ONS) *Statement on the Scope and Standards of Oncology Nursing Practice* (Brant & Wickham, 2004). Clinical indicators in oncology nursing need to be developed and tested, and thresholds for evaluation need to be established. Indicators are needed for high-risk, high-volume clinical activities or problems. Furthermore, indicators are needed for processes of providing nursing care, complications that are nurse-dependent, and nursing-sensitive patient outcomes (Miaskowski, 1989). One way of approaching quality care issues in oncology and other disciplines is to ensure an evidence-based practice (EBP) environment for education, system issues, and performance. Incorporating EBP throughout an organization can be challenging; however, with evidence-based resources such as those offered in the ONS Putting Evidence Into Practice (PEP) initiative, quality improvement activities can be implemented for resolving oncology patient problems. This chapter provides four clinical examples of quality improvement activities facilitated through application of the ONS PEP Resources in a healthcare environment.

Creating an Evidence-Based Practice Environment Through Education

EBP is essential in providing quality patient care. Nurses who are not comfortable with the EBP process may need education and support from both management and EBP nurse experts. Prior to educating nurses, it is important to ask if the organization's philosophy and mission support EBP. If the organization does not support EBP, demonstrating the success of EBP on patient care through small unit-based projects is essential (Fineout-Overholt, Cox, Robbins, & Gray, 2005).

One method for educating oncology nurses about EBP is to teach them how to implement the ONS PEP Resources in practice. Teaching nurses how to identify and carry out evidence-based nursing interventions must be reinforced in daily patient care. The following clinical example describes how two nurse experts delivered an easy and creative method for educating nurses about an evidence-based intervention for preventing infection. The resulting change in practice was measured and documented, both essential evaluation steps for demonstrating a successful practice change (Ingersoll, 2005).

Clinical Example

"Spreading the PEP" Through Unit Bulletin Boards and Staff Team Huddles

Advanced practice nurses (APNs) have a significant responsibility to ensure that clinical practice is evidence-based in their settings. Since the initial distribution of the ONS PEP Resources in 2006, oncology APNs and staff nurses have attempted to use them in clinical practice by seeking effective, realistic integration strategies. The goal is to equip the staff to use the ONS PEP Resources; the challenge is developing practical applications that will successfully foster staff ownership and investment. Ultimately, incorporation of EBP results in positive patient outcomes and promotes nursing as a scientifically based profession.

One strategy developed by clinical nurse specialists (CNSs) in a community oncology program may be duplicated easily in other oncology clinical settings. When evaluating potential strategies for communicating and integrating the ONS PEP Resources, CNSs reviewed the communication structure in the work setting. In addition to the education and administration bulletin boards placed in central staff areas, monthly staff meetings, and the organization's intranet Nurse Communication Portal, the medical oncology nursing staff participate in daily "team huddles" for administrative announcements, clinical updates, and unit operations prior to shift report. These team huddles are mandatory and take about 10 minutes.

Historically, the topic of EBP had not been included in these communication forums. Up until this point, staff nurses had not been accountable for integrating EBP into their daily practice unless it was required through mandatory education or regulatory requirements. Nor was it the norm to discuss the evidence behind clinical decisions or patient goals. The clinical staff nurses had no formal arena in which to address clinical practice issues and questions. To prevent EBP from being just an academic exercise, CNSs wondered if the key was to make it "real" for daily practice.

The following are potential steps to get started.

1. Communicate the importance of EBP/ONS PEP Resources in terms of improving nursing-sensitive patient outcomes, and obtain approval for bulletin boards dedicated to these in central staff areas.
2. Integrate the EBP/ONS PEP bulletin board into the team huddles by reviewing and applying the bulletin board content to relevant patient situations.
3. Establish an EBP/ONS PEP question of the week. Such a question would come from performance improvement initiatives, staff feedback through "Ask your burning clinical question," trends in poor patient outcomes, trends in patient admissions, current organizational or regulatory initiatives (e.g., hand washing, sepsis, pain management), and unit council meetings. The clinical question can be introduced in the team huddle around the EBP/ONS PEP bulletin board, and supporting evidence with practical examples also can be discussed for application in daily practice.
4. As the APNs perform daily clinical rounds, the ONS PEP information can be reinforced in real-time encounters with staff members to assist them in applying the interventions recommended by the ONS PEP Resources into patients' individualized plans of care.

For example, the first EBP question was "How does hand washing impact infection prevention in the patient with cancer?" According to the ONS PEP resource on prevention of infection, hand hygiene using soap and water or an antiseptic hand rub for all patients with cancer and their caregivers is recommended for practice. This intervention supports the organizational hand hygiene initiative to reduce the risk for infections in hospitalized patients. The question was posed in a team huddle, the evidence was reinforced by the ONS PEP bulletin board (see Figure 19-1), and an audit of compliance was posted. Subsequent audits revealed an improvement in staff hand hygiene compliance.

Patty Geddie, MS, RN, AOCNS®
Susan Dempsey-Walls, MN, RN, AOCNS®
Oncology Clinical Nurse Specialists
M.D. Anderson Cancer Center Orlando–Orlando Health
Orlando, FL

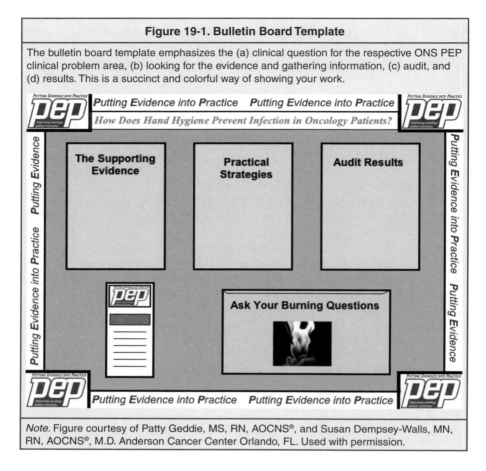

Figure 19-1. Bulletin Board Template

The bulletin board template emphasizes the (a) clinical question for the respective ONS PEP clinical problem area, (b) looking for the evidence and gathering information, (c) audit, and (d) results. This is a succinct and colorful way of showing your work.

Note. Figure courtesy of Patty Geddie, MS, RN, AOCNS®, and Susan Dempsey-Walls, MN, RN, AOCNS®, M.D. Anderson Cancer Center Orlando, FL. Used with permission.

Another strategy to promote an EBP environment through education is a journal club. In an informal setting, the dialogue and enthusiasm for topics in the literature can be explored. Journal clubs can be multidisciplinary and often work best when a moderator leads the discussion. This strategy has benefits for novice nurses in the EBP process, as it provides education and exploration and increases reading habits (Profetto-McGrath, 2005). The ONS PEP topics can be explored further through journal clubs, perhaps focusing on a selected intervention. This also may be an avenue to examine new clinical questions outside of the ONS PEP topics.

Creating an Evidence-Based Practice Environment Through a System Change

Making a successful EBP change may require multiple strategies targeted to individual, group, and organizational levels (Mohide & King, 2003). Implementation of clinical practice guidelines is recognized as a significant change, especially if current practice differs from the guideline recommendations (Grol, 2001; Moulding, Silagy, & Weller, 1999; Solberg et al., 2000). The following are five essential components for guideline implementation (DiCenso et al., 2002).

1. Selection of a high-quality, state-of-the-art, evidence-based guideline
2. Identification and commitment of key stakeholders who can successfully influence implementation
3. Assessment of the environment for guideline implementation readiness
4. Use of multiple proven implementation strategies
5. Evaluation of the guideline implementation

A toolkit by DiCenso et al. for implementation of clinical practice guidelines is available at www.rnao.org.

High-quality, well-developed, practical evidence-based guidelines implemented for managing healthcare problems are seen by practitioners, payers, and policy makers as potentially powerful tools for the achievement of effective and efficient care (Woolf, Grol, Hutchinson, Eccles, & Grinnshaw, 1999). Although the ONS PEP Resources are not defined as guidelines, they are recognized as high-quality, state-of-the-art, evidence-based resources. The following clinical example describes a successful practice change based on the ONS PEP Resources for the prevention of infection. The first four guideline-implementation components are achieved. Evaluation of the change in practice based on the ONS PEP Resources will be needed once the practice change is made throughout the hospital health system.

Clinical Example

Putting PEP Into Practice: Formation of a Neutropenia Improvement Project Team in a Community-Based Hospital

The purpose of the Neutropenia Improvement Project Team was to improve the process for triaging and managing patients with cancer presenting to the emergency department with febrile neutropenia. The team identified multiple delays in patients receiving their first dose of antibiotic therapy and a lack of understanding by emergency department nursing staff regarding management of patients experiencing febrile neutropenia.

The team consisted of the clinical nurse specialist, clinical scholar staff nurses, a clinical pharmacist, and the oncology medical director. Utilizing the ONS PEP resource on prevention of infection and the most recent edition of the National Comprehensive Cancer Network's clinical practice guidelines for neutropenia, the team developed a standardized order set for febrile neutropenia. A neutropenic protocol had already existed at the institution and had recently been revised and updated to reflect EBP standards. After reviewing the protocol, the team decided to take it a step further and develop standing orders that would be reflective of this protocol. The development of a standing order set would allow for quick retrieval of evidence-based care via a one-page document, which ultimately could expedite life-saving interventions. The interdisciplinary team transformed the protocol into a one-page, succinct order set with the inclusion of a nursing care orders section for patients with febrile neutropenia. The ONS PEP resource allowed the team to include evidence-based nursing standards of care for these patients.

Other evidence-based initiatives implemented by the team included

- Implementation of oncology staff and emergency nursing staff educational programs on the topic of febrile neutropenia to help "fast track" the patient from the emergency department to the inpatient oncology unit
- Educational review of nursing management for patients with febrile neutropenia during annual oncology nursing competencies
- Development of standardized discharge instruction forms for neutropenia that are provided to patients upon discharge from the inpatient or outpatient units following chemotherapy
- Provision of ALERT pocket cards (supported by Amgen) that state "I have neutropenia and an infection" to patients upon discharge from the inpatient or outpatient units following chemotherapy that they would then present to emergency room staff.

The project team utilized the ONS PEP Resources in an effort to formulate a standing order set for the management of patients admitted with febrile neutropenia, an oncologic emergency, coupled with intense education aimed at improving outcomes in this patient population. The standing order set has been approved and is being implemented initially at the nurses' hospital and then subsequently throughout the three-hospital health system.

Michele E. Gaguski, RN, MSN, AOCN®, CHPN, APN-C
Oncology Clinical Nurse Specialist
Ocean Medical Center
Brick, NJ

Mary Brandsema, BSN, RN, OCN®
Lani Gernalin, BSN, RN, OCN®
Elizabeth Martinez, BSN, RN, OCN®
Clinical Nursing Staff Scholars
Ocean Medical Center
Brick, NJ

Creating an Evidence-Based Practice Environment Through Performance Evaluation

Performance problems are difficult areas to address, often overlap, and are related to other quality improvement areas. ONS, the Joint Commission, and individual institutions and practices want to provide quality care and, thus, have expectations of staff achieving specific competencies. Competencies are increasingly relevant because of the varied staff caring for patients with cancer and new issues to consider in cancer survivors (Grant, Economou, Ferrell, & Bhatia, 2007; Smith & Lichtveld, 2007). In creative ways, the ONS PEP Resources as applied to clinical problems can lead to development of competencies of nursing staff. The following is a clinical example illustrating the use of the ONS PEP Resources for competency evaluation.

Clinical Example

Competency Testing of the ONS PEP Resource Information

One oncology nurse returned from the 2008 ONS Congress with all four volumes of the ONS PEP Resources. After presenting the idea of making these evidence-based resources the standard of practice to the chief nursing officer, the nurse manager, and the cancer program coordinator, it was decided that the organization would "go live" with the ONS PEP Resources. The clinical coordinator researched the corporate online education program, HealthStream, to see if similar information was available that could be implemented for nursing competencies. A few resources were available, but none that were felt to meet the needs for EBP. Because the policies and procedures were based on ONS standards, the ONS PEP Resources seemed to be a great resource. Why not write a competency using the ONS PEP Resources?

Implementation

It was decided to write a 10-question competency for each volume of the ONS PEP Resources. After completing volume 1, the manager and the cancer program coordinator were asked to take the test. The clinical coordinator wanted the test to be available in a written format and on HealthStream. A lunch-and-learn meeting was provided for the staff to familiarize them with the ONS PEP Resources. The resources and their impact on patient care were discussed, and staff was informed that the materials would be available in the nurses' resource room. The staff was made aware that an educational program was being developed for each of the volumes. The manager, the cancer program coordinator, RNs, licensed practical nurses, nurse technicians, and unit clerks attended the lunch-and-learn meeting.

While reviewing the ONS PEP Resources, it was noticed that they work in conjunction with the hospital core measures in numerous areas, particularly prevention of infection, such as for flu and pneumonia vaccines. This has been a concern for physicians and nurses in the facility. A comment section had recently been placed in the electronic charting system, in the medication documenting section, so that nurses can document a reason why the influenza or pneumonia vaccines were not appropriate at the time (e.g., neutropenia and induction of chemotherapy).

ONS PEP Resources Test

The 10 questions in volume 1 address fatigue, chemotherapy-induced nausea and vomiting, prevention of infection and mucositis, and sleep-wake disturbances. Upon successful completion of each test, the nurse will receive 1 CEU. The question format is multiple choice or yes/no. The ONS PEP categories *Recommended for*

Practice, Likely to Be Effective, Benefits Balanced With Harms, Effectiveness Not Established, Effectiveness Unlikely, Not Recommended for Practice, and *Expert Opinion* are included in the questions.

Summary

Integrating information into educational programs will improve staff knowledge and standard of care for patients. Hospital Corporation of America (HCA) has 169 hospitals in the United States and England and 185,000 employees who could potentially benefit from these competencies. The future goal is to implement EBP standards into the nursing care plans in the hospital's electronic charting system.

Kathy Browne, RN, OCN®
Clinical Coordinator, Medical-Surgical Oncology
North Florida Regional Medical Center
Gainesville, FL

Clinical Example

Using the ONS PEP Process for Other Clinical Problems

The evidence-based principles that were used to create the ONS PEP Resources can be applied to other oncology clinical problems. EBP begins with asking a clinical question. Questions that arise in everyday practice may not always be addressed through the current ONS PEP Resources. Therefore, to provide evidence-based interventions, understanding the evidence-based process is helpful. Using the PICO format (P = patient population, I = intervention or area of interest, C = comparison intervention or comparison group, and O = outcome), the initial step is to ask a clinical question. The second step is to search for the best evidence through a literature search, with systematic reviews or meta-analysis being the highest levels of evidence. Step three is to critically appraise the evidence from the literature search. An evaluation of the evidence then leads to implementing an intervention if the evidence has been sufficient. Lastly, the clinical outcome should be evaluated after implementing the intervention (Fineout-Overholt et al., 2005). Figure 19-2 provides an example of using the PICO model for an unanswered clinical question.

Shanna Henningsen, BSN, RN, OCN®
Lead Nurse, Medical Oncology Unit
University of Toledo Medical Center
Toledo, OH

Janelle M. Tipton, MSN, RN, AOCN®
Oncology Clinical Nurse Specialist
University of Toledo Medical Center
Toledo, OH

Figure 19-2. Example of Using the PICO System

Problem: Several patients with cancer receive platelet transfusions via a peripherally inserted central catheter (PICC) line. Current policy states that platelets are to be infused via gravity drip. Because of the length and gauge of available PICC lines, it is difficult to deliver transfusions in a relatively short time frame. Staff nurses had begun doing peripheral venipunctures on these patients to transfuse the platelets quickly to avoid their expiration. Nurses assumed that platelets would be damaged if administered via infusion pump. Was that true? If not, could we save time and resources and ensure patient comfort if the policy was changed?

P (Patient population): Oncology patients receiving platelet transfusions
I (Intervention): Safety of platelet transfusion via infusion pump
C (Comparison): Gravity drip versus infusion pump administration of platelets
O (Outcome): Ensuring platelet integrity

- Step 1—Develop a question: Is it safe to administer platelets via infusion pump?
- Step 2—Literature search is performed with assistance from blood bank staff resources and infusion pump company.
- Step 3—Critical appraisal of the literature showed that data existed to support a policy change. Platelet integrity is maintained using pumps.
- Step 4—Implement policy change, and communicate to staff and affected individuals.
- Step 5—Evaluation: Change resulted in improved patient satisfaction, improved nursing satisfaction, cost savings for materials, and more efficient use of nursing time.

Promoting Evidence-Based Practice in the Workplace

The clinical examples highlighted in this chapter provide practical ways to ensure that EBP is implemented in education, system change, and performance activities. By providing an EBP environment throughout an organization, quality patient care is a realistic and distinct outcome. Quality improvement can and should be initiated by the involved caregivers. With guidance from APNs, nurse managers, quality improvement staff, and others, the staff can identify care issues and be involved in making changes according to the evidence. Outcomes need to be identified, monitored, and reported to highlight nursing care accomplishments and to recognize the continual need to monitor and improve care. Change can be difficult; however, integrating those involved in the care from the onset can be a learning experience and can expose nursing staff to the quality improvement process.

References

Brant, J.M., & Wickham, R.S. (2004). *Statement on the scope and standards of oncology nursing practice.* Pittsburgh, PA: Oncology Nursing Society.

DiCenso, A., Virani, T., Bajnok I., Borycki, E., Davies, B., Graham, I., et al. (2002). A toolkit to facilitate the implementation of clinical practice guidelines in healthcare settings. *Hospital Quarterly, 5*(3), 55–60.

Fineout-Overholt, E., Cox, J., Robbins, B., & Gray, Y.L. (2005). Teaching evidence-based practice. In B. Melnyk & E. Fineout-Overholt (Eds.), *Evidence-based practice in nursing and healthcare: A guide to best practice* (pp. 407–441). Philadelphia: Lippincott Williams & Wilkins.

Grant, M., Economou, D., Ferrell, B., & Bhatia, S. (2007). Preparing professional staff to care for cancer survivors. *Journal of Cancer Survivorship, 1*(1), 98–106.

Grol, R. (2001). Successes and failures in the implementation of evidence-based guidelines for clinical practice. *Medical Care, 39*(8, Suppl. 2), 1146–1154.

Ingersoll, G.L. (2005). Generating evidence through outcomes management. In B. Melnyk & E. Fineout-Overholt (Eds.), *Evidence-based practice in nursing and healthcare: A guide to best practice* (pp. 299–332). Philadelphia: Lippincott Williams & Wilkins.

Institute of Medicine. (2001). *Crossing the quality chasm: A new health system for the 21st century.* Retrieved September 3, 2008, from http://books.nap.edu/openbook.php?record_id=10027&page=12

Miaskowski, C. (1989). Quality assurance issues in oncology nursing. *Cancer, 64*(Suppl. 1), 285–289.

Mohide, E.A., & King, B. (2003). Building a foundation for evidence-based practice: Experiences in a tertiary hospital. *Evidence-Based Nursing, 6*(4), 100–105.

Moulding, N.T., Silagy, C.A., & Weller, D.P. (1999). A framework for effective management of change in clinical practice dissemination and implementation of clinical practice guidelines. *Quality in Health Care, 8*(3), 177–183.

Profetto-McGrath, J. (2005). Critical thinking and evidence-based practice. *Journal of Professional Nursing, 21*(6), 364–371.

Smith, A.P., & Lichtveld, M.Y. (2007). A competency-based approach to expanding the cancer care workforce. *Medsurg Nursing, 16*(2), 109–117.

Solberg, L.I., Brekke, M.I., Fazio, C.J., Fowles, J., Jacobsen, D.N., Kottke, T.E., et al. (2000). Lessons from experienced guideline implementers: Attend to many factors and use multiple strategies. *Joint Commission Journal of Quality Improvement, 26*(4), 171–188.

Woolf, S.H., Grol, R., Hutchinson, A., Eccles, M., & Grinnshaw, J. (1999). Clinical guidelines, potential benefits, limitations, and harms of clinical guidelines. *BMJ, 318*(7182), 527–530.

Epilogue

Five years ago, when the Oncology Nursing Society (ONS) Putting Evidence Into Practice (PEP) Resources were just a dream, it was never imagined what a huge success these evidence-based resources would be! The resources were first introduced to the ONS membership in 2006, and they continue to be in high demand by members and nonmembers. Numerous presentations have been made both nationally and internationally on the ONS PEP Resources, which speaks to the interest that other organizations have in the initiative.

ONS members have a critical role in developing the ONS PEP Resources. They identify the need for a specific resource and work together as a team composed of advanced practice nurses, staff nurses, and nurse scientists to develop it. We have listened to what our members want, and *Putting Evidence Into Practice: Improving Oncology Patient Outcomes* is a result of your requests. Many members told us that more information was needed about how to measure the effect of evidence-based interventions on patient outcomes. In addition, we were told how challenging it is to carry 16 cards in one's pocket! We hope this book has met both of those needs.

As more scientific evidence is published, the ONS PEP Resources will continue to be updated. I hope that by the next edition of this book, we will have data that demonstrate the positive impact of the ONS PEP Resources on patient outcomes. Data can be collected on a unit or hospital level through quality improvement projects or through a research protocol. If you are collecting information on the impact of the ONS PEP Resources on patient outcomes, please be sure to contact the ONS Research Team at research@ons.org.

I am pleased that you are using this book to "PEP Up Your Practice!"

Paula T. Rieger, MSN, RN, AOCN®, FAAN
ONS Chief Executive Officer

Index

The letter f *after a page number indicates that relevant content appears in a figure; the letter* t, *in a table.*

A

acetaminophen, for pain, 223
acetyl-L-carnitine, for peripheral neuropathy, 244
acupressure, for nausea/vomiting, 74–75
acupuncture
    for depression, 115
    for dyspnea, 144
    for fatigue, 162
    for nausea/vomiting, 71, 75
    for peripheral neuropathy, 247
acustimulation, for nausea/vomiting, 75, 77
acute nausea/vomiting, 71–73. *See also* chemotherapy-induced nausea and vomiting
acute promyelocytic leukemia (APL), bleeding with, 253
adenosine 5' triphosphate (ATP), for fatigue, 163
Adult and Child Sleep Assessment Tools, 286
adult day care, for caregiver strain/burden, 60
air travel precautions, with lymphedema, 189–190
allopurinol, for mucositis, 203
aloe vera, for mucositis, 206
alpha-lipoic acid
    for fatigue, 164–165
    for peripheral neuropathy, 245
alprazolam (Xanax®)
    for anxiety, 44
    for nausea/vomiting, 71
alvimopan, for constipation, 95
American Red Cross, on bleeding control, 262

American Society of Clinical Oncology (ASCO), Quality Oncology Practice Initiative, 11
amifostine
    for diarrhea, 127
    for mucositis, 203
    for peripheral neuropathy, 245
amitriptyline, for depression, 112
amoxicillin, for infection, 184
amphotericin B, 203, 275, 280
anemia, 158
anesthetics, for pain, 226–227
animal-assisted therapy, for fatigue, 162–163
animal encounters, and infection prevention, 278
Anodyne® therapy, for peripheral neuropathy, 248
anorexia
    assessment of, 26
    case study of, 28–29
    definition of, 25
    incidence of, 25
    measurement tools for, 19t
    PEP resource for, 31–35
anorexia-cachexia syndrome. *See* anorexia
antiarrhythmics, for pain, 229
antibiotics
    for infection, 184, 186, 275–276
    for mucositis, 203
anticipatory nausea/vomiting, 71. *See also* chemotherapy-induced nausea and vomiting
anticonvulsants, for pain, 226
antidepressants
    for anxiety, 44

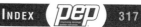

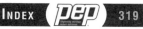

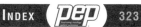